Stedman's

OPHTHALMOLOGY
WORDS

STEDMANS

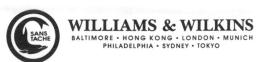

WILLIAMS & WILKINS
BALTIMORE · HONG KONG · LONDON · MUNICH
PHILADELPHIA · SYDNEY · TOKYO

Series Editor: Elizabeth Randolph
Editorial Staff: Terri Koffler, MT
             Linda Galbraith, CMT-ART
Production Manager: Cordelia Slaughter
Cover Design: Carla Frank

Copyright © 1993
Williams & Wilkins
428 East Preston Street
Baltimore, Maryland 21202, USA

Printed in the United States of America

Library of Congress Cataloging-in-Publication Data
Stedman, Thomas Lathrop, 1853–1938.
    Stedman's ophthalmology words.
      p. cm.
    Developed from the database of Stedman's medical dictionary, 25th ed. and supplemented by other sources.
    Includes bibliographical references.
    ISBN 0-683-07952-2
    1. Ophthalmology—Terminology.   I. Stedman, Thomas Lathrop,
1853–1938. Medical dictionary.   II. Title.   III. Title:
Ophthalmology words.
    [DNLM: 1. Ophthalmology—dictionaries. WV 13 S812]
RE20.S7 1992
617.7'0014—dc20
DNLM/DLC
for Library of Congress   92-22886
                                          CIP

95 96
3 4 5 6 7 8 9 10

Contents

Acknowledgments

An important part of our editorial process is the involvement of medical transcriptionists—as advisors, reviewers and/or editors. Terri Koffler, MT, of Littleton, CO did an excellent job of editing and proofing the manuscript, working closely with Linda Galbraith, CMT-ART.

This book also benefitted from the word research and editorial expertise of Catherine Gilliam, CMT, and Sandra Manzo, Transcription Supervisor at the Massachusetts Eye and Ear Infirmary.

Special thanks go to the members of the Williams & Wilkins MT Advisory Board, whose expertise, ideas, and words contribute to the overall quality of this and other Stedman's word books: LaVonne Alexis, CMT; Joan Bachman; Addie M. Garner; Suzanne Minnick, CMT; Susan Pierce, CMT, ART; Laurie J. Spangler, CMT; Harriet Stewart, CMT; and Dorothy Vickers.

Explanatory Notes

Stedman's Ophthalmology Words offers an authoritative assurance of quality and exactness to the wordsmiths of the health care professions—medical transcriptionists, medical editors and copy editors, medical records personnel and the many other users and producers of medical documentation. It can be used to validate both the spelling and accuracy of terminology in ophthalmology. This compilation of over 48,000 entries, fully cross-indexed for quick access, was built from a base vocabulary of 28,000 medical words, phrases, abbreviations, and acronyms. The extensive A–Z list was developed from the database of *Stedman's Medical Dictionary 25ed.*, and supplemented by terminology found in the current medical literature.

Medical transcription is an art as well as a science. Both are needed to correctly interpret a physician's dictation, whose language is a product of education, training, and experience. This variety in medical language means that there are several acceptable ways to express certain terms, including jargon. *Stedman's Ophthalmology Words* provides variant spellings and phrasings for many terms. This, in addition to complete cross-indexing, makes *Stedman's Ophthalmology Words* a valuable resource for determining the validity of ophthalmology terms as they are encountered.

Stedman's Ophthalmology Words includes up-to-date terminology of external and internal diseases of the eye, ocular tumors, neuro-ophthalmology, and lasers. The user will find listed thousands of ocular diseases and syndromes, diagnostic and surgical procedures, and equipment names—including instruments, lenses, implants, dressings, and sutures. Ophthalmologic abbreviations and medications are also included. For a shortcut, an appendix lists terms related to cataract extraction.

Alphabetical Organization

Alphabetization of entries is letter by letter as spelled, ignoring punctuation, spaces, prefixed numbers, Greek letters, or other characters. For example:

acid-fast staining methods
acid formaldehyde hematin
α_1**-acid glycoprotein**
acid hematin

In subentries, the abbreviated singular form or the spelled-out plural form of the noun main entry word is ignored in alphabetization.

Format and Style

All main entries are in **boldface** to speed up location of a sought-after entry, to enhance distinction between main entries and subentries, and to relieve the textual density of the pages.

Irregular plurals and variant spellings are shown on the same line as the singular or preferred form of the word. For example:

macula, pl. **maculae**

Selivanof's reagent, Seliwanow's reagent

Possessive forms that occur in the medical literature are retained in this reference. It should be noted however that equipment and instrument names are shown in the non-possessive. To form the non-possessives advocated by the American Association for Medical Transcription and other groups, simply drop the apostrophe or apostrophe "s" from the end of the word.

Cross-indexing

The word list is in an index-like main entry-subentry format that contains two combined alphabetical listings:

(1) a noun main entry-subentry organization typical of the A-Z section of medical dictionaries like *Stedman's*:

implant
acorn-shaped eye i.
acrylic i.
Allen-Braley i.
Allen orbital i.

detachment
aphakic d.
bullous d.
choroidal d.
ciliochoroidal d.

(2) An adjective main entry-subentry organization, which lists words and phrases as you hear them. The main entries are the adjectives or modifiers in a multi-word term. The subentries are the nouns around which the terms are constructed and to which the adjectives or modifiers pertain:

cicatricial
c. conjunctivitis
c. ectropion
c. entropion
c. mass

orbital
o. abscess
o. adipose tissue
o. akinesia
o. amyloidosis

This format provides the user with more than one way to locate and identify a multi-word term. For example:

forceps
Allen-Braley f.

Allen-Braley
A.-B. forceps
A.-B. implant

solution
dexamethasone s.

dexamethasone
d. solution

It also allows the user to see together all terms that contain a particular descriptor as well as all types, kinds, or variations of a noun entity. For example:

depth
focal d.
d. of focus
sagittal d.

punctal
p. cautery
p. dilator
p. lens
p. occlusion

References

Adams, Ophthalmology word book. Philadelphia: W.B. Saunders, 1991.

Cassin and Solomon. Dictionary of eye terminology, 2nd ed. Gainesville: Triad Publishing, 1990.

Coles, Ophthalmology: a diagnostic text. Baltimore: Williams & Wilkins, 1989.

Journal of cataract and refractive surgery. Baltimore: Williams & Wilkins, 1991.

1992 Ophthalmic drug facts. St. Louis: Facts and Comparisons, 1992.

Seminars in Ophthalmology. Philadelphia: W.B. Saunders, 1991.

Stedman's abbreviations, acronyms & symbols. Baltimore: Williams & Wilkins, 1991.

Stedman's medical dictionary, 25 ed. Baltimore: Williams & Wilkins, 1990.

Stein et al., Ophthalmic terminology, 3rd ed. St. Louis: Mosby-Yearbook, 1992.

Tasman and Jaeger, eds. Duane's clinical ophthalmology. Philadelphia: J.B. Lippincott, 1991.

Tasman and Jaeger, eds. Duane's foundations of clinical ophthalmology. Philadelphia: J.B. Lippincott, 1991.

Your Medical Word Resource Publisher

We strive to provide you with the most up-to-date and accurate word references available. Your use of this word book will prompt new editions, which will be published as often as justified by updates and revisions. We welcome your suggestions for improvements, changes, corrections, and additions—whatever will make this **Stedman's** product more useful to you. Please use the postpaid card at the back of this book and send your recommendations to the Reference Division at Williams & Wilkins.

A
  accommodation
AA
  amplitude of accommodation
AACG
  acute angle-closure glaucoma
AAMD
  atrophic age-related macular
    degeneration
Aarskog syndrome
Aase syndrome
Abadie's
  A. sign
  A. sign of exophthalmic
    goiter
abaissement
A band
Abbe refractometer
abducens
  a. facial paralysis
  a. internuclear neurons
  a. muscle
  a. nerve
  a. palsy
  a. paralysis
abducent nerve (N.VI)
abduct
abducted
abduction
abductor muscles
aberrant
  a. degeneration of third
    nerve
  a. regeneration
  a. regeneration of nerve
aberration
  angle of a.
  chromatic a.
  chromatic lens a.
  color a.
  coma a.
  curvature a.
  dioptric a.
  distantial a.
  distortion a.
  lateral a.
  lens a.
  longitudinal a.
  meridional a.
  monochromatic a.

  newtonian a.
  oblique a.
  optical a.
  regeneration a.
  spherical a.
  spherical lens a.
aberrometer
abetalipoproteinemia
ab externo filtering operation
ability vergence
abiotrophy
  retinal a.
ablation
  panretinal a.
  pituitary a.
  toric a.
ablatio retinae
ablepharia
ablepharon
ablepharous
ablephary
ablepsia, ablepsy
Abney's effect
abnormal
  a. correspondence
  a. harmonious retinal
    correspondence
  a. retinal correspondence
    (ARC)
  a. staining pattern
  a. unharmonious retinal
    correspondence
abnormality
  chromosome a.
  congenital a.
  facial movement a.
  immunologic a.
  intraretinal microvascular a.
    (IRMA)
  lipid a.
  microvascular a.
  platelet a.
  saccadic a.
  vertebrobasilar vascular a.
abrader
  cornea a.
  Howard a.
Abraham
  A. iridectomy laser lens
  A. iridectomy lens

Abraham *(continued)*
 A. iridotomy
 A. iridotomy lens
 A. peripheral button
  iridotomy lens
 A. YAG laser lens
abrasio corneae
abrasion
 central a.
 conjunctival a.
 a. of cornea
 corneal a.
 a. from contact lens
 traumatic corneal a.
abrin
A- & B-scan ultrasonography
abscess, pl. **abscesses**
 corneal a.
 lacrimal a.
 orbital a.
 retrobulbar a.
 ring a.
 a. ring
 subperiosteal a.
 vitreous a.
abscessed
abscessus siccus corneae
abscission
 corneal a.
absent guttata
absolute
 a. accommodation
 a. alcohol
 a. glaucoma
 a. hemianopsia
 a. hyperopia
 a. intensity threshold acuity
 near point a.
 a. scotoma
 a. strabismus
absolutum
 glaucoma a.
absorbable
 a. gelatin film
 a. suture
absorbance
absorbency
absorptance
 radiant a.
absorption
 a. lines
abtorsion
abutted

abutting
AC
 accommodative convergence
 air chamber
 anterior chamber
 AC eye drops
AC/A
 accommodative
  convergence/accommodation
  ratio
acanthamebiasis
Acanthamoeba
 A. keratitis
acanthocytosis
acantholysis
acanthoma
 a. fissuratum
acanthosis
 a. nigricans
ACC
 anterior central curve
Acc
 accommodation
accessoriae
 glandulae lacrimales a.
accessory
 a. fiber
 a. nucleus
 a. organs of eye
accident
 cerebrovascular a. (CVA)
accidental
 a. image
 a. mydriasis
accommodation (A, Acc)
 absolute a.
 amplitude of a. (AA)
 binocular a.
 breadth of a.
 a. of crystalline lens
 esodeviation a.
 esotropia a.
 excessive a.
 a. of eye
 far point of a. (fpa)
 fusion with a.
 iridoplegia a.
 a. of lens
 near point of a. (NPA)
 negative a.
 paralysis of a.
 a. phosphene
 a. phosphene of Czermak

position a.
positive a.
punctum proximum of a.
pupils equal, reactive to light and a. (PERLA)
pupils equal, round, reactive to light and a. (PERRLA)
range of a.
reflex a.
a. reflex
relative a.
residual a.
a. rule
subnormal a.
tonic a.
accommodation-convergence ratio
accommodative
a. asthenopia
a. convergence (AC)
a. convergence/accommodation ratio (AC/A)
a. cyclophoria
a. effort syndrome
a. esodeviation
a. esophoria
a. esotropia
a. palsy
a. spasm
a. squint
a. strabismus
a. target
accommodometer
accreta
cataracta a.
Accugel lens
accumulation
lipid a.
Accutane
ACE
angiotensin-converting enzyme
aceclidine
acetaldehyde
acetaminophen
acetanilid
acetate
cellulose a.
cortisone a.
hydrocortisone a.
medroxyprogesterone a.
phenylmercuric a.
potassium a.

prednisolone a.
sodium a.
acetazolamide
acetic acid
acetohexamide
acetone
Acetonide
acetoxphenylmercury
acetoxycycloheximide (AXM)
acetylcholine
a. chloride
a. receptor antibody level
acetylcholinesterase
acetylcysteine
N-acetyl-β-D-glucosamidase
acetylsalicylic acid
ACG
angle-closure glaucoma
achloropsia
achroacytosis
achromat
achromate
achromatic
a. doublet
a. lens
a. objective
a. perimetry
a. spectacle lens
a. threshold
a. vision
achromatism
achromatopia
achromatopic
achromatopsia, achromatopsy
atypical a.
complete a.
cone a.
incomplete a.
rod a.
typical a.
X-linked a.
achromia
Achromycin
acid
acetic a.
acetylsalicylic a.
amino a.
γ-aminobutyric a. (GABA)
aminocaproic a.
ε-aminocaproic a. (EACA)
arachidonic a.
ascorbic a.
boric a.

acid *(continued)*
    a. burn
    carbolic a.
    disodium
      ethylenediaminete-
      traacetic a.
    ethylenediaminetetraacetic a.
      (EDTA)
    folinic a.
    a. hematin
    hyaluronic a. (HA)
    hydrochloric a.
    lysergic a.
    a. mucopolysaccharide stain
    nalidixic a.
    nicotinic a.
    p-aminobenzoic a. (PAB,
      PABA)
    phosphonoformic a.
    phosphoric a.
    picric a.
    salicylic a.
    sulfuric a.
    tartaric a.
    tranexamic a.
    trichloracetic a.
    valproic a.
acid-fast bacilli
acidophilic adenoma
acidosis
    diabetic a.
acid-resistant penicillin
acid-Schiff stain
aciduria
    amino a.
acinar lacrimal gland
Acinetobacter calcoaceticus
acinus, pl. **acini**
    lacrimal gland a.
aclastic
ACLD
    Association for Children and
    Adults with Learning
    Disabilities
acne
    a. ciliaris
    a. conjunctivitis
    a. rosacea
    a. rosacea
      blepharoconjunctivitis
    a. rosacea conjunctivitis
    a. rosacea corneal ulcer
    a. rosacea keratitis

acnes
    Propionibacterium a.
acorea
acorn-shaped
    a.-s. eye implant
    a.-s. implant
acoustic
    a. nerve
    a. neuroma
    a. spot
acoustical
    a. conductive gel
    a. hollowing
    a. shadowing
    a. sonolucent
acquired
    a. astigmatism
    a. color defect
    a. distichia
    a. entropion
    a. esotropia
    a. immune response
    a. immunodeficiency
      syndrome (AIDS)
    a. jerk nystagmus
    a. melanosis
    a. pendular nystagmus
    a. retinoschisis
acquisita
    epidermolysis bullosa a.
ACR
    Clear Eyes ACR
acridine orange stain
acritochromacy
acrocephalia
acrocephalosyndactyly,
    acrocephalosyndactylia
acrocephaly
acrodermatitis
    a. chronica atrophicans
    a. enteropathica
acrofacial dysostosis
acromegalic habitus
acromegaly
acrospermia
    eccrine a.
acrospiroma
acrosyringium
acrylate
    silicone a.
acrylic
    a. implant
    a. lens

ACS
Alcon Closure System
ACS needle
ACT
alternate cover test
ACTH
adrenocorticotropic hormone
actin
a. filament
actinic
a. conjunctivitis
a. keratitis
a. keratosis
a. ray ophthalmia
a. retinitis
Actinomadura madurae
Actinomyces
Actinomycetales
actinomycin D
actinomycosis
nodules in a.
action
mechanism of a.
mode of a.
primary a.
secondary a.
active pterygium
activity
antimicrobial a.
laser a.
actomyosin ATPase
Acuiometer
Acuity
Mentor BVAT II Video A.
acuity
absolute intensity
threshold a.
best-corrected visual a.
(BVA)
binocular visual a.
a. card procedure
central visual a.
distance a.
distance visual a. (DVA)
grating a.
minimum perceptible a.
minimum separable a.
near visual a. (NVA)
perceptible a.
resolution a.
separable a.
spatial a.
stereo a.

stereoscopic a.
true visual a. (TVA)
Vernier a.
Vernier visual a.
visibility a.
visual a. (VA)
a. visual projector
Acuscan Transducer 400
acute
a. angle-closure glaucoma
(AACG)
a. atopic conjunctivitis
a. catarrhal conjunctivitis
a. catarrhal rhinitis
a. chalazion
a. chronic glaucoma
a. congestive conjunctivitis
a. congestive glaucoma
a. contagious conjunctivitis
a. dacryocystitis
a. diffuse serous choroiditis
a. epidemic conjunctivitis
a. follicular conjunctivitis
a. glaucoma
a. hemorrhagic conjunctivitis
a. hydrops
a. macular neuroretinopathy
a. multifocal placoid
pigment epitheliopathy
(AMPPE)
a. multifocal posterior
pigment epitheliopathy
a. multifocal posterior
placoid pigment
epitheliopathy
a. posterior multifocal
placoid pigment
epitheliopathy (APMPPE)
a. retinal necrosis syndrome
a. spastic entropion
AcuteCare
Becton Dickinson A.
acyanotic heart disease
acycloguanosine
acyclovir
Adams'
A. ectropion
A. operation
A. operation for ectropion
Adapettes
Adapt
adaptation
color a.

adaptation *(continued)*
    dark a.
    light a.
    photopic a.
    retinal a.
    scotopic a.
adaptive immunity
adaptometer
    Collin 140 color a.
    color a.
    Feldman a.
    Goldmann-Weeker dark a.
adaptometry
    dark a.
adaptor
    Sheehy-Urban sliding lens a.
    Zeiss cine a.
Addison's disease
addition
adduct
adducted
adduction
    a. impairment
adductor
    a. muscles
A-dellen
adenine arabinoside (ara-A)
adenocarcinoma
adenohypophysis
adenohypophysitis
    lymphocytic a.
adenoid cystic carcinoma
adenologaditis
adenoma
    acidophilic a.
    basophilic a.
    chromophobe a.
    endocrine-inactive a.
    Fuchs' a.
    invasive a.
    parathyroid a.
    pituitary a.
    pleomorphic a.
    prolactin-secreting a.
    sebaceous a.
    a. sebaceum
adenomectomy
    medical a.
adenopathy
    preauricular a.
adenophthalmia
adenosine
    a. monophosphate (AMP)

    a. triphosphatase (ATPase)
    a. triphosphate (ATP)
adenoviral
    a. keratoconjunctivitis
adenovirus (ADV)
    a. conjunctivitis
adequacy
    blink a.
adherence syndrome
adherens
    leukoma a.
    macula a.
    zonula a.
adherent
    a. cataract
    a. lens
    a. leukoma
adhesion
    thermal a.'s
adhesive
    Brown sterile a.
    cyanoacrylate a.
    cyanoacrylate tissue a.
    a. syndrome
    tissue a.
Adie's
    A. pupil
    A. syndrome
    A. tonic pupil
adipocyte
adiposa
    pseudophakia a.
adipose
    a. body
    a. tissue
aditus orbitae
adjustable suture
adjustment
    intraoperative a.
    postoperative a.
Adler's operation
administration
    intraocular a.
    oral a.
    parenteral a.
    route of a.
adnatum
    ankyloblepharon filiforme a.
adnerval
adneural
adnexa
    ocular a.
    a. oculi

adnexal
adolescent cataract
adrenal
    a. disorder
    a. hypertension
adrenalin
Adrenaline
adrenergic
    a. agent
    a. agonist
    a. blocking agent
β-adrenergic blocking agent
adrenochrome
adrenocorticotropic hormone
  (ACTH)
adrenoleukodystrophy
    neonatal a.
Adriablastina
Adriamycin
Adson forceps
Adsorbocarpine
Adsorbonac
Adsorbotear
adtorsion
adult
    a. inclusion conjunctivitis
    a. medullocpithelioma
adult-onset
    a.-o. cataract
    a.-o. diabetes
adultorum
    blennorrhea a.
ADV
    adenovirus
advancement
    capsular a.
    a. flap
    a. procedure
    tendon a.
adverse reaction
Aebli
    A. corneal scissors
    A. corneal section scissors
aegyptius
aerial haze
aerogenes
    Enterobacter a.
Aeromonas hydrophila
aerosol keratitis
Aerosporin
aeruginosa
    Pseudomonas a.

Aesculap
    A. argon ophthalmic laser
    A. excimer laser
aesthesiometer
afferent
    a. defect
    a. limb
    a. nerve
    a. pupillary defect (APD)
    a. visual symptom
afocal optical system
African eyeworm
africanum
    Mycobacterium a.
aftercataract
    a. bur
aftereffects
afterimage
    complementary a.
    negative a.
    positive a.
    a. test
afterimagery
afterperception
aftervision
against motion
against-the-rule astigmatism
agar
    blood a.
    chocolate a.
    Sabouraud's a.
    Thayer-Martin a.
agenesis
    colossal a.
agent
    adrenergic a.
    adrenergic blocking a.
    β-adrenergic blocking a.
    alkylating a.
    anovulatory a.
    anticholinesterase a.
    antifibrinolytic a.
    antifungal a.
    anti-inflammatory a.
    antimicrobial a.
    antimitotic a.
    antineoplastic a.
    antiplatelet a.
    antiviral a.
    bacteriocidal a.
    bacteriostatic a.
    beta-adrenergic blocking a.
    beta-blocking a.

agent *(continued)*
    chelating a.
    chemotherapeutic a.
    cholinergic blocking a.
    hyperosmotic a.
    hypertonic a.
    hypotensive a.
    immunosuppressive a.
    inhalational a.
    intravenous a.
    parasympatholytic a.
    parasympathomimetic a.
    staining a.
    sympathomimetic a.
    viscosity a.
    wetting a.
ageotrophic nystagmus
age-related
    a.-r. cataract
    a.-r. macular degeneration
    (AMD, ARMD)
    a.-r. ptosis
agglutination
    lid a.
    plasmoid a.
    a. technique
agglutinins
aggregates
aggregation
AGL-400
    Mira AGL-400
aglaucopsia
Agnew
    A. canaliculus knife
    A. keratome
    A. tattooing needle
Agnew's
    A. canthoplasty
    A. operation
Agnew-Verhoeff incision
agnosia
    optic a.
    topographic a.
    visual a.
    visual-spatial a.
agonist
    adrenergic a.
    beta-adrenergic a.
    a. muscle
agonist-antagonist relationship
agranulocytosis
agraphia
    alexia with a.

agraphic
Agrikola
    A. lacrimal retractor
    A. lacrimal sac retractor
    A. refractor
    A. tattooing needle
Agrikola's operation
AGR triad
    aniridia, genitourinary
    abnormalities, and mental
    retardation
Ahlström's syndrome
AHM
    anterior hyaloid membrane
Aicardi's syndrome
AIDS
    acquired immunodeficiency
    syndrome
AIDS-related
    AIDS-r. complex (ARC)
    AIDS-r. retinitis
aileron
aiming beam
AION
    anterior ischemic optic neuritis
    anterior ischemic optic
    neuropathy
air
    a. bubble
    a. cannula
    a. cell
    a. chamber (AC)
    a. cystitome
    a. injection cannula
    intraocular a.
    a. rifle
air-block glaucoma
air-fluid exchange
AIRLens contact lens
air-puff
    a.-p. contact tonometer
    a.-p. noncontact tonometer
    a.-p. tonometer
Airy cylindric lens
Airy disk
Akarpine
AK-Chlor
AK-Cide
AK-Con
AK-Con-A
AK-Dex
AK-Dilate
Aker lens pusher

AK-Fluor
AK-Homatropine
akinesia
    Nadbath's a.
    O'Brien's a. technique
    orbital a.
    retrobulbar a.
    Scheie's a.
    supraorbital a.
    Van Lint a.
akinesis
    pupillary sphincter a.
akinetic
AK-Lor
AK-Mycin
AK-NaCl
AK-Nefrin
AK-Neo-Cort
AK-Neo-Dex
aknephascopia
Akorn
AK-Pentolate
AK-Poly-Bac
AK-Pred
AK-Rinse
AK-Spore
AK-Spore H.C.
AK-Sulf Forte
AK-Taine
AK-Tate
AK-Tracin
AK-Trol
AK-Vaso-A
AK-Vernacon
AKWA Tears
AK-Zol
Alabama-Green needle holder
Alabama University utility forceps
alacrima
ala minor ossis sphenoidalis
alar
Albalon-A Liquifilm
Albalon Liquifilm
Albamycin
albedo
    a. retinae
Albers-Schönberg disease
albescens
    retinitis punctata a.
albicans
    Candida a.

albinism
    autosomal dominant
      oculocutaneous a.
    autosomal recessive
      ocular a.
    Bergsma-Kaiser-Kupfer
      oculocutaneous a.
    Donaldson-Fitzpatrick
      oculocutaneous a.
    localized a.
    Nettleship-Falls X-linked
      ocular a.
    ocular a.
    oculocutaneous a.
    partial a.
    punctate oculocutaneous a.
    tyrosinase-negative type
      oculocutaneous a.
    tyrosinase-positive type
      oculocutaneous a.
    yellow-mutant
      oculocutaneous a.
albinism-hemorrhagic diathesis
albinoidism
    oculocutaneous a.
    punctate oculocutaneous a.
albinotic
    a. fundus
albipunctalis
    fundus a.
albipunctate fundus
Albright's
    A. disease
    A. syndrome
albuginea oculi
albugo
albumin
albuminoid
albuminuric
    a. amaurosis
    a. retinitis
albuminurinicus
    diabetes a.
Alcaine
Alcaine Drop-Tainers
alcian blue stain
Alclear
alcohol
    absolute a.
    cetyl a.
    ethyl a.
    intoxication with a.
    methyl a.

alcohol *(continued)*
nicotinyl a.
phenylethyl a.
polyvinyl a. (PVA)
toxicity of a.
alcoholic amblyopia
alcoholism
Alcon
A. applanation pneumatonograph
A. aspiration
A. aspirator
A. cautery
A. Closure System (ACS)
A. cryoextractor
A. cryophake
A. cryosurgical unit
A. CU-15 4-mil needle
A. disposable drape
A. hand cautery
A. I-knife
A. indirect ophthalmoscope
A. irrigating/aspirating unit
A. irrigating needle
A. knife
A. Microsponge
A. phacoemulsification
A. phacoemulsification unit
A. reverse cutting needle
A. spatula needle
A. suture
A. taper cut needle
A. taper point needle
A. tonometer
A. vitrectomy probe
A. vitrector
Alconefrin
Alder-Reilly phenomenon
Alder's anomaly
Aldomet
aldose reductase
aldosteronism
Alexander-Ballen retractor
Alexander's law
alexia
optical a.
subcortical a.
a. with agraphia
alexic
Alezzandrini's syndrome
alfentanil

Alfonso
A. guarded bur
A. speculum
Alger
A. brush
A. brush rust ring remover
algera
dysopsia a., dysopia a.
Alges bifocal contact lens
algorithm
Alhazen's theories
Alidase
alignment
ocular a.
aliquot
alkali
a. burn
a. burn of cornea
a. burn to eye
a. Congo red stain
Alkaline
isopropyl alcohol Isopto A.
Isopto A.
alkaline
a. burn
a. phosphatase
alkaloid
dissociated a.
ergot a.
undissociated a.
alkaptonuria
alkylating agent
alkyl ether sulfate
allachesthesia
optical a.
allele
allelic polymorphism
Allen
A. cyclodialysis
A. orbital implant
Allen-Barkan forceps
Allen-Barker forceps
Allen-Braley
A.-B. forceps
A.-B. implant
Allen-Burian trabeculotome
Allen's
A. operation
Allen-Schiötz tonometer
Allen-Thorpe
A.-T. goniolens
A.-T. gonioscopic prism
A.-T. lens

Allerest
Allergan
    A. Humphrey laser
    A. Humphrey perimeter
    A. Humphrey
      photokeratoscope
    A. Humphrey refractor
    A. lensometer
    A. lensometer
    A. Medical Optics (AMO)
    A. Medical Optics
      photokeratoscope
allergen
allergic
    a. blepharitis
    a. conjunctivitis
    a. granulomatosis
    a. keratoconjunctivitis
    a. pannus
    a. phlyctenulosis
    a. response
    a. rhinitis
allergica
    iritis recidivans
      staphylococcal a.
allergic keratoconjunctivitis
    staphylococcal a. k.
allesthesia
    visual a.
alligator
    a. scissors
Allis forceps
allograft
    a. corneal rejection
allokeratoplasty
allopathic keratoplasty
allophthalmia
alloplastic donor material
allopurinol
alloxan diabetes
all-Perspex
    a.-P. CQ lens
    a.-P. Kelman Omnifit lens
Allport cutting bur
Allport's operation
all-*trans*-retinal
Almocarpine
Almocetamide
Aloe reading unit
alopecia
    a. areata
    a. orbicularis
Alpar implant

alpha
    a. angle
    a. hemolytic
    a. receptor
alpha-agonist
alpha-antagonist
alphabetical keratitis
Alpha Chymar
alpha-chymotrypsin
    a.-c. cannula
    a.-c. glaucoma
alpha-chymotrypsin-induced
    glaucoma
Alphadrol
alpha-methyldopa
alpha-methyl-*p*-tyrosine
Alpidine
Alport's syndrome
Alström-Hallgren syndrome
Alström-Olsen syndrome
Alström's
    A. disease
    A. syndrome
Alsus-Knapp operation
Alsus' operation
ALT
    argon laser trabeculopexy
alternate
    a. cover test (ACT)
    a. cover-uncover test
    a. day esotropia
    a. day strabismus
alternating
    a. cross-eyes
    a. esotropia
    a. exophoria
    a. exotropia
    a. hypertropia
    a. hypotropia
    a. light test
    a. mydriasis
    a. oculomotor hemiplegia
    a. strabismus
    a. sursumduction
    a. tropia
alternation
Alternative
    Soft Mate Enzyme A.
alternocular
altitudinal
    a. defect
    a. field
    a. field defect

altitudinal *(continued)*
    a. hemianopsia
    a. scotoma
ALTP
    argon laser trabeculoplasty
aluminum
    a. chloride
    a. eye shield
    a. metal
    a. nicotinate
Alvis
    A. curette
    A. fixation forceps
    A. foreign body spud
    A. spud
Alvis-Lancaster sclerotome
Alvis' operation
Alzheimer's disease
AMA
    American Medical Association
amacrinal
amacrine cell
amaurosis
    albuminuric a.
    Burns' a.
    cat's eye a.
    central a.
    a. centralis
    cerebral a.
    congenital a.
    a. congenita of Leber
    diabetic a.
    a. fugax
    gutta a.
    hysteric a.
    intoxification a.
    Leber's a.
    Leber's congenital a.
    a. nystagmus
    a. partialis fugax
    pressure a.
    reflex a.
    saburral a.
    toxic a.
    uremic a.
amaurotic
    a. cat's eye
    a. familial idiocy
    a. idiocy
    a. mydriasis
    a. nystagmus
    a. pupil
    a. pupillary paralysis

ambient
ambiopia
amblyope
amblyopia
    alcoholic a.
    ametropic a.
    anisometric a.
    anisometropic a.
    arsenic a.
    astigmatic a.
    axial a.
    color a.
    a. crapulosa
    crossed a.
    a. cruciata
    deprivation a.
    eclipse a.
    esotropic a.
    ethyl alcohol a.
    ex a.
    a. ex anopia
    a. ex anopsia
    exertional a.
    functional a.
    hysteric a.
    hysterical a.
    index a.
    irreversible a.
    meridional a.
    microstrabismic a.
    nocturnal a.
    nutritional a.
    organic a.
    postmarital a.
    postoperative a.
    quinine a.
    receptor a.
    reflex a.
    refractive a.
    relative a.
    reversible a.
    sensory a.
    strabismic a.
    suppressed a.
    suppression a.
    tobacco a.
    tobacco/alcohol a.
    toxic a.
    traumatic a.
    uremic a.
amblyopiatrics
amblyopic

amblyoscope
    major a.
    Worth a.
Ambrose suture forceps
AMD
    age-related macular degeneration
amebiasis
amelanotic
ameliorate
ameliorated
ameloblastic neurilemoma
Amenabar
    A. capsule forceps
    A. counterpressor
    A. discission hook
    A. iris retractor
    A. lens
    A. lens loupe
    A. loupe
American
    A. Hydron
    A. Hydron instruments
    A. leishmaniasis
    A. Medical Association
    (AMA)
    A. Medical Optics
    A. Medical Optics Baron
    lens
    A. National Standards
    Institute (ANSI)
    A. Optical contrast
    sensitivity system
    A. Optical ophthalmometer
    A. Optical photocoagulator
    A. Society for Testing and
    Materials (ASTM)
ametrometer
ametropia
    axial a.
    curvature a.
    index a.
    position a.
    refractive a.
    transient a.
ametropic amblyopia
Amicar
amifloxacin
amikacin
Amikin
amine
    vasoactive a.'s
amino
    a. acid

    a. acid metabolism
    a. acid metabolism disorder
    a. aciduria
aminoaciduria cataract
***p*-aminobenzoic acid (PAB, PABA)**
γ-aminobutyric acid (GABA)
aminocaproic acid
ε-aminocaproic acid (EACA)
aminoglycoside
aminophylline
4-aminoquinoline
amiodarone
amitriptyline
ammonia alkali burn
ammonium hydroxide alkali burn
Ammon's
    A. canthoplasty
    A. operation
    A. scleral prominence
amnesic color blindness
amnifocal lens
amniocentesis
amniotocele
AMO
    Allergan Medical Optics
    AMO intraocular lens
    AMO YAG 100 laser
amobarbital
amodiaquine
Amoils
    A. cryoextractor
    A. cryopencil
    A. cryophake
    A. cryoprobe
    A. cryosurgical unit
    A. refractor
    A. retractor
amorphous
    a. corneal dystrophy
    a. dystrophy
amotio retinae
amoxicillin
AMP
    adenosine monophosphate
amphamphterodiplopia
amphetamine
amphodiplopia
amphotericin
amphotericin B
amphoterodiplopia
ampicillin

amplitude
    a. of accommodation, a. of convergence (AA)
    convergence a.'s
    divergence a.'s
    a. of fusion
    fusional convergence a.
    fusional divergence a.
    fusion with a.
    vertical fusional vergence a.
AMPPE
    acute multifocal placoid pigment epitheliopathy
ampulla
    a. canaliculi lacrimalis
    a. ductus lacrimalis
    a. of lacrimal canal
    a. of lacrimal duct
ampullae
amputator
    Smith intraocular capsular a.
Amsler
    A. aqueous transplant needle
    A. marker
    A. needle
    A. scleral marker
Amsler's
    A. chart
    A. corneal graft
    A. grid
    A. grid test
    A. operation
    A. test
Amsoft lens
Amvisc
    A. Plus
    A. Plus solution
    A. solution
amyl nitrite
amyloid
    a. corneal degeneration
amyloidosis
    conjunctival a.
    localized a.
    orbital a.
    primary a.
    primary familial a.
    secondary a.
Amytal
ANA
    antinuclear antibody

Anacel
anaclasis
anaerobic
    a. medium
    a. ocular infection
anagioid disk
anaglyph
    a. test
anagnosasthenia
Anagnostakis' operation
analgesia
    a. permeation
    surface a.
analgesic
analmoscope
    Pickford-Nicholson a.
analphalipoproteinemia
analysis
    corneal topographic a.
    linkage a.
    pedigree a.
analyzer, analyzor
    Friedmann visual field a.
    Humphrey field a.
    Humphrey Instruments vision a.
    Humphrey lens a.
    Humphrey visual field a.
    profile a.
    Vision a.
anamorphosis
anaphoria
anaphylactic
    a. conjunctivitis
    a. reaction
anaphylaxis
anastigmatic
    a. lens
anastomosis, pl. **anastomoses**
anatomic
    a. equator
    a. substrate
anatropia
anatropic
ANCA
    antineutrophil cytoplasmic antibody
Ancef
anchor
    a. hook
    a. suture
anchored

anchor/fixation
> Searcy a.

anchoring suture
Andersen's syndrome
Anderson-Fabry disease
Andosky's syndrome
androgen
Anectine
Anel
> A. probe
> A. syringe

Anel's operation
anemia
> aplastic a.
> macrocytic a.
> Mediterranean a.
> microcytic a.
> normocytic a.
> normocytic hypochromic a.
> pernicious a.
> sickle cell a.

anemone cell tumor
anencephaly
anergy
anesthesia
> cornea a.
> exam under a. (EUA)
> general a.
> infraorbital a.
> intraorbital a.
> modified Van Lint's a.
> O'Brien's a.
> orbital a.
> retrobulbar a.
> topical a.
> Van Lint a.

anesthetic
> general a.
> inhalation a.
> local a.
> topical a.

anetoderma
> Jadassohn-type a.

aneuploids
aneuploidy
aneurysm
> arteriovenous a.
> basilar artery a.
> berry a.
> carotid a.
> cavernous sinus a.
> cerebral artery a.
> cirsoid a.

> communicating artery a.
> fusiform a.
> Leber's a.
> Leber's miliary a.
> miliary a.
> ophthalmic artery a.
> a. of orbit
> orbital a.
> racemose a.
> a. of retinal arteriole
> retinal artery a.
> saccular a.
> suprasellar a.

aneurysmal bone cyst
Angelucci's
> A. operation
> A. syndrome

angiitis
angioblastic meningioma
angiodiathermy
angioedema
angioendotheliomatosis
> neoplastic a.

angiogram
> fluorescein a.

angiography
> anterior segment a.
> carotid a.
> cerebral a.
> cerebral radionuclide a.
> digital subtraction a.
> fluorescein a. (FA)
> magnetic resonance a.
> orbital a.
> vertebral a.

angioid
> a. retinal streaks
> a. streak

angiokeratoma
> a. corporis diffusum
> a. corporis diffusum
>   universale
> diffuse a.

**angiolymphoid hyperplasia with
  eosinophilia**
angioma
> cavernous a.
> conjunctival a.
> episcleral a.
> nerve head a.
> orbital a.
> racemose a.

15

angioma *(continued)*
    a. serpinginosum
    spider a.
angiomatosis
    cerebroretinal a.
    encephalofacial a.
    encephalotrigeminal a.
    meningocutaneous a.
    a. of retina
    a. retinae
    retinal a.
    retinocerebellar a.
angiopathia retinae juvenilis
angiopathic retinopathy
angiopathy
    cerebral amyloid a.
angiophakomatosis
angiosarcoma
    orbital a.
angioscopy
    fluorescein fundus a.
angioscotoma
angioscotometry
angiospasm
angiospastic retinopathy
angiotensin
angiotensin-converting enzyme (ACE)
angle
    a. of aberration
    a. of abnormality
    alpha a.
    a. of anomaly, anomaly a.
    a. of anterior chamber
    anterior chamber a.
    a. of aperture
    apical a.
    biorbital a.
    cerebellopontine a.
    chamber a.
    a. of convergence, convergence a.
    critical a.
    deformity a.
    a. of deviation
    a. of direction
    disparity a.
    drainage a.
    a. of eccentricity
    elevation a.
    a. of emergence
    filtration a.

    a. of Fuchs
    gamma a.
    a. of incidence, incident a.
    iridial a.
    iridocorneal a.
    a. of iris
    Jacquart's a.
    kappa a.
    lambda a.
    large kappa a.
    lateral a.
    limiting a.
    medial a.
    meter a.
    minimum separable a.
    minimum visible a.
    minimum visual a.
    ocular a.
    optic a.
    pantoscopic a.
    a. of polarization
    a. recession
    a. of reflection
    refracting a. of prism
    a. of refraction, refraction a.
    space of iridocorneal a.
    a. squint
    a. of squint, squint a.
    a. structure
    visual a.
    wetting a.
    a. width
    zipped a.
angle-closure glaucoma (ACG)
angled
    a. capsule forceps
    a. counterpressor
    a. discission hook
    a. iris hook and IOL dialer
    a. iris retractor
    a. iris spatula
    a. left/right cannula
    a. lens loupe
    a. nucleus removal loupe
    a. probe
    a. suction tube
    a. Vico manipulator
angle-fixated lens
angle-recession glaucoma
angle-supported lens

angling
pantoscopic a.
angor ocularis
Ångström's law
Ångström unit
angular
a. aqueous sinus plexus
a. blepharitis
a. blepharoconjunctivitis
a. conjunctivitis
a. distance
a. gyrus
a. iridocornealis
a. junction of eyelid
a. line
a. oculi lateralis
a. oculi medialis
a. vein
angularis
vena a.
angulated iris spatula
angulation
angulus
a. iridis
a. iridocornealis
a. oculi lateralis
a. oculi medialis
anhidrosis
anhidrotic ectodermal dysplasia
anhydrase
carbonic a.
a. glycerol
anicteric
anionic surfactant
aniridia
traumatic a.
aniridia, genitourinary abnormalities, and mental retardation (AGR triad)
Anis
A. forceps
A. irrigating vectis
A. staple lens
aniseikonia
spectacle-induced a.
aniseikonic lens
anisoaccommodation
anisochromatic
anisocoria
a. contraction
essential a.
anisometric amblyopia
anisometrope

anisometropia
axial a.
myopic a.
refractive a.
anisometropic amblyopia
anisophoria
induced a.
anisopia
anisotropal
anisotropy
ankyloblepharon
external a.
a. filiforme adnatum
a. totale
ankylosing spondylitis
anlage
lacrimal duct a.
anneal
annular
a. bifocal contact lens
a. cataract
a. corneal graft
a. corneal graft operation
a. keratitis
a. macular dystrophy
a. plexus
a. scleritis
a. scotoma
a. staphyloma
a. synechia
a. ulcer
annulus, anulus
a. ciliaris
a. of conjunctiva
a. iridis major
a. iridis minor
a. tendineus communis
a. of Zinn
a. zinnii
anomalopia
anomaloscope
Nagel a.
anomalous
a. correspondence
a. disks
a. fixation
a. retinal correspondence (ARC)
a. trichromatism
a. trichromatopsia
anomaly
Alder's a.
a. angle

anomaly *(continued)*
    Axenfeld's a.
    coloboma a.'s
    congenital a.
    craniofacial a.
    developmental a.
    facial a.'s
    Klippel-Feil a.
    lacrimal angle duct a.
    morning glory a.
    morning glory optic disk a.
    oculocephalic a.
    oculocephalic vascular a.
    osseous a.
    Peter's a.
    Rieger's a.
anophoria
anophthalmia
    consecutive a.
    primary a.
    secondary a.
anophthalmic socket
anophthalmos
    congenital a.
anophthalmus
anopia
    amblyopia ex a.
anopsia
    ex a.
anorexia nervosa
anorthopia
anorthoscope
anotropia
anovulatory agent
anoxia
ANSI
    American National Standards
    Institute
antagonist
    contralateral a.
    folic acid a.
    inhibitional palsy of
    contralateral a.
    ipsilateral a.
antazoline
    a. phosphate and
    naphazoline HCl
antecubital vein
anteflexion of iris
anterior
    a. axial cataract
    a. axial developmental
    cataract

a. axial embryonal cataract
a. axonal embryonal
cataract
camera bulbi a.
camera oculi a.
a. capsule
a. capsulectomy
a. capsule shagreen
a. capsulotomy
a. cataract
a. central curve (ACC)
a. cerebral artery
a. chamber (AC)
a. chamber angle
a. chamber cannula
a. chamber cleavage
syndrome
a. chamber of eye
a. chamber irrigating vectis
a. chamber irrigator
a. chamber lens
a. chamber lymphoma
a. chamber paracentesis
a. chamber reaction
a. chamber sinus
a. chamber synechia scissors
a. chamber tap
a. chamber trabecula
a. chamber tube
a. choroiditis
a. ciliary artery
a. ciliary vein
a. cleavage syndrome
a. conjunctival artery
a. conjunctival vein
a. corneal curvature
a. corneal staphyloma
a. cylinder
a. embryotoxon
a. epithelium corneae
a. focal point
a. hyaloidal fibrovascular
proliferation
a. hyaloid membrane
(AHM)
a. hydrophthalmia
a. ischemic optic neuritis
(AION)
a. ischemic optic
neuropathy (AION)
a. keratoconus
a. knee of von Willebrand
lamina elastica a.

a. lens
a. lens capsule
limiting lamina a.
a. limiting lamina
a. limiting ring
a. lip
a. megalophthalmos
a. megalophthalmus
a. membrane dystrophy
a. mosaic crocodile shagreen
a. ocular segment
a. optical zone (AOZ)
a. peripheral curve (APC)
a. polar cataract
a. pole
a. pole cataract
a. puncture
a. pyramidal cataract
a. scleritis
a. sclerochoroiditis
a. sclerotomy
a. segment
a. segment angiography
a. segment of eye
a. segment necrosis
a. segment sleeve
a. staphyloma
a. symblepharon
a. synechia
a. uveitis
a. visual pathway
a. vitrectomy
anterior chamber (AC)
angle of a. c.
flat a. c.
anteriores
limbal palpebrales a.
vena ciliares a.
anterius
foramen lacerum a.
anteroposterior
a. axis
a. axis of Fick
Anthony orbital compressor
anthrax
antiacetylcholine receptor antibody
Antibiotic
Triple A.
antibiotic
bacteriocidal a.
bacteriostatic a.

broad-spectrum a.
prophylactic a.
antibody, pl. antibodies
antiacetylcholine receptor a.
antilens protein antibodies
antineutrophil cytoplasmic a.
  (ANCA)
antinuclear a. (ANA)
antiphospholipid a.
antiretina a.
complement-fixing a.
cytotoxic a.
HIV-specific antibodies
homotropic a.
indirect fluorescent a. (IFA)
monoclonal a.
stimulatory a.
treponemal a.
antibody-dependent cytotoxic
  hypersensitivity
anticataract drug
anticholinesterase
a. agent
a. inhibitor
anticoagulant
lupus a.
anticomplement immunofluorescence
anticonvulsant
antidepressant
antidote
antidromic conduction
antifibrinolytic agent
antifreeze
antifungal agent
antigen
Australia a. (Au Ag)
early a.
EBV-associated a.
EBV nuclear a.
extractable nuclear a.
hepatitis B surface a.
HLA-A29 a.
HLA-B5 a.
HLA-B7 a.
HLA-B15 a.
HLA-B27 a.
human leukocyte a. (HLA)
Kveim a.
major histocompatibility a.
nuclear a.
rheumatoid-associated
  nuclear a.

antigen *(continued)*
    transplantation a.
    viral capsid a. (VCA)
antigenicity
antiglaucoma surgery
antihistamine
antihyaluronidase
anti-inflammatories
anti-inflammatory agent
antilens protein antibodies
antilewisite
    British a. (BAL)
Antilirium
antimelanoma
antimetabolite
antimetropia
antimicrobial
    a. activity
    a. agent
antimitotic agent
antimongoloid slant
antimuscarinic
antineoplastic agent
antineutrophil cytoplasmic antibody (ANCA)
antinuclear
    a. antibody (ANA)
    a. factor
antiophthalmic
antioxidant enzyme
antiphospholipid antibody
antiplatelet agent
antiprostaglandin
antipsychotic
antipyrine
antireflection coating
antiretina antibody
antisuppression exercise
antiteratogen
antitonic
antitoxin
α_1-**antitrypsin**
antiviral agent
antixerophthalmic
Antley-Bixler syndrome
Anton-Babinski syndrome
Antoni patterns
Anton's
    A. symptom
    A. syndrome
antrophose
anulus (*var. of* annulus)

AO
    AO applanation tonometer
    AO binocular indirect ophthalmoscope
    AO Ful-Vue diagnostic unit
    AO lens
    AO lensometer
    AO Project-O-Chart
    AO Reichert Instruments
    AO Reichert Instruments applanation tonometer
    AO Reichert Instruments binocular indirect ophthalmoscope
    AO Reichert Instruments Ful-Vue diagnostic unit
    AO Reichert Instruments lensometer
    AO Reichert Instruments Project-O-Chart
    AO Reichert lensometer
    AO rotary prism
    AO Vectographic Project-O-Chart slide
aorta
    coarctation of a.
aortic
    a. arch syndrome
    a. hypoperfusion
Aosept
AOZ
    anterior optical zone
A pattern
A-pattern
    A.-p. esotropia
    A.-p. exotropia
    A.-p. strabismus
APC
    anterior peripheral curve
APD
    afferent pupillary defect
Apert
    acrocephalosyndactylia of A.
Apert's
    A. disease
    A. syndrome
aperture
    a. disk
    numerical a. (NA)
    orbital a.
    pupillary a.
apex, pl. **apices**
    corneal a.

a. fracture
orbital a.
a. of prism
aphacia
aphacic
aphacos
aphake
aphakia
binocular a.
extracapsular a.
monocular a.
aphakial, aphakic
aphasia
optic a.
visual a.
aphose
aphotesthesia
aphotic
aphthous-like
aphthous ulcer
apical
a. angle
a. clearance
a. cone
a. radius
a. zone
a. zone of cornea
apices
aplanatic
a. focus
a. lens
aplanatism
aplasia
lacrimal nucleus a.
macular a.
a. of optic nerve
punctum a.
retinal a.
aplastic anemia
APMPPE
acute posterior multifocal
placoid pigment epitheliopathy
apnea
apochromatic
a. lens
a. objective
apocrine
a. gland
a. hydrocystoma
Apollo's disease
aponeurosis
aponeurotic ptosis

apoplectic
a. glaucoma
a. retinitis
apoplexy
occipital a.
pituitary a.
a. of pituitary
retinal a.
apostilb
apparatus
ciliary a.
dioptric a.
Frigitronics cryosurgery a.
Frigitronics nitrous oxide
cryosurgery a.
Golgi a.
lacrimal a.
a. lacrimalis
a. suspensorius lentis
Vactro perilimbal suction a.
appearance
beaten-bronze a.
beaten-copper a.
beaten-metal a.
cobblestone a.
dropped-socket a.
ground-glass a.
mottled a.
salt and pepper a.
spongy a.
squashed-tomato a.
appendage of eye
applamatic tonometer
applanation
a. pressure
tension by a. (TAP)
a. tension (AT)
a. tonometer
a. tonometry
applanometer
applanometry
application
diathermy a.'s
pilot a.
applicator
beta therapy eye a.
Gass dye a.
Gifford a.
Appolionio lens
apposition
approach
Berke's a.
Caldwell-Luc a.

approach *(continued)*
    fornix a.
    Iliff's a.
    limbal a.
    pars plana a.
apraclonidine
apraclonidine HCl
apraxia
    Cogan's a.
    Cogan's congenital
      oculomotor a.
    constructional a.
    a. of gaze
    oculomotor a.
Apresoline
Apt
Aquaflex
    A. contact lens
    A. lens
Aqua-Flow
aqua oculi
Aquasight lens
AquaSite
Aquasonic 100 gel
Aqua-Tears
aqueous
    a. chamber
    a. flare
    a. flow
    a. humor
    a. humor eye
    a. inflow
    a. layer
    a. layer of tear film
    a. outflow
    a. paracentesis
    plasmoid a.
    a. tear deficiency (ATD)
    a. tear layer
    a. transplant needle
    a. vein
aqueous-influx phenomenon
aquocapsulitis
ara-A
    adenine arabinoside
    arabinosyladenine
arabinoside
    adenine a. (ara-A)
    cytosine a. (ara-C)
arabinosyladenine (ara-A)
arabinosylcytosine (ara-C)

ara-C
    arabinosylcytosine
    cytosine arabinoside
arachidonic acid
arachnodactyly
arachnoid
    a. hemorrhage
    a. sheath
arachnoidal cyst
arachnoiditis
    chiasmal a.
    opticochiasmatic a.
Aralen Phosphate
arborescens keratitis
arborescent cataract
arborization
    pattern a.
    a. pattern
ARC
    abnormal retinal correspondence
    AIDS-related complex
    anomalous retinal
      correspondence
    unharmonious ARC
arc
    a. and bowl perimeters
    a. of contact
    contact a.
    nuclear a.
    a. perimeter
    a. perimetry
    a. scotoma
    a. staining
    xenon a.
arcade
    inferior a.
    inferior temporal a.,
      inferotemporal a.
    limbal a.
    major a.
    superior a.
    superior vascular a.
    temporal a.
    vascular a.
arc-flash conjunctivitis
arch
    orbital a.
    Salus' a.
    superciliary a.
    supraorbital a.
arched brow
archery

architecture
    nasal a.
arciform density
arcs
    blue a.
arcuate
    a. Bjerrum's scotoma
    a. commissure
    a. course
    a. defect
    a. field defects
    a. nerve fiber bundle
    a. retinal folds
    a. scotoma
    a. staining
    a. transverse keratotomy
arcus, gen. and pl. **arcus**
    a. adiposus
    a. cornealis, corneal a.
    a. juvenilis, juvenile a.
    a. lipoides
    opaque a.
    a. senilis
    unilateral a.
Arden gratings
area, pl. **areae, areas**
    aspheric lenticular a.
    Bjerrum's a.
    Brodmann's a.
    a. centralis
    a. of conscious regard
    a. cribrosa
    a. of critical definition
    fusion a.
    macular a.
    a. martegiani
    mirror a.
    Panum's fusion a.
    papillary a.
    parastriate a.
    spindle-shaped a.
    visual association a.
areata
    alopecia a.
areflexia
    pupillary a.
areolar
    a. central choroiditis
    a. choroiditis
    a. choroidopathy
argamblyopia
argema
arginine-reduced diet

argon
    a. blue
    a. blue laser
    a. green
    a. green laser
    a. laser
    a. laser coagulator
    a. laser
      endophotocoagulation
    a. laser iridectomy
    a. laser photocoagulation
    a. laser trabeculopexy (ALT)
    a. laser trabeculoplasty
      (ALTP)
argon-fluoride laser
argon-pumped tunable dye laser
Argyll-Robertson
    A.-R. instruments
    A.-R. operation
    A.-R. pupil
    A.-R. pupil sign
argyria
argyriasis
argyrism
Argyrol
Argyrol S.S.
argyrosis
ariboflavinosis
aridosiliculose cataract
aridosiliquata
    cataracta a.
aridosiliquate cataract
Arion's
    A. operation
    A. sling
Aristocort
Aristospan
Arlt
    A. lens
    A. lens loupe
    A. loupe
    A. scoop
Arlt-Jaesche
    A.-J. excision
    A.-J. operation
    A.-J. recessus
    A.-J. sinus
    A.-J. trachoma
Arlt's
    A. disease
    A. epicanthus repair
    A. eyelid repair
    A. line

Arlt's *(continued)*
    A. operation
    A. pterygium
    A. sinus
    A. trachoma
    A. triangle
Armaly-Drance technique
ARMD
    age-related macular degeneration
Arnold
    zygomatic foramen of A.
Arnold-Chiari malformation
arrachement
array
    ordered a.
    radial vessel a.
AR 1000 refractor
arrest
    cardiac a.
arrestin
arrhinencephaly
Arrowhead's operation
Arroyo
    A. encircling suture
    A. expressor
    A. forceps
    A. implant
    A. protector
    A. trephine
Arroyo's
    A. cataract extraction
    A. dacryostomy
    A. keratoplasty
    A. operation
    A. sign
    A. tenotomy
Arruga
    A. capsule forceps
    A. encircling suture
    A. expressor
    A. forceps
    A. implant
    A. lacrimal trephine
    A. lens
    A. needle holder
    A. protector
    A. retractor
    A. trephine
Arruga-Berens operation
Arruga-McCool capsule forceps
Arruga-Moura-Brazil implant
Arruga's
    A. cataract extraction

    A. dacryostomy
    A. keratoplasty
    A. operation
    A. tenotomy
arsenic amblyopia
arterial
    a. circle
    a. circle of greater iris
    a. circle of lesser iris
    a. hypertension
arteriography
    cerebral a.
arteriohepatic dysplasia
arteriola
    a. macularis inferior
    a. macularis superior
    a. medialis retinae
    a. nasalis retinae inferior
    a. nasalis retinae superior
    a. temporalis retinae
    inferior
    a. temporalis retinae
    superior
arteriolar
    a. attenuation
    a. narrowing
    a. nicking
    a. occlusive disease
    a. sclerosis
arteriole
    a. communication
    copper-wire a.
    inferior macular a.
    macular a.
    narrowing of a.
    retinal a.
    silver-wire a.
    a. straightening
    superior macular a.
arteriolosclerosis
arteriolovenous crossings
arteriosclerosis
    cerebral a.
    a. of retina
arteriosclerotic
    a. ischemic optic
    neuropathy
    a. retinopathy
arteriosus
arteriovenous (AV)
    a. aneurysm
    a. communication
    a. crossing defect

a. malformation
a. nicking
a. patterns
a. ratio
a. strabismus syndrome
arteritic ischemic optic neuropathy
arteritis
cranial a.
giant cell a. (GCA)
pseudotemporal a.
temporal a. (TA)
artery
anterior cerebral a.
anterior ciliary a.
anterior conjunctival a.
basilar a.
calcarine a.
carotid a.
central a.
central retinal a. (CRA)
cerebellar a.
cerebral a.
ciliary a.
cilioretinal a.
conjunctival a.
copper-wire a.
corkscrew a.
episcleral a.
ethmoidal a.
hyaline a.
hyalitis a.
hyaloid a.
hypophyseal a.
inferior nasal a.,
  inferonasal a.
inferior temporal a.,
  inferotemporal a.
infraorbital a.
internal carotid a.
lacrimal a.
long ciliary a.
long posterior ciliary a.'s
middle cerebral a.
ophthalmic a.
optic a.
parieto-occipital a.
posterior cerebral a.
posterior ciliary a.
posterior conjunctival a.
retinal a.
short ciliary a.
short posterior ciliary a.
superior nasal a.

superior temporal a.
supraorbital a.
tarsal a.
temporal a.
temporo-occipital a.
thrombosed a.
vertebrobasilar a.
zygomatico-orbital a.
arthritis
juvenile rheumatoid a.
postinfective reactive a.
rheumatoid a.
arthro-ophthalmopathy
hereditary progressive a.-o.
arthropod
Arthus' reaction
articularis
lentis a.
artifact
artifactiously
artifactual
artificial
a. cornea
a. diabetes
a. eye
a. lens
a. pupil
a. silk keratitis
a. tears
a. vision
Artificial Tears
arylsulfatase
A-scan
Cilco Sonometric A-s.
Jedmed A-s.
Jedmed/DGH A-s.
A-s. ultrasonogram
A-s. ultrasonography
Ascaris lumbricoides
Ascher's
A. aqueous-influx
  phenomenon
A. glass-rod phenomenon
A. syndrome
A. vein
Aschner's reflex
Asch septal forceps
Ascon instruments
ascorbic acid
asepsis
aseptic bone necrosis
ash leaf spot

25

As.M.
   myopic astigmatism
as needed (p.r.n.)
aspartylglycosaminuria
aspergillosis
   a. uveitis
Aspergillus
   A. fumigatus
aspheric
   a. cataract lens
   a. contact lens
   a. cornea
   a. lens
   a. lenticular area
   a. spectacle lens
   a. viewing lens
aspherical ophthalmoscopic lens
aspirating/irrigating vectis
aspiration
   Alcon a.
   cataract a.
   a. of cortex
   a. of lens
   a. portal
   vitreous a.
aspirator
   Alcon a.
   Castroviejo a.
   Castroviejo orbital a.
   Cavitron a.
   Cooper a.
   Fibra Sonics phaco a.
   Fink cataract a.
   Kelman a.
   Nugent a.
   Nugent soft cataract a.
   Stat a.
assay
   enzyme-linked
     immunosorbent a. (ELISA)
   immunofluorescent a.
   Lowry's a.
   mucous a.
   Raji cell a.
Assi cannula
Association
   American Medical A.
     (AMA)
   A. for Children and Adults
     with Learning Disabilities
     (ACLD)
   A. of Technical Personnel
     in Ophthalmology (ATPO)

association
   CHARGE a.
Ast.
   astigmatism
asteroid
   a. bodies
   a. hyalitis
   hyaloid a.
   a. hyalosis
asteroides
   Nocardia a.
asthenocoria
asthenometer
asthenope
asthenopia
   accommodative a.
   muscular a.
   nervous a.
   neurasthenic a.
   retinal a.
   tarsal a.
asthenopic
asthma
astigmagraph
astigmagraphic error
astigmatic
   a. amblyopia
   a. axis
   a. clock
   a. dial
   a. dial chart
   a. error
   a. image
   a. keratotomy
   a. lens
astigmatism (Ast.)
   acquired a.
   against-the-rule a.
   asymmetric a.
   compound a.
   compound hyperopic a.
   compound myopic a.
   congenital a.
   corneal a.
   a. correction
   direct a.
   hypermetropic a.
   hyperopic a.
   inverse a.
   irregular a.
   lenticular a.
   mixed a.
   myopic a. (As.M.)

oblique a.
a. of oblique pencils
physiologic a.
radial a.
radical a.
regular a.
residual a.
reversed a.
simple a.
simple hyperopic a.
simple myopic a.
total a.
with-the-rule a.
astigmatometer, astigmometer
astigmatometry, astigmometry
astigmatoscope
astigmatoscopy
astigmia
astigmic
astigmometer (*var. of*
astigmatometer)
astigmometry (*var. of*
astigmatometry)
astigmoscope
astigmoscopy
ASTM
American Society for Testing
and Materials
astrocyte
astrocytic
a. glioma
a. hamartoma
astrocytoma
juvenile pilocytic a.
pilocytic a.
retinal a.
asymmetric
a. astigmatism
a. refractive errors
a. surgery
asymmetry
chromatic a.
asymptomatic
A syndrome
AT
applanation tension
Atabrine
ataxia
cerebellar a.
Friedreich's a.
hereditary cerebellar a.
Marie's a.
ocular a.

Pierre-Marie's a.
vestibulocerebellar a.
ataxia-telangiectasia
a.-t. syndrome
ataxic nystagmus
ATD
aqueous tear deficiency
atenolol
Athens suture spreader
atheroembolism
atheroma
atherosclerosis
ischemic a.
atherosclerotic ischemic neuritis
athetosis
pupillary a.
Atkin lid block
Atkinson
A. block
A. corneal scissors
A. 25-G short curved
cystitome
A. needle
A. retrobulbar needle
A. sclerotome
A. single-bevel blunt-tip
needle
A. tip peribulbar needle
Atkinson's
A. technique
atonia
atonic
a. ectropion
a. entropion
a. epiphora
atopic
a. cataract
a. conjunctivitis
a. dermatitis
a. eczema
a. eczema
keratoconjunctivitis
a. keratoconjunctivitis
a. line
atopy
ATP
adenosine triphosphate
ATPase
adenosine triphosphatase
actomyosin ATPase
ATPO
Association of Technical
Personnel in Ophthalmology

atracurium
Atraloc suture
atresia
    a. iridis
    retinal a.
    tilting lens a.
atretoblepharia
atretopsia
atrial fibrillation
Atropa belladonna
Atropair
atrophia
    a. bulbi
    a. bulborum hereditaria
    a. choroideae et retinae
    a. dolorosa
    a. gyrata
atrophic
    a. age-related macular
      degeneration (AAMD)
    a. degenerative maculopathy
    a. excavation
    a. heterochromia
    a. macular degeneration
    a. polychondritis
    a. rhinitis
atrophicans
    acrodermatitis chronica a.
atrophy
    Behr's a.
    Behr's optic a.
    bow-tie a.
    bow-tie optic a.
    bulbous a.
    central areolar choroidal a.
    cerebral a.
    choriocapillary a.
    chorioretinal a.
    choroidal a.
    choroidal gyrate a.
    choroidal myopic a.
    choroidal secondary a.
    choroidal vascular a.
    congenital optic a.
    consecutive a.
    consecutive optic a.
    diabetic optic a.
    diffuse inflammatory
      eyelid a.
    essential iris a.
    essential progressive a. of
      iris
    Fuchs' a.

glaucomatous a.
gray a.
gyrate a.
gyrate a. of choroid and
  retina
hemifacial a.
heredodegenerative a.
heredofamilial optic a.
infantile optic a.
iris a.
ischemic choroidal a.
ischemic optic a.
juvenile optic a.
Kjer's dominant a.
Kjer's dominant optic a.
Kjer's optic a.
Leber's a.
Leber's hereditary optic a.
Leber's optic a.
linear subcutaneous a.
morning glory optic a.
myopic choroidal a.
neuritic a.
neurogenic iris a.
optic a.
optic nerve a.
a. of optic nerve
periorbital fat a.
peripapillary choroidal a.
peripheral chorioretinal a.
pigmented paravenous
  chorioretinal a.
postinflammatory a.
primary optic a.
progressive choroidal a.
progressive hemifacial a.
Schnabel's optic a.
secondary optic a.
senile a.
simple optic a.
subcutaneous fat a.
tabetic optic a.
traumatic a.
uveal a.
Atropine
    A. Care 1%
    Isopto A.
atropine
    a. conjunctivitis
    prednisolone and a.
    a. and prednisolone
    a. sulfate
    a. sulfate

atropinism
atropinization
Atropisol
attachment
desmosomal cellular a.
MP Video endoscopic
lens a.
vitreoretinal a.
zonular a.
attack
transient ischemic a. (TIA)
attention
a. deficit disorder
a. reflex
attentiveness
visual a.
attenuation
arteriolar a.
attollens aurem
A-tuck
Atwood loupe
atypical
a. achromatopsia
a. coloboma
a. facial pain
a. mycobacteria
^{198}Au
gold-198
Au Ag
Australia antigen
Aubert's phenomenon
audiovisual
auditory
a. oculogyric reflex
a. perceptual disability
a. reflex
aura
aural
a. nystagmus
a. scotoma
auranofin
aurem
attollens a.
Aureomycin
aureus
Staphylococcus a.
auriasis
auricular glaucoma
aurochromoderma
aurothioglucose
aurothioglycanide
auscultation

Aus Jena-Schiötz tonometer
Australia antigen (Au Ag)
autacoid
autoantibodies
autoantibody
autoclaving
autofluorescence
autofunduscope
autofunduscopy
autogenous
a. dermis fat graft
a. donor material
a. fibronectin
a. keratoplasty
autograft
free skin a.
full-thickness a.
skin a.
split-thickness a.
autoimmune
a. demyelination
a. disease
autoimmunity
autokeratometer
autokeratoplasty
autokinesis visible light
autokinetic
a. effect
a. visible light phenomenon
autolysis
automated
a. hemisphere perimeter
a. perimeter
a. perimetry
a. refractor
a. static threshold perimetry
a. trephine
a. visual field
automatic
a. infrared optometer
a. refractor
a. trephine
a. twin syringe injector
autonomic dysautonomia
familial a. d.
autonomic nervous system
auto-ophthalmoscope
auto-ophthalmoscopy
autophagic vacuole
autophagolysosome
Autophoro-Optimeter
Clark A.-O.
Autoplot

Autorefractor-7
    Subjective A.-7
6600 Autorefractor
autorefractor
autoregulation
autosomal
    a. disorder
    a. dominant disease
    a. dominant oculocutaneous
      albinism
    a. dominant trait
    a. dominant vitellirupture
    a. recessive disease
    a. recessive inheritance
    a. recessive ocular albinism
autosome
Autoswitch System
auxiliary
    a. fiber
    a. lens
auxometer
AV
    arteriovenous
    AV crossing defect
    AV nicking
    AV patterns
    AV strabismus syndrome
avascular keratitis
avascular zone
    foveal a. z.
avidin-biotinylated peroxidase
  complex
avirulent
Avit handpiece
avulsion
    a. of caruncula lacrimalis
    a. of eyelid
    facial nerve a.
a-wave test
awl
    lacrimal a.
    Mustarde a.
axanthopsia
Axenfeld-Krukenberg spindle
Axenfeld's
    A. anomaly
    A. follicular conjunctivitis
    A. loop
    A. nerve loop
    A. syndrome
axes
axial
    a. amblyopia

    a. ametropia
    a. anisometropia
    a. cataract
    a. chamber
    a. embryonal cataract
    a. fusiform cataract
    a. fusiform developmental
      cataract
    a. hyperopia
    a. illumination
    a. length
    a. length of eye
    a. light
    a. myopia
    a. partial childhood cataract
    a. point
    a. proptosis
    a. ray of light
    a. tomography
    a. view
axillary cataract
axis, pl. axes
    anteroposterior a.
    astigmatic a.
    a. bulbi externus
    a. bulbi internus
    cylinder a.
    a. of cylindric lens (x)
    a. of Fick
    Fick's a.
    a. fixation
    frontal a.
    geometric a.
    hypothalamic-pituitary-
      thyroid a.
    lens a.
    a. lentis
    longitudinal a.
    ocular a.
    a. oculi externa
    a. oculi interna
    optical a.
    a. opticus
    orbital a.
    principal optic a.
    pupillary a.
    sagittal a.
    secondary a.
    vertical a.
    visual a.
Axisonic II ultrasound
AXM
    acetoxycycloheximide

axometer
axon
>   fiber layer of a.
>   nerve fiber a.'s
axonal
>   a. loss
>   a. transport
axonometer
axoplasm
axoplasmic
>   a. flow
>   a. stasis
>   a. transport
Ayer chalazion forceps
Ayerst instruments

Azar
>   A. curved cystitome
>   A. lens
>   A. lens-holding forceps
>   A. lens-manipulating hook
>   A. lid speculum
azathioprine
azidothymidine (AZT)
azlocillin
azotemia
azotemic retinitis
AZT
>   azidothymidine
Azulfidine

babesiosis
baby Barraquer needle holder
Baciguent
bacillary layer
Bacille bilié de Calmette-Guérin
  (BCG)
Bacillus
    B. cereus
    B. pyocyaneus
bacillus, pl. bacilli
    acid-fast bacilli
    b. Calmette-Guérin
      vaccination
    gonococcal b.
    Koch-Weeks b.
    pneumococcal b.
    Staphylococcus b.
    streptococcal b.
    tubercle b.
    Weeks' b.
bacitracin
    zinc b.
    b. zinc
bacitracin, neomycin, polymixin B,
  and hydrocortisone
bacitracin, neomycin, and
  polymyxin B
back
    b. surface toric contact lens
    b. vertex power
background
    b. diabetic retinopathy
    b. illumination
    b. retinopathy
    tigroid b.
Backhaus clamp
Backhaus' syndrome
bacteria
    gram-negative b.
    gram-positive b.
bacterial
    b. blepharoconjunctivitis
    b. conjunctivitis
    b. corneal ulcer
    b. culture
    b. disease
    b. endophthalmitis
    b. infection
    b. keratitis

    b. ulcer
    b. uveitis
bactericide
bacterid
bacteriocidal
    b. agent
    b. antibiotic
bacteriostatic
    b. agent
    b. antibiotic
Bacticort
Bactrim
Badal lensmeter
Badal's operation
Baer's nystagmus
bag
    capsular b.
    palpebral adipose b.'s
baggy eyelid
Bagley-Wilmer expressor
Bagolini lens
Bagolini's
    B. striated glasses test
    B. test
Bahn spud
Bailey
    B. chalazion forceps
    B. foreign body remover
    B. lacrimal cannula
Bailey-Lovie
    B.-L. Log Mar chart
    B.-L. Near Test
    B.-L. visual acuity chart
Bailliart
    B. goniometer
    B. ophthalmodynamometer
    B. ophthalmoscope
Baird chalazion forceps
BAL
  British antilewisite
balance
    meridional b.
    muscular b.
balanced
    b. saline solution (BSS)
    b. salt solution (BSS)
Baldex
balding the limbus
Balint's syndrome

ball
ice b.
Pinky b.
retinal ice b.
Super Pinky b.
ballast
prism b.
b. prism
ballasted contact lens
Ballen-Alexander
B.-A. forceps
B.-A. orbital retractor
Baller-Gerold syndrome
Ballet's
B. disease
B. sign
balloon
b. cell formation
Honan b.
Lincoff b.
ballottement
ocular b.
balsam
Canada b.
Bamatter's syndrome
band
#40 b.
A b.
cellophane-like b.
ciliary body b.
circling b.
encircling b.
H b.
b. keratitis
keratitis b.
b. keratopathy
M b.
Mach's b.
scleral b.
silicone b.
Storz b.
traction b.
Watzke b.
Z b.
zonular b.
bandage
binocle b.
binocular b.
Borsch b.
b. contact lens
Elastoplast b.
b. lens
monocular b.

pressure b.
b. scissors
bandelette
keratitis b.
bandpass function
band-shaped
b.-s. keratitis
b.-s. keratopathy
Bangerter
B. iris spatula
B. method of pleoptic
B. muscle forceps
Bangerter's pterygium operation
Bangla Joy conjunctivitis
bank
eye b.
b. keratitis
Banner
B. enucleation snare
B. forceps
B. snare enucleator
bar
Berens prism b.
horizontal prism b.'s
b. prism
b. reader
skiascopy b.
Bárány's
B. caloric test
B. sign
barbital
barbiturate
Bardelli's lid ptosis operation
Bardet-Biedl
B.-B. syndrome
Bard-Parker
B.-P. blade
B.-P. forceps
B.-P. keratome
B.-P. knife
B.-P. razor
B.-P. trephine
Bard's sign
bare
b. lymphocyte syndrome
b. scleral technique
baring of the blind spot
barium flint
Barkan
B. goniolens
B. gonioscopic lens
B. goniotomy knife
B. goniotomy lens

B. infant implant
B. iris forceps
B. knife
B. light
Barkan-Cordes linear cataract operation
Barkan's
 B. double cyclodialysis operation
 B. goniotomy operation
 B. membrane
 B. operation
Barlow's syndrome
Barnes-Hind
 B.-H. contact lens cleaning and soaking solution
 B.-H. wetting solution
Baron-Bietti syndrome
Baron lens
barrage
 double-row diathermy b.
Barraquer
 B. bladebreaker
 B. cannula
 B. cilia forceps
 B. conjunctival forceps
 B. corneal dissector
 B. corneal forceps
 B. corneal utility forceps
 B. cryolathe
 B. curved holder
 B. erysiphake
 B. eye shield
 B. forceps
 B. hemostatic mosquito forceps
 B. implant
 B. iris scissors
 B. irrigator spatula
 B. keratoplasty knife
 B. knife
 B. lens
 B. microkeratome
 B. needle
 B. needle carrier
 B. needle holder
 B. razor bladebreaker
 B. sable brush
 B. scissors
 B. shield
 B. spatula
 B. speculum
 B. sweep

B. trephine
B. vitreous strand scissors
B. wire speculum
Barraquer-Colibri speculum
Barraquer-DeWecker scissors
Barraquer-Krumeich
 B.-K. Swinger refractive
 B.-K. test
Barraquer-Krumeich-Swinger retractor
Barraquer's
 B. enzymatic zonulolysis operation
 B. keratomileusis operation
 B. method
 B. operation
 B. zonulolysis
Barraquer-Vogt needle
Barraquer-von Mondach capsule forceps
Barr body
barred distortion
barrel distortion
Barré's signs
Barrie-Jones
 canaliculodacryorhinostomy operation
Barrier
 B. drape
 B. Phaco Extracapsular Pack
 B. sheet
barrier
 blood b.
 blood-aqueous b.
 blood-ocular b.
 blood-optic nerve b.
 blood-retinal b.
 epithelial b.
 ocular b.
 posterior capsular zonular b.
Barrio's operation
Barron
 B. epikeratophakia trephine
 B. trephine
Bartel spectacles
Bartholin syndrome
basal
 b. cell
 b. cell carcinoma
 b. cell carcinoma of eyelid
 b. cell nevus
 b. cell nevus syndrome

basal *(continued)*
    b. choroid
    b. ciliary body
    b. coil
    b. encephalocele
    b. ganglion
    b. iridectomy
    b. junction
    b. lamina
    b. lamina of choroid
    b. lamina of ciliary body
    b. laminar drusen
    b. layer
    b. ophthalmoplegia
    b. secretion
    b. tear secretion
basalis
    b. choroideae lamina
    b. corporis ciliaris lamina
base in, base-in prism (BI)
base
    cilia b.
    b. curve
    vitreous b.
baseball lens
base-down prism
Basedow's disease
base-in prism (BI)
basement
    b. membrane
    b. membrane dystrophy
base out, base-out prism (BO)
base-out prism (BO)
base up, base-up prism
base-up prism (BU)
basic
    b. esotropia
    b. exotropia
basilar
    b. artery
    b. artery aneurysm
    b. impression
basket
    Schultz fiber b.'s
basket-style scleral supporter speculum
Basol-S
basophil
basophilic
    b. adenoma
    b. reaction
    b. staining
Bassen-Kornzweig syndrome

Basterra's operation
BAT
    Brightness Acuity Test
bathomorphic
Batten-Mayou
    B.-M. disease
    B.-M. syndrome
Batten's
    B. ceroid lipofuscinosis
    B. disease
    B. syndrome
battered-baby syndrome
battered-child syndrome
Battle's sign
Baumgarten's gland
Bausch & Lomb
    B. & L. keratometer
    B. & L. Optima lens
Bausch-Lomb-Thorpe slit lamp
bay
    junctional b.
    lacrimal b.
Bayadi lens
Baylisascaris procyonis
bayonet forceps
BB gun
BB shot forceps
B cell
BCG
    Bacille bilié de Calmette-Guérin
BCNU
    bischloroethylnitrosourea
    carmustine
B-D needle
beading
    retinal venous b.
beaked forceps
Béal's
    B. conjunctivitis
    B. syndrome
beam
    aiming b.
    convergent b.'s
    divergent b.'s
    helium neon b.
    HeNe b.
    proton b.
    b. scatter
Beard-Cutler operation
Beard knife
Beard's operation
bear tracks
beaten-bronze appearance

beaten-copper appearance
beaten-metal appearance
Beaupre
    B. cilia forceps
    B. forceps
Beaver
    B. blade
    B. cataract cryoextractor
    B. cryoextractor
    B. discission blade
    B. eye blade
    B. goniotomy needle knife
    B. handle
    B. keratome
    B. knife
    B. Ocu-1 curved cystitome
    B. scleral Lundsgaard blade
Beaver-Lundsgaard blade
Beaver-Okamura blade
Beaver-Ziegler
    B.-Z. blade
    B.-Z. needle blade
Bechert
    B. 7mm lens
    B. nucleus rotator
Bechert-Kratz cannulated nucleus
retractor
Bechert-McPherson angled tying
forceps
Bechterew's disease
Becker
    B. corneal section
    spatulated scissors
    B. goniogram
    B. gonioscopic prism
Becker-Park speculum
Beckerscope binocular microscope
Becton Dickinson AcuteCare
bed
    capillary b.
    retinal capillary b.
    stromal b.
bedewing
    b. of cornea
    corneal b.
    epithelial b.
    b. to wet
bee
    b. polarization
    b. sting
Beebe
    B. lens
    B. loupe

Beer
    B. blade
    B. canaliculus knife
    B. cataract knife
    B. knife
Beer's
    B. Collyrium
    B. law
    B. operation
Behçet's
    B. disease
    B. skin puncture test
    B. syndrome
Behr's
    B. atrophy
    B. disease
    B. optic atrophy
    B. pupil
    B. syndrome
Bekhterev's
    B. nystagmus
    B. reflex
    B. sign
Belin double-ended needle holder
belladonna
    Atropa b.
Bell crysiphake
Bellows
    B. cryoextractor
    B. cryophake
Bell's
    B. palsy
    B. phenomenon
    B. reflex
bell-shaped curve
belly
    muscle b.
    b. of muscle
    b. of pterygium
belonoskiascopy
Belz lacrimal sac rongeur
Benadryl
Benazol
Bence-Jones protein
bench
    optical b.
bendazac
bender
    Watt stave b.
bending power
Benedict's
    B. operation
    B. orbit operation

Benedikt's syndrome
bengal
rose b.
benign
b. concentric annular macular dystrophy
b. dyskeratosis
b. mucosal pemphigoid
b. paroxysmal positional vertigo (BPPV)
b. paroxysmal postural vertigo
b. tumor
Bennett
B. cilia forceps
B. forceps
benoxinate
b. hydrochloride
Benson's disease
bent
b. blunt blade
b. blunt needle
b. 22-gauge needle
benzalkonium
b. chloride
benzene
b. hexachloride
benzoate
sodium b.
benzodiazepine
benzoquinone
benzoylmethylecgonine
Béraud's valve
berberine
Bercovici wire lid speculum
Berens
B. blade
B. cataract knife
B. conical implant
B. corneal dissector
B. corneal transplant forceps
B. corneal transplant scissors
B. corneoscleral punch
B. dilator
B. electrode
B. everter
B. expressor
B. forceps
B. glaucoma knife
B. hook
B. implant

B. iridocapsulotomy scissors
B. keratome
B. keratoplasty knife
B. lens loupe
B. lid everter
B. lid retractor
B. marking calipers
B. muscle clamp
B. muscle forceps
B. orbital compressor
B. partial keratome
B. prism
B. prism bar
B. ptosis forceps
B. ptosis knife
B. punch
B. pyramidal implant
B. refractor
B. retractor
B. scissors
B. scleral hook
B. spatula
B. speculum
B. sterilizing case
B. suturing forceps
B. test object
B. tonometer
Berens'
B. operation
B. pinhole and dominance test
B. pterygium transplant operation
B. sclerectomy operation
B. three-character test
Berens-Rosa
B.-R. implant
B.-R. scleral implant
Berens-Smith
B.-S. cul-de-sac restoration
B.-S. operation
Berens-Tolman ocular hypertension indicator
Berger's
B. sign
B. space
B. symptom
Bergmeister
papilla of B.
Bergmeister's papilla
Bergsma-Kaiser-Kupfer oculocutaneous albinism
beriberi

Berke
- B. clamp
- B. forceps
- B. lid everter
- B. ptosis forceps

Berke-Krönlein orbitotomy

Berkeley
- B. Bioengineering
- B. Bioengineering bipolar cautery
- B. Bioengineering brass scleral plug
- B. Bioengineering infusion terminal port
- B. Bioengineering mechanized scissors
- B. Bioengineering ocutome
- B. Bioengineering ptosis forceps
- B. Bioengineering stiletto

Berke-Motais operation

Berke's
- B. approach
- B. operation
- B. ptosis

Berlin's
- B. disease
- B. edema

Berman
- B. foreign body locator
- B. localizer
- B. locator

Bernard-Horner syndrome

Bernard's syndrome

Bernell
- B. grid
- B. tangent screen

Bernheimer's fibers

berry aneurysm

Berry's circle

Bertel's position

besiclometer

best-corrected
- b.-c. vision
- b.-c. visual acuity (BVA)

Best's
- B. degeneration
- B. disease
- B. vitelliform dystrophy
- B. vitelliform macular dystrophy

beta
- b. blockers
- b. hemolytic
- b. radiation
- b. receptor
- b. therapy eye applicator

beta-adrenergic
- b.-a. agonist
- b.-a. blocking agent

beta-blocking agent

Betadine

Betagan

Betagen

betalysin

betamethasone

betaxolol
- b. hydrochloride

Bethke's
- B. iridectomy
- B. operation

Betoptic

Betoptic S

Bettman-Noyes fixation forceps

beveled-edge lens

Bezold-Brücke phenomenon

BI
- base in
- base-in prism

Bianchi's
- B. sign
- B. valve

Biber-Haab Dimmer
- B.-H.-D. corneal dystrophy
- B.-H.-D. degeneration
- B.-H.-D. dystrophy

bicarbonate
- sodium b.

bicentric
- b. grinding
- b. lens
- b. spectacle lens

Bick's procedure

biconcave
- b. contact lens
- b. lens

biconvex lens

bicoronal scalp flap

bicurve contact lens

bicylindrical lens

Bidwell's ghost

Bielschowsky-Jansky
- B.-J. disease
- B.-J. syndrome

Bielschowsky-Lutz-Cogan syndrome

Bielschowsky-Parks head-tilt three-
  step test
Bielschowsky's
  B. disease
  B. head-tilt test
  B. operation
  B. phenomenon
  B. sign
  B. strabismus
  B. test
  B. three-step, head-tilt test
Biemond's syndrome
Bietti lens
Bietti's
  B. crystalline corneoretinal
    dystrophy
  B. dystrophy
  B. keratopathy
  B. syndrome
  B. tapetoretinal degeneration
bifixation
bifocal, pl. bifocals
  cement b.
  b. cement
  b. contact lens
  curved-top b.
  Emerson's one-piece
    segment b.
  executive b.
  b. fixation
  flat top b.
  Franklin b.
  Ful-Vue b.
  fused b.
  glass b.
  b. glasses
  invisible b.
  Kryptok b.
  b. lens
  Morck's cement b.
  Nokrome b.
  one-piece b.
  Panoptic b.
  plastic b.
  progressive-add b.
  round top b.
  Schnaitmann's b.
  b. segment
  b. spectacle lens
  b. spectacles
  straight-line b.
  Ultex b.
  Univis b.

bifoveal fixation
bifurcation
big blind spot syndrome
Bigliano tonometer
bilaminar membrane
bilateral
  b. cyst
  b. hemianopsia
  b. homonymous altitudinal
    defect
  b. homonymous
    hemianopsia
  b. sporadic retinoblastoma
  b. strabismus
  b. uveitis
bimedial recession
binary cord
binasal
  b. field
  b. field defect
  b. hemianopsia
  b. quadrant fields
Binkhorst
  B. collar stud lens implant
  B. four-loop iris-fixated
    implant
  B. four-loop iris-fixated lens
  B. four-loop lens
  B. implant
  B. intraocular lens
  B. iridocapsular lens
  B. irrigating cannula
  B. lens
  B. tip
  B. two-loop intraocular lens
    implant
  B. two-loop lens
Binkhorst-Fyodorov lens
binocle
  b. bandage
  b. dressing
binocular
  b. accommodation
  b. aphakia
  b. bandage
  b. depth perception
  b. diplopia
  b. disparities
  b. dressing
  b. eye patch
  b. field
  b. fixation
  b. fixation forceps

b. fusion
b. hemianopsia
b. heterochromia
b. imbalance
b. indirect
b. indirect ophthalmoscope
b. indirect ophthalmoscopy
b. loupe
b. luster
b. ophthalmoscope
b. parallax
b. perimetry
b. polyopia
b. rivalry
b. single vision (BSV)
b. strabismus
b. vision
b. visual acuity
binocularity
Binocular Visual Acuity Test (BVAT)
binoculus
binophthalmoscope
binoscope
bioavailability
biochemical genetics
biochrome test
Bioengineering
Berkeley B.
Biomatrix ocular implant
biometric ruler
biomicroscope
b. slit lamp
biomicroscopy
slit-lamp b.
Biomydrin
Bio-Optics
B.-O. camera
B.-O. specular microscope
B.-O. telescope system
Bio-Pen
B.-P. biometric ruler
biophotometer
Biophysic
B. laser
B. Medical laser
B. Medical YAG laser
biopsy
temporal artery b.
biopter test
Bio-Rad
B.-R. Laboratory
biorbital angle

Biotic-O
biperiden
bipolar
b. cautery
b. cells
b. cone
b. forceps
b. giant
b. retinal cell
b. rod
biprism applanation tonometer
biprong muscle marker
Birbeck granules
Birch-Harman irrigator
Birch-Hirschfeld
B.-H. entropion operation
B.-H. lamp
Birch lamp
bird
bird face
birdshot
b. chorioretinitis
b. chorioretinopathy
b. choroiditis
b. retinochoroiditis
b. retinochoroidopathy
b. retinopathy
b. spot
birefractive
birefringence
corneal b.
birefringent
Birkhauser
B. chart
B. test chart
Birk-Mathelone micro forceps
Birks
B. Mark II Colibri forceps
B. Mark II forceps
B. Mark II grooved forceps
B. Mark II groove forceps
B. Mark II hook
B. Mark II instruments
B. Mark II Instruments micro cross-action holder
B. Mark II Instruments micro trabeculectomy scissors
B. Mark II micro cross-action holder
B. Mark II micro lock-type needle holder

41

Birks *(continued)*
B. Mark II micro needle-
holder forceps
B. Mark II micro push/pull
B. Mark II micro spatula
B. Mark II micro
trabeculectomy scissors
B. Mark II needle holder
B. Mark II push/pull
B. Mark II push/pull
spatula
B. Mark II spatula
B. Mark II straight forceps
B. Mark II suture-tying
forceps
B. Mark II toothed forceps
Birks-Mathelone micro forceps
birth trauma
bischloroethylnitrosourea (BCNU)
Bishop-Harman
B.-H. anterior chamber
cannula
B.-H. anterior chamber
irrigator
B.-H. bladebreaker
B.-H. cannula
B.-H. forceps
B.-H. foreign body forceps
B.-H. irrigating/aspirating
unit
B.-H. irrigator
B.-H. knife
B.-H. Superblade
B.-H. tissue forceps
Bishop-Peter tendon tucker
Bishop tendon tucker
bishydroxycoumarin
Bi-Soft lens
Bisolvon
bispherical lens
bitemporal
b. disparity
b. field defect
b. fugax hemianopsia
b. hemianopic scotoma
b. hemianopsia
bithermal caloric stimulation
biting rongeur
bitoric
b. contact lens
b. lenses

Bitot's
B. patches
B. spot
Bitumi monobjective microscope
Bjerrum
B. scope
B. scotometer
B. screen
Bjerrum's
B. area
B. scotoma
B. sign
BKS Refractive System
black
b. braided nylon suture
b. braided silk suture
b. braided suture
b. cataract
b. cornea
b. eye
b. limb
b. reflex
b. silk sling suture
b. sunburst
b. sunburst sign
black-ball hyphema
blackfly
blackout
visual b.
blade
#15 b.
#15 Bard-Parker b.
Bard-Parker b.
Beaver b.
Beaver discission b.
Beaver eye b.
Beaver-Lundsgaard b.
Beaver-Okamura b.
Beaver scleral
Lundsgaard b.
Beaver-Ziegler b.
Beaver-Ziegler needle b.
Beer b.
bent blunt b.
Berens b.
broken razor b.
Castroviejo b.
Castroviejo razor b.
Cooper Surgeon-Plus
Ultrathin b.
CooperVision Surgeon-Plus
Ultrathin b.
Curdy b.

Curdy-Hebra b.
Dean b.
diamond b.
diamond-dusted knife b.
b. gauge
Gill b.
Gill-Hess b.
Grieshaber b.
GS-9 b.
GSA-9 b.
Hebra b.
Hoskins razor fragment b.
Katena double-edged
 sapphire b.
Keeler retractable b.
Knapp b.
b. knife
Lange b.
Martinez corneal trephine b.
McPherson-Wheeler b.
Micra double-edged
 diamond b.
microvitreoretinal b.
miniature b.
MVB b.
MVR b.
Myocure b.
myringotomy b.
razor b.
replaceable b.
Scheie b.
scleral b.
Sharpoint V-lance b.
Sichel b.
Sputnik Russian razor b.
Superblade No. 75 b.
trephine b.
UltraThin surgical b.
V-lance b.
Wheeler b.
Ziegler b.
bladebreaker
Barraquer b.
Barraquer razor b.
Bishop-Harman b.
Castroviejo b.
Castroviejo-style mini b.
I-tech Castroviejo b.
b. knife
razor b.
Swiss b.
Troutman b.
Vari b.

blade/knife
V-lance b./k.
Blair
B. head drape
B. retractor
B. stiletto
Blairex
B. sterile saline
B. System
Blair's
B. epicanthus repair
B. operation
blanching
blank
contact lens b.
semifinished b.
b. spot
Blasius' lid flap operation
Blaskovics'
B. canthoplasty operation
B. dacryostomy operation
B. flap
B. inversion of tarsus
 operation
B. lid operation
B. operation
B. tarsectomy
Blaskovics-Berke ptosis
Blastomyces dermatitidis
blastomycosis
North American b.
Blatt's operation
Blaydes
B. corneal forceps
B. forceps
B. lens-holding forceps
bleaching powder
blear eye
bleb
conjunctival b.
b. cup
encapsulated b.
endothelial b.
filtering b.
iron-leaking b.
leaking b.
leaking filtering b.
nonleaking b.
postcataract b.
bleb-associated endophthalmitis
bleed
subarachnoid b.
vitreal b.

Blefcon
Blenderm
    B. tape
    B. tape dressing
blennophthalmia
blennorrhagica
    keratoderma b.
blennorrhea
    b. adultorum
    b. conjunctivalis
    inclusion b.
    neonatal inclusion b.
    b. neonatorum
blenorrheal conjunctivitis
Bleph
Bleph-10
    B.-10 Liquifilm
    B.-10 S.O.P.
Blephamide
    B. S.O.P.
blepharadenitis
blepharal
blepharectomy
blepharedema
blepharelosis
blepharism
blepharitis
    b. acarica
    allergic b.
    angular b.
    b. angularis
    chlamydial b.
    b. ciliaris
    ciliary b.
    clostridial b.
    coliform b.
    b. conjunctivitis
    contact b.
    demodectic b.
    diplobacillary b.
    eczematoid b.
    b. follicularis
    fungal b.
    herpes simplex b.
    marginal b.
    b. marginalis
    meibomian b.
    nonulcerative b.
    b. oleosa
    parasitic b.
    b. parasitica
    pediculous b.
    b. phthiriatica

    pustular b.
    rickettsial b.
    b. rosacea
    seborrheic b.
    b. sicca
    b. squamosa
    squamous b.
    squamous seborrheic b.
    staphylococcal b.
    streptococcal b.
    b. ulcerosa
    viral b.
blepharoadenitis
blepharoadenoma
blepharoatheroma
blepharochalasis
    b. forceps
    Krieker's b.
    b. repair
blepharochromidrosis
blepharoclonus
blepharocoloboma
blepharoconjunctivitis
    acne rosacea b.
    angular b.
    bacterial b.
    chronic b.
    b. Moraxella lacunata
    b. rosacea
    staphylococcal b.
    b. vaccinia
blepharodiastasis
blepharokeratoconjunctivitis
blepharomelasma
blepharoncus
blepharopachynsis
blepharophimosis
    epicanthus b.
    b. inversus
    b. ptosis syndrome
    b. syndrome
blepharophyma
blepharoplast
blepharoplastic
blepharoplasty
    Davis-Geck b.
blepharoplegia
blepharoptosis, blepharoptosia
    b. adiposa
    false b.
    b. repair
blepharopyorrhea

blepharorrhaphy
    Elschnig's b.
blepharospasm, blepharospasmus
    essential b.
    hemifacial b.
    primary infantile
      glaucoma b.
    symptomatic b.
blepharospasm-oromandibular
  dystonia
blepharosphincterectomy
blepharostat
    McNeill-Goldmann b.
blepharostenosis
blepharosynechia
blepharotomy
blepharoxysis
Blessig-Iwanoff, Blessig-Ivanov
    B.-I. cyst
    B.-I. microcyst
Blessig's
    B. cyst
    B. groove
    B. lacuna
blind
    color b.
    legally b.
    b. reflex
    b. spot
    b. spot enlargement
    b. spot of Mariotte
    b. spot reflex
    b. spot syndrome
blinding
    b. disease
    b. glare
blindness
    amnesic color b.
    blue b.
    Bright's b.
    cerebral b.
    color b.
    concussion b.
    cortical b.
    cortical psychic b.
    day b.
    deuton color b.
    eclipse b.
    electric light b.
    epidemic b.
    factitious b.
    flash b.
    flight b.

    functional b.
    green b.
    hysterical b.
    Ishihara's test for color b.
    legal b.
    letter b.
    mind b.
    miner's b.
    moon b.
    night b.
    note b.
    nutritional b.
    object b.
    postoperative b.
    protan color b.
    psychic b.
    red b.
    red-green b.
    river b.
    snow b.
    solar b.
    soul b.
    stationary night b.
    syllabic b.
    b. test
    text b.
    total b.
    transient b.
    twilight b.
    word b.
    yellow b.
blind-spot projection technique
blink
    b. adequacy
    b. inadequacy
    b. reflex
blinking
Blink-N-Clean
Blinx
Bloch-Stauffer syndrome
Bloch-Sulzberger syndrome
block
    aphakic pupillary b.
    Atkin lid b.
    Atkinson b.
    ciliary b.
    ciliovitreal b.
    ciliovitrectomy b.
    facial b.
    lid b.
    modified Van Lint b.
    Nadbath b.
    Nadbath facial b.

block *(continued)*
    b. nerve
    nerve b.
    O'Brien b.
    O'Brien lid b.
    posterior peribulbar b.
    pupil b.
    pupillary b.
    regional b.
    retrobulbar b.
    retrobulbar lid b.
    Smith modification of Van
      Lint lid b.
    Spaeth b.
    Stahl caliper b.
    Tanne corneal cutting b.
    Van Lint b.
    Van Lint-Atkinson lid
      akinetic b.
    vitreous b.
blockade
    pharmacological b.
blockage
    internal b.
    b. nystagmus
blocker
    calcium channel b.
blocking of lens blank
blond fundi
blood
    b. agar
    b. barrier
    b. cyst
    b. dyscrasia
    b. factor (M)
    b. lipids
    b. loss
    b. pressure cuff
    b. reflux
    retinal b.
    b. staining of cornea
    b. viscosity
blood-and-thunder retinopathy
blood-aqueous barrier
blood-influx phenomenon
blood-ocular barrier
blood-optic nerve barrier
blood-retinal barrier
bloodshot
blood staining
    corneal b. s.

blooming
    b. of lens
    b. spectacle lens
blotchy positive staining
blot hemorrhage
blown pupil
blow-out
    b.-o. fracture
    b.-o. fracture of orbit
blue
    b. arcs
    argon b.
    b. blindness
    b. cataract
    b. cone
    b. cone monochromasy
    b. cone monochromatism
    b. line
    methylene b.
    b. nevus
    Prussian b.
    b. sclera
    b. spike
    b. spot
    b. vision
blue-dot cataract
blue-field entoptic phenomenon
blue-green argon laser
Blumenthal irrigating cystitome
blunt
    b. needle
    b. trauma
blur
    b. and clear exercise
    optical b.
    b. pattern
    b. point
    spectacle b.
    b. spot
    b. zone
blurring of vision
blush
    red b.
B lymphocyte
B-mode handpiece
B.N.P.
BO
    base out
    base-out prism
board
    cutting b.
boat hook

bobbing
    inverse ocular b.
    ocular b.
    reverse b.
Boberg-Ans
    B.-A. implant
    B.-A. lens
    B.-A. lens implant
Bochdalek's valve
Bodian
    B. lacrimal pigtail probe
    B. mini lacrimal probe
Bodkin thread holder
body, pl. **bodies**
    adipose b.
    asteroid bodies
    Barr b.
    basal ciliary b.
    basal lamina of ciliary b.
    cellular inclusion bodies
    ciliary b.
    colloid b.
    copper foreign bodies
    cystoid b.
    cytoid b.
    Dutcher bodies
    electromagnetic removal of
      foreign b.
    Elschnig b.
    embryonal
      medulloepithelioma of
      ciliary b.
    external geniculate b.
    foreign b. (FB)
    geniculate b.
    Goldmann-Larson foreign b.
    Guarnieri's inclusion b.
    Halberstaedter-Prowazek
      inclusion b.
    Hassall-Henle bodies
    Hassall's b.
    Henderson-Patterson
      inclusion b.
    Henle's b.
    Hensen's b.
    hyaline bodies
    hyaloid b.
    inclusion b.
    intracytoplasmic inclusion b.
    intraocular foreign b.
    intraorbital foreign b.
    Landolt's b.
    lateral geniculate b. (LGB)

    lenticular b.
    lenticular fossa of
      vitreous b.
    Lewy b.
    Lipschütz inclusion b.
    multivesicular bodies
    nigroid b.
    pigmented layer of
      ciliary b.
    pituitary b.
    Prowazek-Greeff b.
    Prowazek-Halberstaedter b.
    Prowazek's inclusion b.
    psammoma bodies
    racquet bodies
    refractile b.
    removal of foreign b.
    Rosenmüller's b.
    Rucker b.
    Russell bodies
    Schaumann's inclusion
      bodies
    sclerotomy removal of
      foreign b.
    trachoma b.
    vitreous b.
    vitreous foreign b.
    wartlike bodies
    Weibel-Palade bodies
Boeck's sarcoid
boggy edema
Böhm's operation
Bohr's model
Boil-n-Soak
bolster
bolus dressing
bombé
    b. configuration
    iris b.
Bonaccolto
    B. forceps
    B. fragment forceps
    B. jeweler forceps
    B. magnet tip forceps
    B. monoplex orbital implant
    B. orbital implant
    B. scleral ring
    B. trephine
    B. utility forceps
Bonaccolto-Flieringa
    B.-F. operation
    B.-F. scleral ring

Bonaccolto-Flieringa *(continued)*
    B.-F. scleral ring operation
    B.-F. vitreous operation
bone
    b. cyst
    ethmoid b.
    foramen of sphenoid b.
    frontal b.
    glandular fossa of frontal b.
    b. graft
    lacrimal b.
    lacrimal sulcus of
      lacrimal b.
    maxillary b.
    orbital b.
    orbital arch of frontal b.
    orbital border of
      sphenoid b.
    orbital plane of frontal b.
    orbital plate of ethmoid b.
    orbital plate of frontal b.
    orbital sulci of frontal b.
    orbital wing of sphenoid b.
    palatine b.
    petrous b.
    b. punch
    b. rongeur
    sphenoid b.
    b. spicule
    supraorbital arch of
      frontal b.
    supraorbital margin of
      frontal b.
    temporal b.
    b. trephine
    uncinate process of
      lacrimal b.
    zygomatic b.
bone-biting
    b.-b. forceps
    b.-b. punch
    b.-b. trephine
Bonn
    B. forceps
    B. iris forceps
    B. iris scissors
    B. micro iris hook
    B. suturing forceps
Bonnet-deChaume-Blanc syndrome
Bonnet's
    B. capsule
    B. enucleation operation
    B. operation

Bonnier's syndrome
bony cataract
Bonzel's
    B. blood staining of cornea
    B. operation
boomerang-shaped lesion
borate
    sodium b.
border
    corneoscleral b.
    rolled up epithelium with
      wavy b.
    b. tissue of Jacoby
Bores
    B. axis marker
    B. twist fixation ring
boric
    b. acid
    b. acid solution
borosilicate crown
Borrelia
    B. burgdorferi
    B. novyi
    B. recurrentis
borreliosis
    Lyme b.
Borsch
    B. bandage
    B. dressing
Borthen's iridotasis operation
Boruchoff forceps
Bossalino's blepharoplasty
    operation
Boston
    B. Advance cleaner
    B. Advance conditioning
      solution
    B. Advance reconditioning
      drops
    B. cleaner
    B. conditioning solution
    B. contact lens
    B. reconditioning drops
    B. trephine
Boston's sign
both eyes (OU)
bottlemaker's cataract
botulinum
    Clostridium b.
botulinum toxin
botulinum toxin type A
botulism
botulismotoxin

Botvin
    B. forceps
    B. iris forceps
Botvin-Bradford enucleator
bouche de tapir
bougie
boule
bound-down muscle
bounding
    b. mydriasis
    b. pupil
bouquet of Rochon-Duvigneaud
Bourneville's disease
boutons
    b. en passant
    b. terminaux
Bovie
    B. cautery
    B. electrocautery unit
    B. electrosurgical unit
    B. retinal detachment unit
    B. unit
    B. wet-field cautery
bovied
bovis
    Mycobacterium b.
bow
Bowen's disease
Bower's disease
bowl
    lenticular b.
Bowman
    B. cataract needle
    B. lacrimal probe
    B. needle
    B. needle stop
    B. probe
    B. stop needle
    B. tube
Bowman's
    B. lamina
    B. layer
    B. membrane
    B. muscle
    B. operation
    B. zone
bowstring
bow-tie
    b.-t. atrophy
    b.-t. hypoplasia
    b.-t. knot
    b.-t. optic atrophy
    b.-t. stitch

boxcarring
box measurement
Boyce needle holder
Boyd
    B. implant
    B. orbital implant
Boyden's chamber technique
Boyd's
    B. operation
    B. zone
Boynton needle holder
Boys-Smith laser lens
Bozzi's foramen
BPPV
    benign paroxysmal positional
    vertigo
brachial
    b. arch syndrome
    b. plexus
    b. plexus palsy
brachium
    b. conjunctiva
    conjunctival b.
brachycephaly
brachymetropia
brachymetropic
brachytherapy
    radioactive plaque b.
Bracken
    B. anterior chamber cannula
    B. cannula
    B. fixation forceps
    B. forceps
    B. iris forceps
    B. irrigating/aspirating unit
Bracken's effect
Bradford snare enucleator
braided
    black b. suture
    b. silk suture
    b. Vicryl suture
braid effect
Braid's
    B. effect
    B. strabismus
Brailey's operation
braille
brailler
    Perkins b.
brain
    b. cortex
    b. damage
    b. dysfunction

brain *(continued)*
    b. stem
    b. tumor
    b. tumor headache
brain-heart infusion broth
brainstem, brain stem
    b. dysfunction
Braley's sign
branch
    b. retinal artery occlusion
    (BRAO)
    b. retinal vein occlusion
    (BRVO)
    b. vein occlusion
Branchamella catarrhalis
BRAO
    branch retinal artery occlusion
brasiliensis
    Nocardia b.
brass scleral plug
Brawley
    B. refractor
    B. retractor
Brawner
    B. implant
    B. orbital implant
brawny
    b. edema
    b. scleritis
    b. tenonitis
    b. trachoma
Brayley
    polymorphic macular
      degeneration of B.
Brazilian ophthalmia
breadth of accommodation
break
    conjunctival b.
    giant retinal b.
    iatrogenic b.
    iatrogenic retinal b.
    b. point
    retinal b.
    b. in retinal integrity
breakdown
    optical b.
    surface b.
breakpoint
    fusion b.
breakthrough
    vitreous hemorrhage b.
breakup
    b. phenomenon

    b. time (BUT)
    b. time of tear
    b. time test
breves
    nervi ciliares b.
Brevital
Brickner's sign
bridge
    b. coloboma
    comfort b.
    keyhole b.
    b. pedicle flap
    b. pedicle flap operation
    saddle b.
    b. of spectacles
    b. suture
Bridge's operation
bridle suture
Briggs' strabismus operation
brightness
    b. difference threshold
Brightness Acuity Test (BAT)
Bright's
    B. blindness
    B. disease
    B. eye
bright-sense
British
    B. antilewisite (BAL)
    B. N system
    B. Standards Institution
      optotype set
Britt
    B. argon/krypton laser
    B. argon laser
    B. argon pulsed laser
    B. BL-12 laser
    B. krypton laser
    B. pulsed argon laser
brittle
    b. cornea syndrome
    b. diabetes
brittle-bone disease
broad-beta disease
broad-spectrum antibiotic
broad thumbs and broad toes
    syndrome
Broca's
    B. plane
    B. visual plane
Brockhurst's technique
Broders' grading
Brodmann's area

broken razor blade
Brolene
Brombach's perimeter
bromhexine
bromide
    demecarium b.
    demecariumdemecarium b.
    pancuronium b.
Bromley's foreign body operation
bromocriptine
bromvinyldeoxyuridine (BVDU)
Bronson-Magnion
    B.-M. eye magnet
    B.-M. forceps
    B.-M. magnet
Bronson-Park speculum
Bronson's foreign body removal
    operation
Bronson-Turner foreign body
    locator
Bronson-Turz
    B.-T. refractor
    B.-T. retractor
bronze diabetes
bronzing
    nuclear b.
Brooke's tumor
broth
    brain-heart infusion b.
brow
    arched b.
    b. fixation
    b. tape
Brown-Beard technique
brown cataract
Brown-Dohlman Silastic corneal
    implant
Brown-McLean syndrome
Brown-Pusey corneal trephine
Brown's
    B. syndrome
    B. tendon
    B. tendon sheath syndrome
    B. vertical retraction
        syndrome
Brown sterile adhesive
broxyquinoline
Brucella
brucellosis
Bruchner's test
Bruch's
    B. gland

    B. layer
    B. membrane
Brücke-Bartley phenomenon
Brücke's
    B. fiber
    B. lens
    B. muscle
    B. tunic
Bruining forceps
bruit
    carotid b.
brunescent cataract
brush
    Alger b.
    Barraquer sable b.
    Haidinger b.
    Thomas b.
Brushfield's spot
Brushfield-Wyatt syndrome
BRVO
    branch retinal vein occlusion
B-scan
    B-s. ultrasonogram
    B-s. ultrasonography
BSS
    balanced saline solution
    balanced salt solution
BSV
    binocular single vision
BU
    base-up prism
bubble
    air b.
    Chamber's sterile
        adhesive b.
    gas b.
    intraocular gas b.
buckle
    choroid b.
    encircling b.
    encircling band for
        scleral b.
    encircling silicone b.
    prominent b.
    scleral b.
Bückler's
    B. I dystrophy
    B. II dystrophy
    B. III dystrophy
buckling
    b. choroid
    Custodis' scleral b.

buckling *(continued)*
    b. sclera
    scleral b.
budding yeast cell
Budge
    ciliospinal center of B.
Budinger's blepharoplasty operation
Buerger's disease
Buettner-Parel
    B.-P. cutter
    B.-P. vitreous cutter
buffer
buffered formaldehyde
buffy coat
bufilcon A
build-up implant
bulbar
    b. conjunctiva
    b. cyanosis
    b. fascia
    b. paralysis
    b. sheath
bulb of eye
bulbi
    atrophia b.
    camera vitrea b.
    capsula b.
    cholesterosis b.
    cyanosis b.
    endothelium camerae
      anterioris b.
    fascia b.
    fascia lata musculares b.
    fascia musculares b.
    lacertus musculi recti
      lateralis b.
    melanosis b.
    musculi b.
    musculus obliquus
      inferior b.
    musculus obliquus
      superior b.
    musculus rectus inferior b.
    musculus rectus lateralis b.
    musculus rectus medialis b.
    siderosis b.
    Tenon's fascia b.
    trochlea musculi obliqui
      superioris b.
    tunica fibrosa b.
    tunica interna b.
    tunica senoria b.
    tunica vasculosa b.

    xanthelasmatosis b.
    xanthomatosis b.
bulbocapnine
bulbous atrophy
bulbus, gen. and pl. **bulbi**
    b. oculi
bulge
    vitreous b.
bulla, pl. **bullae**
    epithelial b.
    ethmoid b.
    b. ethmoidalis cavinasi
    b. ethmoidalis ossis
    b. ossea
bulldog clamp
Buller
    B. eye shield
    B. shield
bullosa
    concha b.
    epidermolysis b.
    keratitis b.
    recessive dystrophic
      epidermolysis b.
bullosis
bullosum
    erythema multiforme b.
bullous
    b. detachment
    b. disorder
    b. keratopathy
    b. pemphigoid
bull's
    b. eye
    b. eye macular lesion
    b. eye maculopathy
    b. eye retinopathy
bullular canal
Bumke's pupil
bundle
    arcuate nerve fiber b.
    b. of Drualt
    Drualt's b.
    inferior arcuate b.
    maculopapillary b.
    maculopapular b.
    nerve b.
    nerve fiber b.
    papillomacular b.
    papillomacular nerve
      fiber b.
    paracentral nerve fiber b.
    superior arcuate b.

Bunge evisceration spoon
Bunker implant
Bunsen grease spot-photometer
Bunsen-Roscoe law
buphthalmia, buphthalmos,
  buphthalmus
bupivacaine
bupranolol
bur
  aftercataract b.
  Alfonso guarded b.
  Allport cutting b.
  Burwell b.
  corneal b.
  corneal foreign body b.
  cutting b.
  diamond b.
  foreign body b.
  lacrimal sac b.
  Storz corneal b.
  Worst corneal b.
  Yazujian b.
Burch
  B. calipers
  B. pick
  B. tendon tucker
Burch-Greenwood
  B.-G. tendon tucker
  B.-G. tucker
Burch-Lester speculum
Burch's
  B. evisceration operation
  B. eye evisceration
    operation
burgdorferi
  Borrelia b.
buried
  b. drusen
  b. suture
Burkitt's lymphoma
burn
  acid b.
  alkali b.
  alkaline b.
  ammonia alkali b.
  ammonium hydroxide
    alkali b.
  chemical b.
  corneal b.
  corneal alkali b.
  laser b.
  radiation b.
  retinal b.

  solar b.
  thermal b.
  ultraviolet b.
burnetii
  Coxiella b.
Burns' amaurosis
Burow's flap operation
Burr
  B. butterfly needle
  B. corneal ring
  B. silicone button
Burr's cornea
burst
  laser b.
Burton lamp
Burwell bur
Busacca's nodule
busulfan
BUT
  breakup time
butacaine
Butazolidin
Butcher's conjunctivitis
butterfly
  b. dystrophy
  b. macular dystrophy
  b. needle
butterfly-shaped pigment epithelial
  dystrophy
button
  Burr silicone b.
  collar b.
  corneal b.
  corneoscleral b.
  Graether collar-b.
  silicone b.
buttonholed
buttonhole iridectomy
button-tip manipulator
butyl
  b. cyanoacrylate
  b. cyanoacrylate glue
butyrate
  cellulose b.
  cellulose acetate b. (CAB)
butyrophenone
Buzzi's operation
BV100 needle
BVA
  best-corrected visual acuity
BVAT
  Binocular Visual Acuity Test

BVDU
    bromvinyldeoxyuridine
b wave
Byron Smith's
    B. S. ectropion operation

B. S. lazy T correction
B. S. operation

C
carbon
cathodal
cathode
Celsius
centigrade
contraction
cylinder
cylindrical lens
cytidine
large calorie
CAB
cellulose acetate butyrate
cable temple
cabufocon A
caecum
punctum c.
caecutiens
Onchocerca c.
caerulea
cataracta c.
café au lait spots
caffeine
Caffey's disease
CAHEA
Committee on Allied Health
Education and Accreditation
Cairn's
C. operation
C. trabeculectomy
caisson's disease
calcareous
c. cataract
c. conjunctivitis
c. degeneration
c. degeneration of cornea
c. deposit
calcarine
c. artery
c. cortex
c. fissure
calciferol
calcification
conjunctival c.
lamellar c.
optic disk drusen c.
sellar c.
calcific band keratopathy

calcinosis, Raynaud's phenomenon, esophageal motility disorder, sclerodactyly, and telangiectasia (CREST)
calcitriol
calcium
c. carbonate chalk
c. channel blocker
c. deposition
c. embolus
c. ethylenediaminetetraacetate
c. hydroxide
c. hypochlorite
c. salts
calcium-containing opacities
calcoaceticus
Acinetobacter c.
calcofluor white stain (CFW)
calculation
lens power c.
power c.
calculus, gen. and pl. calculi
lacrimal c.
Caldwell-Luc
C.-L. approach
C.-L. operation
Caldwell's view
Caldwell-Waters view
Calhoun-Hagler
C.-H. lens extraction operation
C.-H. lens needle
C.-H. needle
C.-H. operation
Calhoun-Merz needle
Calhoun needle
Calibri forceps
caliculus ophthalmicus
caligation
caligo
c. corneae
c. lentis
c. pupilla
calipers
Berens marking c.
Burch c.
Castroviejo c.
Green c.
Jameson c.

calipers *(continued)*
    John Green c.
    Machemer c.
    Stahl c.
    Storz c.
    surgical c.
    Thomas c.
    Thorpe c.
    Thorpe-Castroviejo c.
Callahan
    C. fixation forceps
    C. lens loupe
Callahan's operation
Callender's
    C. cell type classification
    C. classification
callosum
    corpus c.
    splenium of corpus c.
Calmette-Guérin
    Bacille bilié de C.-G.
    (BCG)
Calmette's ophthalmoreaction
caloric
    c. intake
    c. nystagmus
    c. test
    c. testing
caloric-induced nystagmus
calotte
calvaria
Cambridge low-contrast gratings
camera, pl. **camerae, cameras**
    Bio-Optics c.
    c. bulbi anterior
    c. bulbi posterior
    Canon CF-60U fundus c.
    Canon CF-60Z fundus c.
    Canon fundus c.
    Carl Zeiss fundus c.
    Coburn c.
    CooperVision c.
    Docustar fundus c.
    fundus c.
    Garcia-Ibanez c.
    hand-held fundus c.
    House-Urban-Pentax c.
    Kowa c.
    Kowa RC-XV fundus c.
    c. lucida
    Nikon Retinopan fundus c.
    c. obscura
    c. oculi

    c. oculi anterior
    c. oculi posterior
    Olympus fundus c.
    Reichert c.
    retinal c.
    Retinopan 45 c.
    Topcon c.
    c. vitrea bulbi
    Zeiss fundus c.
    Zeiss-Nordenson fundus c.
cAMP
    cyclic adenosine monophosphate
Campbell
    iris retraction syndrome
      of C.
    C. refractor
    C. retractor
    C. slit lamp
campimeter
    stereo c.
campimetry
Campodonico's
    C. canal
    C. operation
CAM stimulator
camsylate
    trimethaphan c.
Canada balsam
canal
    ampulla of lacrimal c.
    bullular c.
    Campodonico's c.
    central c.
    ciliary c.
    Cloquet's c.
    Dorello's c.
    ethmoid c.
    Ferrein's c.
    Fontana's c.
    Hannover's c.
    Hovius' c.
    hyaloid c.
    infraorbital c.
    lacrimal c.
    Lauth's c.
    nasal c.
    nasolacrimal c.
    c. of Nuck
    optic c.
    orbital c.
    Petit's c.
    ruffed c.
    c. of Schlemm

Schlemm's c.
scleral c.
scleroticochoroidal c.
semicircular c.'s
Sondermann's c.
c. of Stilling
supraciliary c.
supraoptic c.
supraorbital c.
tarsal c.
zygomaticofacial c.
zygomaticotemporal c.
canalicular
  c. disorder
  c. duct
  c. laceration
  c. pathway
  c. scissors
canaliculi
canaliculitis
canaliculodacryocystostomy
canaliculodacryorhinostomy
canaliculorhinostomy
canaliculum
canaliculus, pl. **canaliculi**
  common c.
  inferior c.
  c. infraorbitalis opticus
  c. lacrimalis
  lacriman c.
  c. rod and suture
  stenosis c.
  superior c.
  upper c.
canalis
  c. hyaloideus
  c. opticus
cancer
cancer-associated retinopathy
cancrum nasi
candela (cd)
  c. laser
  c. laser lithotriptor
Candida
  C. albicans
candidal
  c. conjunctivitis
  c. endophthalmitis
  c. keratitis
  c. uveitis
candidemia

candidiasis
  c. conjunctivitis
  mucocutaneous c.
candle
  German Hefner c.
  c. wax drippings
candle-meter
candle-power
canicola fever
canis
  Toxocara c.
canities
  c. circumscripta
cannabis
cannula
  air c.
  air injection c.
  alpha-chymotrypsin c.
  angled left/right c.
  anterior chamber c.
  Assi c.
  Bailey lacrimal c.
  Barraquer c.
  Binkhorst irrigating c.
  Bishop-Harman c.
  Bishop-Harman anterior
    chamber c.
  Bracken c.
  Bracken anterior chamber c.
  Castroviejo cyclodialysis c.
  cyclodialysis c.
  De LaVega vitreous
    aspirating c.
  double
    irrigating/aspirating c.
  Drews c.
  Drews irrigating c.
  Fasanella lacrimal c.
  Galt aspirating c.
  Gans c.
  Gans cyclodialysis c.
  Gass c.
  Gass cataract aspirating c.
  Gass vitreous aspirating c.
  Ghormley double c.
  Gills double irrigating-
    aspirating c.
  Gills double Luer-Lok c.
  Gills irrigating-aspirating c.
  Gills-Welsh aspirating c.
  Gills-Welsh double-barreled
    irrigating-aspirating c.

cannula *(continued)*
    Gills-Welsh irrigating-aspirating c.
    Gills-Welsh olive-tip c.
    Girard irrigating c.
    Goldstein c.
    goniotomy knife c.
    Heyner c.
    Heyner double c.
    Hilton self-retaining infusion c.
    Hilton sutureless infusion c.
    Hoffer forward-cutting knife c.
    infusion c.
    iris hook c.
    irrigating c.
    irrigating/aspirating c.
    I-tech c.
    Jensen-Thomas irrigating-aspirating c.
    Johnson double c.
    J-shaped irrigating/aspirating c.
    Kara cataract-aspirating c.
    Karickhoff double c.
    Keeler-Keislar lacrimal c.
    Kelman c.
    Kelman cyclodialysis c.
    Klein curved c.
    Kraff cortex c.
    lacrimal c.
    Lewicky threaded infusion c.
    liquid vitreous-aspirating c.
    Look I/A coaxial c.
    Maumenee goniotomy knife c.
    Maumenee knife goniotomy c.
    McIntyre-Binkhorst irrigating c.
    McIntyre coaxial c.
    Moehle c.
    Moncrieff c.
    Oaks double straight c.
    Oaks straight c.
    O'Gawa cataract-aspirating c.
    O'Gawa two-way aspirating c.
    O'Malley-Heintz infusion c.
    Packo pars plana c.

    Pearce coaxial irrigating/aspirating c.
    Peczon I/A c.
    Pierce coaxial irrigating/aspirating c.
    Pierce I/A c.
    Randolph cyclodialysis c.
    reel aspiration c.
    Roper alpha-chymotrypsin c.
    Rowsey fixation c.
    Scheie anterior chamber c.
    Scheie cataract-aspirating c.
    self-retaining infusion c.
    self-retaining irrigating c.
    Shepard incision irrigating c.
    Shepard radial keratotomy irrigating c.
    side port c.
    sidewall infusion c.
    Simcoe double c.
    Simcoe II PC double c.
    Simcoe reverse aperture c.
    Simcoe reverse irrigating-aspirating c.
    Steriseal disposable c.
    Swets goniotomy knife c.
    Tenner lacrimal c.
    Thomas c.
    Thomas irrigating-aspirating c.
    Thurmond nucleus-irrigating c.
    Troutman c.
    Tulevech c.
    two-way cataract-aspirating c.
    Ulanday double c.
    Veirs c.
    VISCOFLOW c.
    Visitec 1624 irrigating/aspirating c.
    Visitec irrigating/aspirating c.
    vitreous-aspirating c.
    Weil lacrimal c.
    Welsh c.
    Welsh cortex stripper c.
    Welsh flat olive-tip double c.
    Welsh olive-tip c.
    Wergeland double c.
    West lacrimal c.

Canon
- C. Autoref R1
- C. CF-60U fundus camera
- C. CF-60Z fundus camera
- C. fundus camera
- C. refractor

Canon's perimeter
Cantelli's sign
canthal
- c. hypertelorism
- c. ligament
- c. raphe
- c. tendon

canthaxanthin
canthaxanthine crystalline retinopathy
canthectomy
canthi
canthitis
cantholysis
canthomeatal
canthopexy
canthoplasty
- Agnew's c.
- Ammon's c.
- Imre's lateral c.

canthorrhaphy
- Elschnig's c.

canthotomy
- external c.
- lateral c.

canthus, pl. canthi
- inner c.
- lateral c.
- medial c.
- outer c.

cap
- compliance c.
- corneal c.
- Gelfilm c.

capacity
- vital c. (VC)

capillary
- c. bed
- c. hemangioma
- c. hemangioma of eyelid
- c. lumen
- c. nonperfusion
- c. phase
- c. plexus

capita
capitis
- tinea c.

capsaicin
capsid
capsitis
capsula
- c. bulbi
- c. lentis

capsular
- c. advancement
- c. bag
- c. cataract
- c. debris
- c. exfoliation syndrome
- c. fixation
- c. glaucoma
- c. support

capsular-zonular
capsulatum
- *Histoplasma* c.

capsule
- anterior c.
- anterior lens c.
- Bonnet's c.
- crystalline c.
- curling of c.
- exfoliation of c.
- exfoliation of lens c.
- c. forceps
- c. forceps technique
- c. fragment forceps
- c. fragment spatula
- leaves of c.
- lens c.
- c. of lens
- ocular c.
- c. polisher
- Tenon's c.

capsulectomy
- anterior c.

capsulitis
capsulolenticular cataract
capsulorrhexis
- c. forceps
- Kraff-Utrata c.

capsulotome
- Darling c.

capsulotomy
- anterior c.
- Castroviejo's c.
- Darling's c.
- posterior c.
- c. scissors
- triangular c.

capsulotomy *(continued)*
Vannas c.
Verhoeff-Chandler c.
capture
iris c.
pupillary c.
caput, gen. **capitis**, pl. **capita**
c. medusae
Carbacel
Carbachol
Isopto C.
carbachol
carbacholine
carbamazepine
carbenicillin
Carbocaine
carbohydrate metabolism
carbolate
carbolic acid
carbomer 934 P
carbomycin
carbon (C)
c. arc lamp
c. dioxide
c. dioxide laser
c. dioxide retention
c. monoxide
c. monoxide retinopathy
c. tetrachloride
carbonate
lithium c.
sodium c.
carbonic
c. anhydrase
c. anhydrase inhibitor
carboxymethylcellulose sodium
Carcholin
carcinoma
adenoid cystic c.
basal cell c.
embryonal c.
epidermoid c.
c. of eyelid
meibomian gland c.
metastatic c.
radiation-induced c.
sebaceous cell c.
signet-ring c.
squamous cell c.
carcinomatosis
meningeal c.
card
flash picture c.'s

reading c.'s
Sherman c.
Sloan reading c.
Snellen reading c.'s
stigmatometric test c.
Teller acuity c.'s
test c.
cardiac
c. arrest
c. glycoside
c. monitor
c. valvular disease
cardinal
c. direction of gaze
c. field test
c. ocular movements
c. point
c. position
c. position of gaze
c. suture
Cardio-Green
cardiopharyngioma
cardiovascular disease
Cardona
C. corneal prosthesis forceps
C. corneal prosthesis trephine
C. fiberoptic diagnostic lens
C. focalizing fundus implant
C. focalizing fundus lens implant
C. goniofocalizing implant
C. laser
C. threading forceps
Cardrase
carinii
Pneumocystis c.
Carlo Traverso maneuver (CTM)
Carl Zeiss
C. Z. fundus camera
C. Z. instruments
C. Z. lens
C. Z. lensometer
C. Z. tonometer
C. Z. YAG laser
C. Z. Zeiss laser
carmustine (BCNU)
carnosus
pannus c.
β-carotene
carotid
c. aneurysm
c. angiography

c. artery
c. artery insufficiency
c. artery occlusion
c. artery stenosis
c. bruit
c. cavernous fistula
c. cavernous sinus fistula
c. embolus
c. endarterectomy
c. ischemia
c. obstruction
c. occlusive disease
c. occlusive disease
    retinopathy
Carpenter's syndrome
Carpine
    E C.
    Isopto C.
    P.V. C.
carrier
    Barraquer needle c.
    minus c.
CAR syndrome
Cartella
    C. eye shield
    C. shield
carteolol
Carter
    C. sphere
    C. sphere introducer
Carter's operation
cartilage
    central c.
    ciliary c.
    palpebral c.
    tarsal c.
Cartrol
caruncle
    epicanthus c.
    lacrimal c.
caruncula
    lacrimal c.
    c. lacrimalis
carunculae
    trichosis c.
caruncular papilloma
Casanellas' lacrimal operation
case
    Berens sterilizing c.
    Contique contact lens c.
    Fine corneal carrying c.
    c. group
    c. history

index c.
trial c.
caseating
    c. orbital granuloma
    c. tubercle
case-control study
caseosa
    rhinitis c.
caseous necrosis
Casey's operation
Caspar
    C. ring
    C. ring opacity
cast
    hyaline c.
    c. molding
    c. resin lens
Castallo
    C. refractor
    C. retractor
    C. speculum
Castroviejo
    C. acrylic implant
    C. angled keratome
    C. anterior synechia scissors
    C. aspirator
    C. blade
    C. bladebreaker
    C. blade holder
    C. calipers
    C. capsule forceps
    C. clip
    C. clip-applying forceps
    C. compressor
    C. corneal dissector
    C. corneal-holding forceps
    C. corneal scissors with
      inside stop
    C. corneal section scissors
    C. corneal transplant
      marker
    C. corneal transplant
      scissors
    C. corneal transplant
      trephine
    C. corneoscleral forceps
    C. corneoscleral punch
    C. cyclodialysis cannula
    C. cyclodialysis spatula
    C. discission knife
    C. double-ended spatula
    C. electrokeratotome
    C. enucleation snare

Castroviejo *(continued)*
    C. erysiphake
    C. fixation forceps
    C. forceps
    C. implant
    C. improved trephine
    C. iridocapsulotomy scissors
    C. keratome
    C. keratoplasty scissors
    C. knife
    C. lacrimal dilator
    C. lacrimal sac probe
    C. lens loupe
    C. lens spoon
    C. lid clamp
    C. lid forceps
    C. lid retractor
    C. mucotome
    C. needle holder
    C. orbital aspirator
    C. punch
    C. razor blade
    C. refractor
    C. retractor
    C. scissors
    C. scleral fold forceps
    C. scleral marker
    C. scleral shortening clip
    C. sclerotome
    C. snare
    C. snare enucleator
    C. spatula
    C. speculum
    C. suture forceps
    C. suturing forceps
    C. synechia scissors
    C. synechia spatula
    C. trephine
    C. twin knife
    C. tying forceps
    C. vitreous aspirating needle
    C. wide grip handle forceps
Castroviejo-Arruga forceps
Castroviejo-Barraquer needle holder
Castroviejo-Colibri forceps
Castroviejo-Galezowski dilator
Castroviejo-Kalt needle holder
Castroviejo's
    C. anterior synechia
    C. capsulotomy
    C. iridectomy
    C. iridotomy
    C. keratectomy

    C. mini-keratoplasty
    C. operation
    C. radial iridotomy
Castroviejo-Scheie
    C.-S. cyclodiathermy
    C.-S. cyclodiathermy
        operation
Castroviejo-style mini bladebreaker
Castroviejo-Vannas capsulotomy
    scissors
catadioptric
Catalano
    C. corneoscleral forceps
    C. forceps
    C. intubation set
    C. muscle hook
    C. tying forceps
catalase
Catalin
cataphoria
    mature c.
cataplexy
Catapres
cataract
    adherent c.
    adolescent c.
    adult-onset c.
    age-related c.
    aminoaciduria c.
    annular c.
    anterior c.
    anterior axial c.
    anterior axial
        developmental c.
    anterior axial embryonal c.
    anterior axonal
        embryonal c.
    anterior polar c.
    anterior pole c.
    anterior pyramidal c.
    arborescent c.
    aridosiliculose c.
    aridosiliquate c.
    c. aspirating needle
    c. aspiration
    atopic c.
    axial c.
    axial embryonal c.
    axial fusiform c.
    axial fusiform
        developmental c.
    axial partial childhood c.
    axillary c.

black c.
blue c.
blue-dot c.
bony c.
bottlemaker's c.
brown c.
brunescent c.
calcareous c.
capsular c.
capsulolenticular c.
central c.
cerulean c.
cheesy c.
choroidal c.
Christmas tree c.
complete c.
complete congenital c.
complicated c.
concussion c.
congenital c.
contusion c.
copper c.
Coppock c.
coralliform c.
coronary c.
cortical c.
cortical spokes c.
corticosteroid-induced c.
c. couching
couching of c.
crystalline c.
cuneiform c.
cupuliform c.
cystic c.
dendritic c.
dermatogenic c.
developmental c.
diabetic c.
diabetic-osmotic c.
diffuse c.
dilacerated c.
disk-shaped c.
drug-induced c.
dry-shelled c.
early mature c.
electric c.
electric shock c.
embryonal c.
embryonal nuclear c.
embryonic c.
embryopathic c.
evolutional c.

extracapsular extraction
  of c.
extraction of c.
c. extraction
extraction of
  extracapsular c.
extraction of
  intracapsular c.
c. extraction operation
fibroid c., fibrinous c.
flap operation c.
Fleischer's c.
floriform c.
fluid c.
furnacemen's c.
fusiform c.
galactose c.
galactosemia c.
general c.
glassblower's c.
c. glasses
glassworker's c.
glaucomatous c.
gray c.
green c.
Green's c.
hard c.
heat-generated c.
heat-ray c.
hedger c.
heterochromia c.
heterochromic c.
hook-shaped c.
hypermature c.
hypocalcemic c.
hypoglycemic c.
immature c.
incipient c.
infantile c.
infrared c.
intracapsular extraction
  of c.
intumescent c.
irradiation c.
c. irradiation
juvenile c.
juvenile developmental c.
c. knife
c. knife guard
Koby's c.
lacteal c.
lamellar c.
lamellar developmental c.

cataract *(continued)*
    lamellar zonular
      perinuclear c.
    c. lens
    lenticular c.
    life-belt c.
    lightning c.
    c. mask ring
    c. mask shield
    mature c.
    membranous c.
    metabolic c.
    metabolic syndrome c.
    milky c.
    mixed c.
    morgagnian c.
    Morgagni's c.
    myotonic c.
    myotonic dystrophy c.
    naphthalinic c.
    c. needle
    c. nigra
    nuclear c.
    nuclear developmental c.
    nutritional deficiency c.
    O'Brien's c.
    osmotic c.
    overripe c.
    partial c.
    pear c.
    c. pencil
    perinuclear c.
    peripheral c.
    pisciform c.
    poisoning degenerative c.
    polar c.
    posterior polar c.
    posterior subcapsular c.
      (PSC)
    postinflammatory c.
    prematurity c.
    presenile c.
    primary c.
    probe c.
    progressive c.
    puddler's c.
    punctate c.
    pyramidal c.
    radiation c.
    reduplicated c.
    reduplication c.
    ring form congenital c.
    ring-shaped c.

    ripe c.
    rubella c.
    sanguineous c.
    saucer-shaped c.
    secondary c.
    sedimentary c.
    senescent c.
    senescent cortical
      degenerative c.
    senescent nuclear
      degenerative c.
    senile c.
    senile nuclear sclerotic c.
    senile sclerotic c.
    c. senilis
    shaped c.
    sideratic c.
    siderosis c.
    siliculose c.
    snowflake c.
    snowstorm c.
    Soemmering's ring c.
    soft c.
    spear c.
    spear developmental c.
    c. spectacles
    c. spindle
    spindle c.
    spirochetiform c.
    spoke-like sutural c.'s
    c. spoon
    spurious c.
    stationary c.
    stellate c.
    steroid-induced c.
    subcapsular c.
    sugar c.
    sugar-induced c.
    sunflower c.
    supranuclear c.
    c. surgery
    sutural c.
    sutural developmental c.
    syndermatotic c.
    syphilitic c.
    tetany c.
    thermal c.
    total c.
    toxic c.
    traumatic c.
    traumatic degenerative c.
    tremulous c.
    umbilicated c.

vascular c.
Vogt's c.
Vogt-type c.
c. with Down syndrome
x-ray c.
x-ray-induced c.
zonular c.
zonular pulverulent c.

cataracta
    c. accreta
    c. adiposa
    c. aridosiliquata
    c. brunescens ⁓
    c. caerulea
    c. centralis pulverulenta
    c. cerulea
    c. complicata
    c. congenita membranacea
    c. coronaria
    c. dermatogenes
    c. electrica
    c. fibrosa
    c. membranacea accreta
    c. neurodermatica
    c. nigra
    c. nodiformis
    c. ossea

cataractogenesis
cataractogenic drug
cataractous
Catarase
catarrh
    sinus c.
    spring c.
    vernal c.

catarrhal
    c. conjunctivitis
    c. corneal ulcer
    c. marginal ulceration
    c. ophthalmia
    c. ulcerative keratitis

catarrhalis
    Branchamella c.

catatonic pupil
catatropic image
caterpillar-hair ophthalmia
caterpillar ophthalmia
Catford visual acuity test
catgut suture
cathepsin D
cathepsin G
catheter
    French c.

Lincoff balloon c.
red rubber c.

catheterization
    c. of lacrimal duct
    c. of lacrimonasal duct

cathodal (C)
cathode (C)
    c. ray tube (CRT)

cations
catoptric
catoptroscope
cat's
    c. cry syndrome
    c. eye
    c. eye amaurosis
    c. eye effect
    c. eye pupil
    c. eye reflex
    c. eye syndrome

cat-scratch
    c.-s. disease
    c.-s. fever

cautery
    Alcon c.
    Alcon hand c.
    Berkeley Bioengineering
      bipolar c.
    bipolar c.
    Bovie c.
    Bovie wet-field c.
    Codman wet-field c.
    Concept disposable c.
    Concept hand-held c.
    disposable c.
    eraser c.
    Fine micropoint c.
    Geiger c.
    Gonin c.
    Hildreth c.
    Ishihara I-Temp c.
    I-Temp c.
    Khosia c.
    Mentor wet-field c.
    Mira c.
    Mueller c.
    NeoKnife c.
    c. operation
    ophthalmic c.
    Op-Temp c.
    Op-Temp disposable c.
    Parker-Heath c.
    pencil c.
    phacoemulsification c.

cautery *(continued)*
    Prince c.
    punctal c.
    Rommel c.
    Rommel-Hildreth c.
    Scheie c.
    Scheie ophthalmic c.
    scleral c.
    Todd c.
    Valilab c.
    von Graefe c.
    Wadsworth-Todd c.
    wet-field c.
    Wills c.
    Ziegler c.

cava
    superior vena c.

cavern
    Schnabel's c.

cavernous
    c. angioma
    c. hemangioma
    c. sinus
    c. sinus aneurysm
    c. sinus fistula
    c. sinus syndrome
    c. sinus thrombosis

caviae
    Nocardia c.

cavinasi
    bulla ethmoidalis c.

cavitation

Cavitron
    C. aspirator
    C. I/A handpiece
    C. irrigating/aspirating unit
    C. irrigation/aspiration system
    C. unit

Cavitron-Kelman
    C.-K. irrigating/aspirating unit
    C.-K. irrigation/aspiration system

cavity
    laser c.
    opening of orbital c.
    optic papilla c.
    orbital c.
    vitreous c.

CBC
    complete blood count

cc
    with correction

CCF
    critical corresponding frequency

C/D
    cup-to-disk ratio

cd
    candela

CD-5 needle

CDCR
    conjunctivodacryocystorhinostomy

cecal

Ceclor

cecocentral scotoma

cefaclor

cefadroxil

cefazaflur

cefazolin

cefoperazone

ceforanide

cefotaxime

cefsulodin

ceftazidime

ceftizoxime

ceftriaxone

cefuroxime

Celestone

cell
    air c.
    amacrine c.
    B c.
    basal c.
    bipolar c.'s
    bipolar retinal c.
    budding yeast c.
    clump c.
    cluster of retinoblastoma c.
    cone c.
    conjunctival epithelial c.
    conjunctival goblet c.
    corneal c.
    endoneural c.'s
    endothelial c.
    epithelial c.
    epithelioid c.
    ethmoid air c.
    fat c.'s
    fiber c.'s
    flare and c.
    c. and flare (C&F)
    foam c.'s
    foreign body c.

ganglion c.
ghost c.'s
giant c.
giant epithelial c.
glial c.
goblet c.
helper/inducer T c.
horizontal c.'s
inflammatory c.'s
Langerhans' c.
Langhans' giant c.'s
Leber's c.
leukemic c.'s
lipid c.
c. lysis
M c.'s
mast c.
membrane lipid c.
meningeal c.'s
mesenchymal c.'s
metaplastic epithelial c.'s
c.'s of Mueller
Mueller's c.
multinucleated epithelial c.
multinucleated giant c.
multinucleated giant
  epithelial c.
mural c.
myoepithelial c.'s
myoid visual c.
nests and strands of c.'s
neural crest c.
perineural c.
photoreceptor c.
pigment c.'s
plasma c.
polygonal pigmented c.'s
polyhedral c.'s
Reed-Sternberg c.
reticulum c.
retinal visual c.'s
retinoblastoma c.
rod c.
satellite c.'s
Schwann's c.'s
sebaceous c.
somatic c.
spindle c.'s
spindle-shaped c.'s
squamous c.
stem c.
suppressor T c.
Touton's c.

Touton's giant c.'s
visual c.
vitreal c.'s
water c.
Wedl c.'s
wet c.
white c.'s
wing c.
X c.
Y c.

cell-mediated
  c.-m. hypersensitivity
  c.-m. immunity (CMI)
  c.-m. toxicity
cellophane
  c. maculopathy
  c. retinopathy
cellophane-like band
Cellufluor
Cellufresh
cellula
cellulae lentis
cellular
  c. cooperation
  c. debris
  c. inclusion bodies
cellularity
cellulitis
  herpes simplex c.
  orbital c.
  periorbital c.
  preseptal c.
celluloid frame
cellulosa
  tela c.
cellulose
  c. acetate
  c. acetate butyrate (CAB)
  c. acetate butyrate contact
    lens
  c. acetate frame
  c. butyrate
  hydroxyethl c.
  c. nitrate
  c. nitrate frame
Celluvisc
Celsius (C)
Celsus'
  C. lid
  C. operation
  C. spasmodic entropion
    operation

Celsus-Hotz
    C.-H. entropion
    C.-H. operation
cement
    bifocal c.
    c. bifocal
    Morck's c.
center
    gaze c.
    geometric c.
    horizontal gaze c.
    optic c.
    optical c.
    pontine gaze c. (PGC)
    rotation c.
    c. of rotation
    c. of rotation distance
    vertical gaze c.
centering ring
centigrade (C)
centigray
centistoke
centrad
Centra-Flex lens
centrage
central
    c. abrasion
    c. amaurosis
    c. angioplastic retinitis
    c. angioplastic retinopathy
    c. angiospastic retinitis
    c. angiospastic retinopathy
    c. areolar choroidal atrophy
    c. areolar choroidal dystrophy
    c. areolar choroidal sclerosis
    c. areolar pigment epithelial dystrophy
    c. artery
    c. canal
    c. cartilage
    c. cataract
    c. chorioretinitis
    c. choroidal sclerosis
    c. choroiditis
    c. cloudy corneal dystrophy
    c. cloudy dystrophy
    c. cloudy dystrophy of François
    c. cloudy parenchymatous dystrophy
    c. corneal ulcer
    c. disk-shaped retinopathy

    c. edema
    c. edema of cornea
    c. fields
    c. fixation
    c. fovea
    c. fovea of retina
    c. fusion
    c. illumination
    c. iridectomy
    c. island of vision
    c. keyhole of vision
    c. light
    c. nervous system (CNS)
    c. nystagmus
    c. pigmentary retinal dystrophy
    c. posterior curve (CPC)
    c. posterior curve of contact lens
    c. reflex stripe
    c. retina
    c. retinal artery (CRA)
    c. retinal artery occlusion (CRAO)
    c. retinal degeneration
    c. retinal vein (CRV)
    c. retinal vein occlusion (CRVO)
    c. scotoma
    c. scotoma syndrome
    c. serous chorioretinopathy
    c. serous choroidopathy
    c. serous retinitis
    c. serous retinochoroidopathy
    c. serous retinopathy (CSR)
    c. speckled corneal dystrophy
    c. speckled dystrophy
    c. stellate laceration
    c. suppression
    c. thickness
    c. thickness of contact lens
    c. ulcer
    c. vein
    c. vision
    c. visual acuity
    c. yellow point
centralis
    area c.
    fovea c.
centrally-fixing eye
centraphose

centration
centriole
centripetally
centroblast
centrocecal scotoma
centromere
centroperipheral
cephalgia
cephalic
cephalo-orbital
cephalosporin
Cephalosporium
cephalothin
ceramidase
ceramide
    trihexosyl c.
ceratectomy
cerbrotendinous xanthomatosis
cerclage
    c. operation
cerebellar
    c. artery
    c. astrocytoma tumor
    c. ataxia
    c. cortex
    c. disease
    c. dysfunction
    c. hemisphere
    c. hemorrhage
    c. notch
    c. tonsil
    c. vermis
cerebellomedullary
cerebellopontine
    c. angle
    c. angle tumor
cerebelloretinal
cerebellospinal
cerebellotegmental
cerebellothalamic
cerebellum
cerebral
    c. amaurosis
    c. amyloid angiopathy
    c. angiography
    c. arteriography
    c. arteriosclerosis
    c. artery
    c. artery aneurysm
    c. atrophy
    c. blindness
    c. cortex
    c. cortex reflex

c. diplopia
c. dyschromatopsia
c. infarction
c. layer of retina
c. palsy
c. phycomycosis
c. ptosis
c. radionuclide angiography
c. stratum of retina
c. ventricle
cerebri
    pseudotumor c.
cerebritis
cerebrohepatorenal syndrome
cerebro-ocular
cerebro-ophthalmic
cerebropupillary reflex
cerebroretinal angiomatosis
cerebrosidosis
cerebrospinal fluid (CSF)
cerebrovascular accident (CVA)
cerebrovasculature
cerebrum
cereus
    Bacillus c.
ceroid lipofuscinosis
cerulean cataract
ceruloplasmin
cervical
    c. ganglion
    c. lesion
    c. manipulation
    c. nystagmus
    c. vascular disease
cervicitis
cervico-ocular reflex
cervico-oculo-acoustic syndrome
Cestan-Chenais syndrome
Cestan's syndrome
Cetamide
    Isopto C.
cetanol
Cetapred
    Isopto C.
Cetazol
cetyl alcohol
cetylpyridinium chloride
CF
    counting fingers
C&F
    cell and flare
CFW
    calcofluor white stain

chagrin
    peau de c.
chain
    fenestrated c.
chalaza
chalazion, pl. **chalazia**
    acute c.
    c. clamp
    collar-stud c.
    c. curette
    Desmarres' c.
    c. forceps
    Meyhoeffer's c.
    c. trephine
chalcosis
    cornea c.
    c. lentis
chalk
    calcium carbonate c.
chalkitis
Challenger
    C. digital applanation
      tonometer
    C. tonometer
chamber
    air c. (AC)
    c. angle
    anterior c. (AC)
    anterior c. of eye
    aqueous c.
    axial c.
    closed c.
    depth of c.
    eye c.
    flat c.
    flat anterior c.
    hydrometric c.
    post c.
    posterior c. (PC)
    quiet c.
    reformation of c.
    shallow c.
    shallowing of c.
    sterile adhesive bubble c.
    vitreous c.
    vitreous c. of eye
chamber-deepening glaucoma
Chamber's sterile adhesive bubble
chamfer
chancroid
Chandler
    C. forceps
    C. iris forceps

Chandler's
    C. iridectomy
    C. operation
    C. syndrome
    C. vitreous operation
Chandler-Verhoeff
    C.-V. lens extraction
    C.-V. operation
change
    cortical c.
    fatty c.
    Keith-Wagener c.'s (KW)
    KW c.'s
    nuclear c.'s
    senile choroidal c.
    trophic c.
changer
    Galilean magnification c.
    Littmann galilean
      magnification c.
channel
    scleral c.
Chan wrist rest
Charcot-Marie-Tooth disease
Charcot's triad
CHARGE
    coloboma, heart defects, atresia
    choanae, retarded growth,
    genital hypoplasia, and ear
    anomalies
    CHARGE association
    CHARGE syndrome
Charles
    C. anterior segment sleeve
    C. contact lens
    C. Flute needle
    C. infusion sleeve
    C. intraocular lens
    C. irrigating/aspirating unit
    C. irrigating contact lens
    C. irrigating lens
    C. needle
    C. vacuuming needle
    C. vitrector with sleeve
Charles-Bonnet syndrome
Charles' lensectomy
Charlin's syndrome
chart
    Amsler's c.
    astigmatic dial c.
    Bailey-Lovie Log Mar c.
    Bailey-Lovie visual acuity c.
    Birkhauser c.

Birkhauser test c.
color c.
Donders' c.
Duane's accommodation c.
E c.
eye c.
Ferris' c.
Guibor's c.
illiterate eye c.
kindergarten eye c.
Lancaster-Regan dial 1 c.
Lancaster-Regan dial 2 c.
Landolt's c.
Landolt's broken-ring c.
Lebensohn's c.
Lebensohn's reading c.
Lebensohn's visual acuity c.
pedigree c.
Pelli-Robson c.
picture c.
Randot's c.
reading c.
Regan's c.
Reuss' color c.
Snellen's c.
sunburst dial c.
University of Waterloo c.
vectograph c.
Chavasse glass
checkerboard field
check ligament
Chédiak-Higashi
    C.-H. disease
    C.-H. syndrome
cheek
    c. clamp
    c. flap
cheese wire
cheesy cataract
cheiroscope
chelated
chelating agent
chelator
chelonei
    Mycobacterium c.
chemical
    c. burn
    c. conjunctivitis
    c. diabetes
    c. injury
chemically
    c. treated lens
    c. treated spectacle lens

chemodectoma
chemokinesis
chemosis
chemotactic
chemotaxis
chemotherapeutic agent
chemotherapy
chemotic
chemotio
cherry-red
    c.-r. macula
    c.-r. spot
    c.-r. spot in macula
    c.-r. spot myoclonus
        syndrome
Cheyne's nystagmus
Chiari's malformation
chiasm
    optic c.
chiasma
    c. opticum
    c. syndrome
chiasmal
    c. arachnoiditis
    c. compression
    c. disease
    c. dysplasia
    c. glioma
    c. metastasis
    post c.
    c. sulcus
    c. syndrome
chiasmapexy
chiasmatic
    c. cisterna
    c. field defects
    c. syndrome
chiasmometer
Chiba eye needle
Chibroxin
chickenpox
chief fiber
Chievitz
    C. fiber layer
    fiber layer of C.
    C. layer
    transient layer of C.
chin
    c. depression
    c. elevation
chiroscope
chisel
    cornea c.

chisel *(continued)*
    Freer c.
    lacrimal sac c.
    West c.
    West lacrimal sac c.
chi-squared test
Chlamydia
    C. psittaci
    C. trachomatis
chlamydial
    c. blepharitis
    c. conjunctivitis
    c. disease
    c. infection
chloasma
Chloracol
chloral hydrate
chlorambucil
chloramphenicol
chlordiazepoxide
chlorhexidine
chloride
    acetylcholine c.
    aluminum c.
    benzalkonium c.
    cetylpyridinium c.
    edrophonium c.
    hexamethonium c.
    methacholine c.
    quaternary ammonium c.
    sodium c.
    tetraethylammonium c.
chlorine
chlorisondamine
chloroacetophenone
chlorobutanol
Chlorofair
chloroform
chlorolabe
chloroma
Chloromycetin
Chloromycetin hydrocortisone
Chloromyxin
chlorophane
chloropia
chloroprocaine
chloropsia
Chloroptic S.O.P.
chloroquine
    c. keratopathy
    c. retinopathy
chlorpheniramine

chlorphentermine
chlorpromazine
chlorpropamide
chlorprothixene
chlortetracycline
chlorthalidone
Chlor-Trimeton
choanal polyp
chocolate
    c. agar
    c. cyst
choked
    c. disk
    c. optic disc
    c. reflex
cholesteatoma
cholesterinosis
cholesterol
    c. emboli of retina
    c. embolus
    c. ester
    c. granuloma
    c. plaque
cholesterolosis
cholesterosis
    c. bulbi
cholinergic
    c. blocking agent
    c. mechanism
    c. pupil
chondrocyte
Chondrodystrophia calcificans congenita punctata
chondrodystrophy
chondroitin
    hyaluronate sodium with c.
    c. sulfate
    c. sulfate media
    c. sulfate and sodium hyaluronate
chondroma
chondrosarcoma
chord
    c. diameter
    c. incision
    c. length
chordoma
chorea
    Sydenham's c.
choriocapillaris
    lamina c.
    membrana c.

choriocapillary
  c. atrophy
  c. layer
choriocele
chorioid
chorioidea
chorionic vesicle
chorioretinal (C/R)
  c. atrophy
  c. coloboma
  c. degeneration
  c. granuloma
chorioretinitis
  birdshot c.
  central c.
  luetic c.
  peripheral c.
  sclerosing panencephalitis c.
  c. sclopetaria
  senile c.
  syphilitic c.
  toxoplasmosis c.
  viliginous c.
chorioretinopathy
  birdshot c.
  central scrous c.
  disciform c.
  serous c.
choristoma
  epibulbar limbal dermoid c.
  osseous c.
  c. tumor
choroid
  basal c.
  basal lamina of c.
  c. buckle
  buckling c.
  c. coloboma
  contusion of c.
  crescent c.
  c. fissure
  knuckle of c.
  reattachment of c.
  vascular lamina of c.
  c. vein
choroidal
  c. atrophy
  c. cataract
  c. coloboma
  c. detachment
  c. dystrophy
  c. edema
  c. flush

  c. fold
  c. granuloma
  c. gyrate atrophy
  c. hemangioma
  c. hemorrhage
  c. hyperfluorescence
  c. infiltration
  c. ischemia
  kissing c.'s
  c. lesion
  c. melanoma
  c. membrane
  c. myopic atrophy
  c. neoplasm
  c. neovascularization (CNV)
  c. neovascular membrane
  c. nevus
  c. primary sclerosis
  c. ring
  c. rupture
  c. scan
  c. sclerosis
  c. secondary atrophy
  c. tap
  c. vascular atrophy
  c. vascular occlusion
  c. vessel
choroidea
choroideae
  complexus basalis c.
  lamina vasculosa c.
  tapetum c.
choroidectomy
choroideremia
choroiditis
  acute diffuse serous c.
  anterior c.
  areolar c.
  areolar central c.
  birdshot c.
  central c.
  diffuse c.
  disseminated c.
  Douvas' honeycombed c.
  Doyne's c.
  Doyne's familial
    honeycombed c.
  Doyne's honeycombed c.
  exudative c.
  focal c.
  Föerster's c.
  geographic peripapillary c.
  c. guttata senilis

choroiditis *(continued)*
    guttata senilis c.
    histoplasmic c.
    Holthouse-Batten
      superficial c.
    Hutchinson-Tays central
      guttate c.
    Jensen's c.
    Jensen's juxtapapillaris c.
    juxtapupillary c.
    macular c.
    metastatic c.
    multifocal c.
    c. myopia
    nongranulomatous c.
    posterior c.
    proliferative c.
    recurrent c.
    senescent macular
      exudative c.
    senile macular exudative c.
    c. serosa
    serosa c.
    serpiginous c.
    suppurative c.
    syphilitic c.
    Tay's c.
    toxoplasmic c.
    traumatic c.
choroidocapillaris
    lamina c.
choroidocyclitis
choroidoiritis
choroidopathy
    areolar c.
    central serous c.
    Doyne's honeycombed c.
    geographic c.
    geographic helicoid
      peripapillary c.
    guttate c.
    helicoid c.
    inner punctate c.
    myopic c.
    senile guttate c.
    serpiginous c.
choroidoretinal dystrophy
choroidoretinitis
choroidosis
choroidovaginal vein
Choyce
    C. implant
    C. intraocular lens

    C. lens
    C. lens-inserting forceps
    C. Mark VIII implant
    C. Mark VIII lens
Christmas tree cataract
chromatic
    c. aberration
    c. asymmetry
    c. dispersion
    c. lens aberration
    c. perimetry
    c. spectrum
    c. vision
chromaticities
    complementary c.
chromatin
    nuclear c.
chromatism
chromatometer
chromatopsia
chromatoptometer
chromatoptometry
chromatoskiameter
chromic
    c. catgut suture
    c. collagen suture
    c. gut suture
    c. myopia
    c. suture
chromodacryorrhea
chromometer
chromophane
chromophobe adenoma
chromophore
chromoretinopathy
chromoscope
chromoscopy
chromosomal duplication
chromosome
    c. abnormality
    c. deletion
    c. mapping
    X c.
    Y c.
chromostereopsis
chronic
    c. angle-closure glaucoma
    c. blepharoconjunctivitis
    c. catarrhal conjunctivitis
    c. catarrhal rhinitis
    c. conjunctivitis
    c. cyclitis
    c. dacryocystitis

c. endophthalmitis
c. follicular conjunctivitis
c. glaucoma
c. granulomatous disease
c. narrow-angle glaucoma
c. open-angle glaucoma (COAG)
c. progressive external ophthalmoplegia (CPEO)
c. progressive ophthalmoplegia
c. serpiginous ulcer
c. simple glaucoma
c. superficial keratitis
chrysarobin
chrysiasis
chrysoderma
Churg-Strauss syndrome
Chvostek's sign
chylomicron
Chymar
Alpha C.
chymotrypsin
α-chymotrypsin
α-chymotrypsin-induced glaucoma
Ciaccio's gland
Cibasoft
C. contact lens
C. lens
Cibathin lens
Cibis
C. electrode
C. needle
C. ski needle
Cibis'
C. conjunctivitis
C. ectropion
C. entropion
C. liquid silicone procedure
C. operation
C. pemphigoid
cibisotome
cicatrices
cicatriceum
ectropion c.
entropion c.
cicatricial
c. conjunctivitis
c. ectropion
c. entropion
c. mass
c. pemphigoid

c. retinopathy of prematurity
c. retrolental fibroplasia
c. strabismus
cicatrix, pl. **cicatrices**
cystoid c.
filtering c.
cicatrization
cicatrizing
c. conjunctivitis
Cilco
C. argon laser
C. Frigitronics
C. Frigitronics laser
C. Hoffer Laseridge
C. Hoffer Laseridge laser
C. intraocular lens
C. krypton laser
C. lens forceps
C. MonoFlex multi-piece PMMA intraocular lens
C. perimeter
C. Sonometric A-scan
C. Ultrasound Unit
C. vitrector
C. YAG laser
Cilco/Lasertek
C. A/K laser
C. argon laser
C. krypton laser
Cilco-Simcoe II lens
Cilco-Sonometrics lens
cilia
c. base
c. ectopia
c. forceps
ciliare
corpus c.
ciliares
plicae c.
processus c.
ciliaris
acne c.
annulus c.
blepharitis c.
corona c.
corpus c.
fibrae circulares musculi c.
fibrae longitudinales musculi c.
fibrae meridionales musculi c.
fibrae radiales musculi c.

ciliaris *(continued)*
 gangliosus c.
 c. muscle
 musculus c.
 orbicularis c.
 pars plana corporis c.
 pars plicata corporis c.
 radix oculomotoria
  ganglii c.
 radix sympathica ganglii c.
 striae c.
 zona c.
 zonula c.
ciliariscope
ciliarotomy
ciliary
 c. apparatus
 c. artery
 c. blepharitis
 c. block
 c. block glaucoma
 c. body
 c. body band
 c. body coloboma
 c. canal
 c. cartilage
 c. crown
 c. disk
 c. epithelium
 c. flush
 c. folds
 c. ganglion
 c. ganglionic plexus
 c. gland
 c. hyperemia
 c. injection
 c. ligament
 c. margin
 c. margin of iris
 c. muscle
 c. nerve
 c. procedure
 c. processes
 c. reflex
 c. region
 c. ring
 c. spasm
 c. staphyloma
 c. sulcus
 c. vein
 c. vessel
 c. zone
 c. zonule

ciliate
ciliated
ciliectomy
ciliochoroidal
 c. detachment
 c. effusion
ciliodestructive surgery
cilioequatorial fiber
ciliogenesis
cilioposterocapsular fiber
cilioretinal
 c. artery
 c. vein
cilioscleral
ciliosis
ciliospinal
 c. center of Budge
 c. reflex
ciliotomy
ciliovitreal block
ciliovitrectomy
 c. block
cilium, pl. cilia
cillo
cillosis
Ciloxan
cimetidine
cinch
cinching operation
cincture
cinema eye
cine-magnetic resonance imaging
Cine-Microscope
ciprofloxacin
circadian heterotropia
circinata
 retinitis c.
circinate
 c. exudate
 retinal c.
 c. retinitis
 c. retinopathy
circle
 arterial c.
 Berry's c.
 c. of confusion
 c. diffusion
 c. of dispersion
 c. dissipation
 episcleral arterial c.
 c. of greater iris
 c. of Haller
 Hovius' c.

c. of least confusion
least diffusion c.
c. of lesser iris
Minsky's c.
Vieth-Muller c.
c. of Willis
Zinn-Haller arterial c.
Zinn's c.
circlet
Zinn's c.
circling band
circular
c. ciliary muscle
c. ciliary muscle fiber
c. dichroism
c. fiber
c. nystagmus
c. synechia
circulated
moon c.
circulation
conjunctival c.
episcleral c.
retinal c.
sludging of c.
circulus
c. arteriosus halleri
c. arteriosus iridis major
c. arteriosus iridis minor
c. vasculosus nervi optici
c. zinnii
circumbulbar
circumcorneal injection
circumduction
c. hyperphoria
circumferential
circumlental space
circumocular
circumorbital
circumpapillary
circumscribe
circumscribed episcleritis
circus senilis
cirrhosis
cirsoid aneurysm
cirsomphalos
cirsophthalmia
cirsophthalmus
cisplatin
cis-platinum
cis-**retinal**
cisterna
chiasmatic c.

cisternography
Citelli rongeur
citrate
potassium c.
sodium c.
CL
contact lens
clamp
Backhaus c.
Berens muscle c.
Berke c.
bulldog c.
Castroviejo lid c.
chalazion c.
cheek c.
cross-action c.
cross-action towel c.
Desmarres lid c.
Erhardt c.
Gladstone-Putterman
entropion c.
Gladstone-Putterman
transmarginal rotation
entropion c.
Jones towel c.
Moria-France
dacryocystorhinostomy c.
mosquito c.
muscle c.
Prince c.
Prince muscle c.
Putterman levator
resection c.
Putterman-Mueller
blepharoptosis c.
Putterman ptosis c.
Robin chalazion c.
Schaedel cross-action
towel c.
serrefine c.
clarity
optical c.
Clark
C. Autophoro-Optimeter
C. capsule fragment forceps
C. speculum
Clark-Verhoeff capsule forceps
Clarvisan
classical congenital esophoria
classification
Callender's c.
Callender's cell type c.
Duane's c.

classification *(continued)*
    Keith-Wagener c.
    Keith-Wagener-Barker c.
    LeFort c.
    Leishman's c.
    MacCallan's c.
    Scheie's c.
    Shaffer-Weiss c.
    Tessier's c.
    Wagener-Clay-Gipner c.
Claude-Bernard-Horner syndrome
Claude's syndrome
claudication
    jaw c.
Clayman
    C. guide
    C. intraocular lens
    C. lens
    C. lens-holding forceps
    C. lens implant forceps
    C. lens-inserting forceps
    C. posterior chamber lens
Clayman-Knolle irrigating lens
  loop
Clean
    Gel C.
    Sila C.
cleaner
    Boston c.
    Boston Advance c.
    enzymatic c.
    enzyme c.
    gas-permeable daily c.
    Lens Plus daily c.
    Opti-Zyme enzymatic c.
    ProFree/GP weekly
      enzymatic c.
    ReNu Effervescent
      enzymatic c.
    ReNu Thermal enzymatic c.
    Sensitive Eyes daily c.
    Soflens enzymatic contact
      lens c.
    Soft Mate Enzyme Plus c.
    Soft Mate Hands Off
      daily c.
    Ultrazyme enzymatic c.
    Vision Care enzymatic c.
Clean-N-Soak
Clean-N-Stow
cleanup
    cortical c.

Clear
    C. Eyes
    C. Eyes ACR
    Lens C.
clearance
    apical c.
clear windows
Cleasby
    C. spatula
    C. spatulated needle
Cleasby's
    C. iridectomy operation
    C. operation
cleavage syndrome
cleft
    corneal c.
    cortical c.
    cyclodialysis c.'s
    excessive cyclodialysis c.'s
    facial c.
    c. syndrome
clefting
    cortical c.
    Tessier's c.
Clens
Clerf needle holder
clerical spectacles
Clerz 2
click phenomenon
climatic
    c. droplet keratopathy
    c. keratopathy
clindamycin
clinical
    c. genetics
    c. trial
Clinitex
    C. Charles
      endophotocoagulator probe
    C. photocoagulator
    C. photomydriasis
clinocephaly
clinometer
clinoscope
clioquinol
clip
    Castroviejo c.
    Castroviejo scleral
      shortening c.
    double tantalum c.
    Federov four-loop iris c.
    Friedman c.

Friedman tantalum c.
Halberg trial c.
holding c.
Janelli c.
lens c.
Platina c.
scleral shortening c.
tantalum c.
trial c.
two-way towel c.
clip-applying forceps
clivus
clock
astigmatic c.
c. dial
clock-mechanism esotropia
clofazimine
Clomid
clomiphene
clonality
clonidine
C loop
C-loop posterior chamber lens
Cloquet's canal
closed
c. chamber
eyelids sutured c.
c. loop
c. surgery
c. surgery on eye
closed-angle glaucoma
closed circuit television
closed-eye surgery
closed-funnel vitreoretinopathy
closed-loop system
closed-system pars plana vitrectomy
clostridial blepharitis
Clostridium
C. botulinum
C. perfringens
C. tetani
closure
crow-foot c.
forced-eye c.
wound c.
clotrimazole
clouding
corneal c.
feathery c.
Cloudman mouse melanoma
cloudy cornea
clove-hitch suture

cloxacillin
clump
c. cell
vortex-like c.'s
clumped
c. pigmentation
c. retinal pigment
clumping
pigment c.
pigmentary rarefaction and c.
cluster
c. headache
macular c.'s
c. of pigmented spots
c. of retinoblastoma cell
CMD
cystoid macular degeneration
CME
cystoid macular edema
CMI
cell-mediated immunity
CN
cranial nerve
CNS
central nervous system
CNV
choroidal neovascularization
CO_2
CO_2 laser
CO_2 Sharplan laser
COAG
chronic open-angle glaucoma
coagulate
coagulating electrode
coagulation
disseminated intravascular c.
c. factor
light c.
Meyer-Schwickerath light c.
coagulator
argon laser c.
Evergreen Lasertek c.
Grieshaber micro-bipolar c.
Laserflex c.
Meyer-Schwickerath c.
Walker c.
coagulum
coalesce
coalesced
coalescing
coal-mining lensectomy
coarctate retina

coarctation of aorta
coarse punctate staining
coastal erysipelas
coast erosion
coat
    buffy c.
    sclerotic c.
    uveal c.
coated Vicryl suture
coating
    antireflection c.
    color c.
    edge c.
    c. of lens
    c. material
    mirror c.
    proteinaceous c.
    RLX c.
    c. for spectacle lens
Coats'
    C. disease
    C. retinitis
    C. ring
    C. white ring
coaxial illumination
cobalt
    c. blue filter
    c. therapy
cobblestone
    c. appearance
    c. conjunctivitis
    c. degeneration
    c. papilla
    c. retinal degeneration
Coburn
    C. camera
    C. intraocular lens
    C. irrigation/aspiration
        system
    C. irrigation/aspiration unit
    C. lens
    C. lensometer
    C. refractor
    C. tonometer
Coburn-Meditec
Coburn-Rodenstock
    C.-R. lamp
    C.-R. slit lamp
cocaine
    c. hydrochloride
    c. methylphenidate
    c. test

cocci
    gram-positive c.
Coccidioides immitis
Coccidioides skin test
coccidioidomycosis
Cochet-Bonnet esthesiometer
cochleopupillary reflex
Cockayne's syndrome
co-contraction syndrome
codeine
Codman/Micra
Codman wet-field cautery
codominance
coefficient
    correlation c.
    c. of facility of outflow
    c. of outflow
    c. of variation
Coerens tumor
Coffin-Lowry syndrome
Cogan-Boberg-Ans
    C.-B.-A. implant
    C.-B.-A. lens implant
Cogan-Reese syndrome
Cogan's
    C. apraxia
    C. congenital oculomotor
        apraxia
    C. corneal dystrophy
    C. disease
    C. dystrophy
    C. interstitial keratitis
    C. microcystic corneal
        epithelial dystrophy
    C. microcystic dystrophy
    C. microcystic epithelial
        corneal dystrophy
    C. sign
    C. syndrome
cognition
cognoscibile
    minimum c.
cogwheel
    c. movement
    c. ocular movements
    c. pupil
    c. pursuit
    c. pursuit movement
cogwheeling
Cohan
    C. corneal forceps
    C. needle holder
Cohan-Barraquer microscope

Cohan-Vannas iris scissors
Cohan-Westcott scissors
Cohen corneal forceps
Cohen's syndrome
Coherent
    C. 920 argon/dye laser
    C. 900 argon laser
    C. 920 argon laser
    C. dye laser
    C. krypton laser
    C. 7910 laser
    C. Medical YAG laser
    C. radiation argon/krypton
      laser
    C. radiation argon model
      800 laser
    C. radiation Fluorotron
cohort study
coil
    basal c.
    electromagnetic scleral
      search c.
    scleral search c.
coin gauge
cold-opposite, warm-same (COWS)
Coleman retractor
Coleman Taylor IOL forceps
colforsin
coli
    Escherichia c.
Colibri
    C. forceps
    C. micro forceps
coliform
    c. blepharitis
    c. organism
colistin
collagen
    c. bandage lens
    c. disease
    c. fibers
    c. lamellae
    c. and rheumatoid-related
      disease
    c. shield
    c. vascular disease
collagenase inhibitor
collagenolytic trabecular ring
collagenous trabecular ring
collar button
collarette
collar-stud chalazion

colliculus
    superior c.
Collier
    tucked lid of C.
Collier's sign
collimated
collimator
Collin-Beard operation
Collin 140 color adaptometer
Collins' syndrome
colliquation
    discrete c.
colliquative
    discrete c.
collodion dressing
colloid
    c. body
    c. cyst
    c. deposits
colloidal silver
collyria
Collyrium
    Beer's C.
    C. eye drops
    C. for Fresh Eyes
Colmascope
coloboma
    c. anomalies
    atypical c.
    bridge c.
    chorioretinal c.
    choroid c.
    c. of choroid
    choroidal c.
    ciliary body c.
    complete c.
    congenital optic nerve c.
    dysplastic c.
    eyelid c.
    fissure c.
    Fuchs' c.
    Fuchs' inferior c.
    Fuchs' spot c.
    c. of fundus
    c. iridis, iris c.
    c. of iris
    c. of lens
    c. lentis
    c. lobuli
    macular c.
    optic c.
    optic nerve c.
    c. of optic nerve

coloboma *(continued)*
    c. palpebrale
    peripapillary c.
    c. of retina
    c. retinae
    retinochoroidal c.
    typical c.
    vitreous c.
    c. of vitreous
coloboma, heart defects, atresia choanae, retarded growth, genital hypoplasia, and ear anomalies (CHARGE)
colobomata
colobomatous
    c. cyst
    c. microphthalmia
color
    c. aberration
    c. adaptation
    c. adaptometer
    c. amblyopia
    c. blind
    c. blindness
    c. chart
    c. coating
    c. comparison
    complementary c.
    confusion c.'s
    c. confusion
    c. constancy
    c. contrast
    c. defect
    deviant c.
    c. discrimination
    c. disk
    end-point c.
    eye c.
    c. fusion
    incidental c.
    metameric c.
    c. mixing
    Munsell's c.
    opponent c.
    c. perception
    c. perimetry
    primary c.
    pure c.
    reflected c.'s
    saturated c.
    c. saturation
    c. scotoma

    c. sense
    simple c.
    solid c.
    c. spectrum
    c. test
    c. theory
    c. triangle
    c. vision (VC)
    c. vision test
    c. washout
colorimeter
colossal agenesis
colposcope
    Zeiss c.
column
    ocular dominance c.'s
columnar layer
Coly-Mycin S
coma
    c. aberration
Comberg
    C. contact lens
    C. lens
    C. localization
Comberg's foreign body operation
Combiline System
combination
    sulfonamide and decongestant c.
    sulfonamide and steroid c.
combined
    c. dystrophy of Fuchs'
    c. fracture
    c. glaucoma
combined-mechanism glaucoma
comedo pattern
comet scotoma
Comfort
    C. drops
    C. Tears
comfort bridge
comitance
comitant
    c. exodeviation
    c. exophoria
    c. exotropia
    c. heterotropia
    c. squint
    c. strabismus
comminuted orbital fracture
commissura
    c. palpebrarum lateralis

c. palpebrarum medialis
c. palpebrarum nasalis
c. palpebrarum temporalis
commissurae opticae
commissure
arcuate c.
c. of Gudden
Gudden's c.
interthalamic c.
Meynert's c.
optic c.
palpebral c.
posterior c.
posterior chiasmatic c.
supraoptic c.
commitant vertical deviation
**Committee on Allied Health
Education and Accreditation
(CAHEA)**
common
c. canaliculus
c. tendinous ring
commotio retinae
communicating artery aneurysm
communication
arteriole c.
arteriovenous c.
communis
annulus tendineus c.
comparison
color c.
c. eyepiece
compatibility
compensated
c. glaucoma
c. segment
compensating eyepiece
compensatory
c. head posture
c. posture
complement
c. component
c. fixation test
c. system
complementary
c. afterimage
c. chromaticities
c. color
complement-fixing
c.-f. antibody
complete
c. achromatopsia
c. blood count (CBC)

c. cataract
c. coloboma
c. congenital cataract
c. hemianopsia
c. iridectomy
c. iridoplegia
complex
AIDS-related c. (ARC)
avidin-biotinylated
peroxidase c.
c. ectropion
Golgi's c.
immune c.
major histocompatibility c.
(MHC)
c. motion tomography
triple symptom c.
complexus basalis choroideae
compliance cap
complicata
cataracta c.
complicated cataract
component
complement c.
quick left/right c.
composition of spectacle lens
compound
c. astigmatism
c. eye
Hurler-Scheie c.
c. hyperopic astigmatism
c. lens
c. myopic astigmatism
c. nevus
quaternary ammonium c.
silver c.
c. spectacles
c. vesicle
compression
chiasmal c.
c. cyanosis
c. dressing
limbal c.
c. molding
prechiasmal c.
c. retinopathy
c. suture
compressive
c. defect
c. nystagmus
c. optic nerve defect
compressor
Anthony orbital c.

compressor *(continued)*
    Berens orbital c.
    Castroviejo c.
    orbital c.
    orbital enucleation c.
computed
    c. perimetry
    c. tomography (CT)
    c. tomography scan
computerized photokeratoscope
Computon Microtonometer
concave
    c. cylinder
    c. lens
    c. mirror
    c. reflecting surface
    c. spectacle lens
concavity
concavoconcave lens
concavoconvex lens
concentric
    c. constriction
    c. folds
    c. lesion
    c. stria
concentrically
Concept
    C. disposable cautery
    C. hand-held cautery
concha bullosa
conclination
concomitance
concomitant
    c. exophoria
    c. heterotropia
    c. strabismus
concretion
    conjunctival c.
concussion
    c. blindness
    c. cataract
    c. injury
    c. of the retina
condensate
condensing lens
condition
    null c.
    predisposing c.
conduction
    antidromic c.
cone
    c. achromatopsia
    apical c.

    bipolar c.
    blue c.
    c. cell
    c. degeneration
    c. dysfunction
    c. dystrophy
    c. fiber
    c. function
    c. granule
    layer of rods and c.'s
    McIntyre truncated c.
    c. monochromacy
    monochromatic c.
    c. monochromatism
    c. monochromats
    muscle c.
    ocular c.
    c. opsin
    pedicle c.
    c. photopigments
    retinal c.
    Rochon-Duvigneaud bouquet
      of c.'s
    rods and c.'s
    triad of retinal c.
    twin c.
    c. vision
    visual c.
cone-rod
    c.-r. degeneration
    c.-r. dystrophy
configuration
    bombé c.
    Kratz-Sinskey loop c.
    vacuolar c.
    whorl-like c.
confluent
conformer
    eye implant c.
    Fox c.
    McGuire c.
    silicone c.
    Universal c.
confrontation
    c. fields
    c. method
    c. visual field test
confrontational
confusion
    circle of c.
    circle of least c.
    color c.
    c. colors

congenital c.
visual c.
congenita
dyskeratosis c.
myotonia c.
congenital
c. abducens facial paralysis
c. abducens nerve palsy
c. abnormality
c. amaurosis
c. anomaly
c. anophthalmos
c. astigmatism
c. brain malformation
c. bulbar paralysis
c. cataract
c. cleft of iris
c. confusion
c. conus
c. crescents
c. dacryocele
c. dacryocystitis
c. dermoid
c. dermoid of limbus
c. dichromatism
c. disorder
c. dystrophic ptosis
c. dystrophy
c. dysversion
c. ectropion
c. endothelial dystrophy
c. entropion
c. esophoria
c. esotropia
c. facial diplegia
c. fibrous syndrome
c. glaucoma
c. heart disease
c. hemianopsia
c. hemolytic jaundice
c. hereditary corneal
dystrophy
c. hereditary endothelial
corneal dystrophy
c. hereditary endothelial
dystrophy
c. heterochromia
c. hypophosphatasia
c. ichthyosis
c. impatency
latent c.
c. lens dislocation
c. lens opacities

c. leukoderma
c. leukopathia
c. limbal corneal dermoid
c. limbal corneal dermoid
tumor
c. macular degeneration
c. medullated optic nerve
fibers
c. melanocytosis
c. melanosis oculi
c. nasolacrimal duct
obstruction
c. nystagmus
c. ocular melanocytosis
c. oculodermal
melanocytosis
c. oculofacial paralysis
c. oculomotor nerve palsy
c. optic atrophy
c. optic nerve coloboma
c. optic nerve pit
c. pterygium
c. ptosis
c. retinal folds
c. retinoschisis
c. rubella syndrome
c. superior oblique
underaction
c. syphilis
c. syphilitic conjunctivitis
c. toxoplasmosis
congested vessels
congestion
c. of conjunctiva
deep c.
superficial c.
transient c.
congestive glaucoma
Congo red
congruent points
congruity
congruous
c. field defect
c. hemianopsia
c. homonymous hemianopic
scotoma
coni
conical
c. cornea
c. implant
c. protrusion
conjugacy
object/image c.

conjugate
  c. deviation
  c. deviation of eyes
  c. disparity
  c. foci
  c. focus
  c. gaze
  c. movement
  c. movement of eyes
  c. nystagmus
  c. ocular movements
  c. paralysis
  c. point
conjugately
conjunctiva, gen. and pl. **conjunctivae**
  annulus of c.
  brachium c.
  bulbar c.
  congestion of c.
  emphysema of c.
  epitheliosis desquamativa
    conjunctivae
  Föerster's c.
  c. forceps
  glandulae mucosae
    conjunctivae
  leptotrichosis c.
  palpebral c.
  plica semilunaris
    conjunctivae
  c. retractor
  saccus conjunctivae
  sebaceous gland of c.
  semilunar folds of c.
  siderosis conjunctivae
  c. spreader
  tela c.
  temporal bulbar c.
  tunica c.
  xerosis conjunctivae
**conjunctiva-associated lymphoid
tissue**
conjunctival
  c. abrasion
  c. amyloidosis
  c. angioma
  c. artery
  c. bleb
  c. brachium
  c. break
  c. calcification
  c. circulation
  c. concretion

  c. contusions
  c. crystals
  c. cul-de-sac
  c. cyst
  c. deposits
  c. dermoids
  c. discharge
  c. dysplasia
  c. edema
  c. epithelial cell
  c. exudate
  c. flap
  c. fold
  c. follicle
  c. gland
  c. goblet cell
  c. goblet cell densities
  c. graft
  c. granuloma
  c. hemangioma
  c. hemorrhage
  c. hyperemia
  c. impression cytology
  c. incision
  c. injection
  c. laceration
  c. limbus
  c. lipodermoid
  c. lithiasis
  c. lymphangioma
  c. lymphoid tumor
  c. melanoma
  c. melanotic lesion
  c. membrane
  c. necrosis
  c. nevus
  c. nodule
  c. papilla
  c. papilloma
  c. patch graft
  c. phlyctenulosis
  c. pigmented nevus
  c. reaction
  c. recession
  c. reflex
  c. ring
  c. sac
  c. scarring
  c. scissors
  c. scrapings
  c. semilunar folds
  c. slough
  c. smear

c. staining
c. tear
c. ulcer
c. varix
c. vein
c. xerosis
conjunctivales
  glandulae c.
  glandulae ciliares c.
  glandulae sebaceae c.
  venae c.
  venae anteriores c.
  venae posteriores c.
conjunctivalis
  nodulus c.
  saccus c.
conjunctiva-Muller muscle excision
conjunctiviplasty
conjunctivitis
  acne c.
  acne rosacea c.
  actinic c.
  acute atopic c.
  acute catarrhal c.
  acute congestive c.
  acute contagious c.
  acute epidemic c.
  acute follicular c.
  acute hemorrhagic c.
  adenovirus c.
  adult inclusion c.
  allergic c.
  anaphylactic c.
  angular c.
  arc-flash c.
  c. arida
  atopic c.
  atropine c.
  Axenfeld's follicular c.
  bacterial c.
  Bangla Joy c.
  Béal's c.
  blenorrheal c.
  blepharitis c.
  Butcher's c.
  calcareous c.
  candidal c.
  candidiasis c.
  catarrhal c.
  chemical c.
  chlamydial c.
  chronic c.
  chronic catarrhal c.

chronic follicular c.
Cibis' c.
cicatricial c.
cicatrizing c.
cobblestone c.
congenital syphilitic c.
contact c.
contagious granular c.
croupous c.
diphtheritic c.
diplobacillary c.
eczematous c.
Egyptian c.
Elschnig's c.
epidemic c.
erythema multiforme c.
exanthematous c.
factitious c.
follicular c.
giant papillary c. (GPC)
gonococcal c.
gonorrheal c.
gout c.
granular c.
hay fever c.
hemorrhagic c.
herpes simplex c.
herpes zoster c.
immunological c.
inclusion c.
infantile purulent c.
infectious c.
Koch-Weeks c.
lacrimal c.
lagophthalmia c.
larval c.
c. ligneous
ligneous c.
lithiasis c.
c. medicamentosa
meibomian c.
membranous c.
meningococcus c.
microbiallergic c.
c. molluscum
molluscum c.
Morax-Axenfeld c.
mucopurulent c.
c. necroticans infectiosus
necrotic infectious c.
neisserial c.
neonatal c.
neonatal inclusion c.

conjunctivitis *(continued)*
    newborn c.
    c. nodosa
    nodular c.
    nonatopic allergic c.
    ocular vaccinia c.
    oculoglandular c.
    papillary c.
    Parinaud's c.
    Parinaud's oculoglandular c.
    Pascheff's c.
    c. petrificans
    phlyctenular c.
    pinkeye c.
    pneumococcal c.
    prairie c.
    pseudomembranous c.
    pseudovernal c.
    purulent c.
    Reiter's disease c.
    rubeola c.
    Samoan c.
    Sanyal's c.
    scrofulous c.
    shipyard c.
    simple c.
    simple acute c.
    Singapore epidemic c.
    snow c.
    spring c.
    springtime c.
    squirrel plague c.
    staphylococcal c.
    swimming pool c.
    Thygeson's chronic
      follicular c.
    toxic c.
    toxic follicular c.
    toxicogenic c.
    trachoma inclusion c.
    trachomatous c.
    tuberculosis c.
    tularemic c., c. tularensis
    unilateral c.
    uratic c.
    vernal c.
    viral c.
    Wegener's granulomatosis c.
    welder's c.
    Widmark's c.
    Wucherer's c.
    c. xeroderma pigmentosum

conjunctivochalasis
conjunctivodacryocystorhinostomy
  (CDCR)
conjunctivodacryocystostomy
conjunctivoma
conjunctivoplasty
conjunctivorhinostomy
conjunctivotarsal
conjunctivo-Tenon's flap
Con-Lish polishing method
connection
    Luer c.'s
    synaptic c.
connective
    c. tissue
    c. tissue disorder
    c. tissue membrane
connector
    McIntyre nylon cannula c.
Conn syndrome
conoid
    c. lens
    c. lenses
    c. of Sturm
    Sturm's c.
conomyoidin
conophthalmus
Conradi's syndrome
Conrad's
    C. operation
    C. orbital blowout fracture
      operation
consanguinity
consecutive
    c. anophthalmia
    c. atrophy
    c. esotropia
    c. exotropia
    c. optic atrophy
consensual
    c. light reflex
    c. light response
    c. pupillary response
    c. reaction
Consept
    Soft Mate C.
constancy
    color c.
constant
    c. esotropia
    c. exophoria
    c. hypertropia
    c. hypotropia

c. monocular tropia
c. nystagmus
c. strabismus
constricted pupil
constriction
    concentric c.
    focal c.
constructional apraxia
consummatum
    glaucoma c.
Contact
    C. A- and B-scan
contact
    arc of c.
    c. arc
    c. bandage lens
    c. blepharitis
    c. burns of globe
    c. conjunctivitis
    c. dermatitis
    c. dermatoconjunctivitis
    eye c.
    c. glasses
    haptic c.
    c. illumination
    c. lens (CL)
    c. lens blank
    c. lens chord diameter
    c. lens curve
    c. lens diameter
    c. lens height
    c. lens overwearing
      syndrome
    c. lens thickness
    c. lens vertex power
    c. low-vacuum lens
    c. method
contact lens (CL)
    AIRLens c. l.
    annular bifocal c. l.
    aphakic c. l.
    aspheric c. l.
    c. l. blank
    cellulose acetate butyrate c.
      l.
    contour c. l.
    decentration of c. l.
    disposable c. l.
    double slab-off c. l.
    c. l. for drug administration
    Dyer nomogram system of
      ordering c. l.

    extended-wear c. l. (EWCL)
    finished c. l.
    c. l. flat
    flexible-wear c. l.
    fluorocarbon in c. l.
    gas-permeable c. l.
    Korb c. l.
    lenticular c. l.
    lenticular-cut c. l.
    loose c. l.
    microthin c. l.
    minus carrier c. l.
    polymethyl methacrylate c.
      l.
    prism ballast c. l.
    prolonged-wear c. l.
    rigid gas-permeable c. l.
      (RGP)
    scratched c. l.
    semifinished c. l.
    silicone c. l.
    silicone acrylate c. l.
    single-cut c. l.
    Soper cone c. l.
    steep c. l.
    thickness of c. l.
    tight c. l.
    toric c. l
    toroidal c. l.
    wetting angle of c. l.
    X chrom c. l.
    zone of c. l.
contactologist
contactology
contactoscope
contagiosa
    impetigo c.
contagiosum
    ecthyma c.
    keratitis molluscum c.
    molluscum c.
contagious granular conjunctivitis
content
    orbital c.
    water c.
contiguity
contiguous
    c. fibers
    c. pattern
Contino's
    C. epithelioma
    C. glaucoma

continuous
> c. fiber
> c. laser

continuous-wave argon laser
Contique contact lens case
contour
> c. contact lens
> corneal c.
> edge c.
> eyelid c.
> c. interaction
> c. lens
> scalloped c.'s
> c. stereo test

contraceptive
> oral c.

contracted socket
contraction (C)
> anisocoria c.
> c. of cyclitic membrane
> c. and liquefaction
> c. of pupil
> pupillary c.
> pupillary sphincter c.'s
> vermiform c.'s
> vitreous c.

contracture
> socket c.

contralateral
> c. antagonist
> c. eye
> c. synergist

contrast
> color c.
> c. discrimination
> gallium citrate c.
> long-scale c.
> low c.
> c. material
> c. media
> c. sensitivity
> short-scale c.
> simultaneous c.
> successive c.
> c. visualization

contrecoup injury
control
> c. group
> supranuclear c.

contusion
> c. angle glaucoma
> c. cataract
> c. of choroid

> conjunctival c.'s
> corneal c.
> c. of eye
> c. glaucoma
> c. of globe
> c. of orbit
> vitreoretinal c.

conular
conus, pl. **coni**
> congenital c.
> distraction c.
> c. distraction
> inferior c.
> lateral oblique c.
> myopic c.
> c. of optic disk
> c. shell type eye implant
> supertraction c.
> c. supertraction
> underlying c.

conventional
> c. outflow
> c. shell implant

converge
convergence
> accommodative c. (AC)
> amplitude of c.
> c. amplitudes
> angle of c.
> c. angle
> c. excess
> excess esotropia c.
> far-point c.
> far point of c.
> fusional c.
> c. insufficiency
> c. insufficiency exotropia
> near point of c. (NPC)
> negative c.
> c. nystagmus
> c. paralysis
> c. point
> c. position
> positive c.
> proximal c.
> punctum proximum of c. (PP)
> range of c.
> relative c.
> c. retraction nystagmus
> c. spasm
> tonic c.

unit of c.
voluntary c.
convergence-evoked nystagmus
convergency reflex
convergent
    c. beams
    c. deviation
    c. exercises
    c. light
    c. ray
    c. squint
    c. strabismus
    c. wavefront
converging
    c. lens
    c. meniscus
    c. meniscus lens
    c. ray
convergiometer
convex
    high c.
    c. lens
    low c.
    c. mirror
    c. plano lens
    c. reflecting surface
    c. spectacle lens
convexity
convexoconcave lens
convexoconvex lens
convulsion
Conway lid retractor
Cook speculum
Cooper
    C. aspirator
    C. blade fragment
    C. I&A Unit
    C. implant
    C. irrigating/aspirating unit
    C. laser
    C. 2000 laser
    C. 2500 laser
    C. Laser Sonics laser
    C. Surgeon-Plus Ultrathin
      blade
cooperation
    cellular c.
Cooper's operation
CooperVision
    C. argon laser
    C. balanced salt solution
    C. camera

C. Diagnostic Imaging
  refractor
C. fragmatome
C. I/A machine
C. imaging perimeter
C. irrigating/aspirating unit
C. irrigating needle
C. irrigation/aspiration unit
C. laser
C. microscope
C. ocutome
C. perimeter
C. photokeratoscope
C. PMMA-ACL Flex lens
C. refractive
  photokeratoscope
C. refractive surgery
  photokeratoscope
C. spatulated needle
C. Surgeon-Plus Ultrathin
  blade
C. ultrasonography
C. ultrasound
C. vitrector
C. YAG laser
Copeland
    C. implant
    C. intraocular lens
    C. pan chamber lens
    C. radial panchamber
      intraocular lens
    C. radial panchamber UV
      lens
    C. retinoscope
    C. streak retinoscope
Copeland's retinoscopy
copiopia
copolymer
copper
    c. cataract
    c. deposition
    c. foreign bodies
    c. metabolism
copper-wire
    c.-w. arteriole
    c.-w. artery
    c.-w. effect
    c.-w. reflex
copper wiring
Coppock cataract
coquille plano lens
Coracin
coralliform cataract

Corbett spud
Corboy
 C. hemostat
 C. needle holder
cord
 binary c.
 spinal c.
 white c.
Cordarone
cordless monocular indirect
 ophthalmoscope
core
 nerve c.
 c. vitrectomy
corecleisis, coreclisis
corectasia, corectasis
corectome
corectomedialysis
corectomy
corectopia
coredialysis
corediastasis
corelysis
coremorphosis
corenclisis
corcometer
coreometry
coreoplasty
corepexy
corepraxy
corestenoma
 c. congenitum
coretomedialysis
coretomy
corkscrew
 c. artery
 c. visual field defect
cornea, gen. **corneae**
 c. abrader
 abrasio corneae
 abrasion of c.
 abscessus siccus corneae
 alkali burn of c.
 c. anesthesia
 anterior epithelium corneae
 apical zone of c.
 arcus corneae
 arcus lipoides corneae
 artificial c.
 aspheric c.
 bedewing of c.
 black c.
 blood staining of c.

Bonzel's blood staining
 of c.
Burr's c.
calcareous degeneration
 of c.
caligo corneae
central edema of c.
c. chalcosis
c. chisel
cloudy c.
conical c.
degeneration of c.
deturgescence of c.
diameter of c.
donor c.
dystrophia adiposa corneae
dystrophia endothelialis
 corneae
dystrophia epithelialis
 corneae
dystrophy of c.
edema of c.
endothelial cell surface
 of c.
epithelium anterius corneae
epithelium posterius corneae
facies anterior corneae
facies posterior corneae
c. farinata
fistula of c.
flat c.
floury c.
c. globosa
c. guttata
guttata of c.
c. guttate lesion
infiltrates in c.
lamina limitans anterior
 corneae
lamina limitans posterior
 corneae
lash abrasion of c.
lattice dystrophy of c.
lead incrustation of c.
limbus of c.
liquor corneae
marginal degeneration of c.
meridian of c.
c. opaca
opalescent c.
oval c.
phthisis c.
pigmented line of c.

c. plana
c. plana congenita familiares
posterior conical c.
posterior epithelium of c.
recurrent erosion of c.
rust ring of c.
c. sensitivity
spherical c.
substantia propria corneae
sugar-loaf c.
superficial line of c.
ulceration of c.
c. urica
c. verticillata
c. verticullata
Vogt's c.
white ring of c.
xerosis of c.

cornea-holding forceps
corneal

c. abrasion
c. abscess
c. abscission
c. alkali burn
c. apex
c. arcus
c. astigmatism
c. bedewing
c. birefringence
c. blood staining
c. bur
c. burn
c. button
c. cap
c. cell
c. cleft
c. clouding
c. contact lens
c. contour
c. contusion
c. corpuscle
c. crystals
c. curette
c. curvature
c. cyst
c. debrider
c. decompensation
c. deep opacity
c. degeneration
c. dehydration
c. dellen
c. dendrite
c. deposits

c. deturgescence
c. diameter
c. dissector
c. distortion
c. dysgenesis
c. dysplasia
c. dystrophy
c. dystrophy of
  Waardenburg-Jonkers
c. ectasia
c. edema
c. endothelial dystrophy
c. endothelial guttate
  dystrophy
c. endothelial pigmentary
  dispersion
c. endothelium
c. enlargement
c. epithelium
c. erosion
c. crysiphake
c. facet
c. fascia lata spatula
c. filament
c. fissure
c. fistula
c. fixation forceps
c. foreign body bur
c. full-thickness
c. furrow degeneration
c. graft
c. graft operation
c. graft spatula
c. graft step
c. guttata
c. guttate dystrophy
c. guttering
c. hook
c. implant
c. incision
c. inferior limbal
c. infiltrate
c. inlays
c. iron line
c. keratitis
c. knife
c. knife dissector
c. laceration
c. lamella
c. lamellar groove
c. leakage
c. lens
c. light reflex

corneal *(continued)*
  c. light shield
  c. limbus
  c. line
  c. luster
  c. marginal furrow
  c. melt
  c. meridian
  c. microscope
  c. mushroom
  c. nebula
  c. needle
  c. neovascularization
  c. nerve
  c. opacification
  c. opacity
  c. optical density
  c. pachometer
  c. pannus
  c. pellucid
  c. perforation
  c. phlyctenulosis
  c. prosthesis forceps
  c. prosthesis trephine
  c. protrusion
  c. punch
  c. punctate infiltrate
  c. punctate lesion
  c. reflection
  c. reflex
  c. ring
  c. scar
  c. scarring
  c. scissors
  c. section spatulated scissors
  c. sensation
  c. spatulated scissors
  c. splinter forceps
  c. spot
  c. staining
  c. staining test
  c. staphyloma
  c. stria
  c. stroma
  c. stromal dystrophy
  c. substance
  c. surgery
  c. thinning
  c. topographic analysis
  c. topography
  c. transplant
  c. transplantation
  c. transplant centering ring
  c. transplant marker
  c. trauma
  c. trepanation
  c. trephine
  c. tube
  c. ulcer
  c. vascularization
  c. velum
  c. vortex dystrophy
  c. xerosis
cornealis
  rima c.
Corneascope
corneitis
Cornelia de Lange syndrome
corneoblepharon
corneodysgenesis
corneoiritis
corneomandibular reflex
corneomental reflex
corneopterygoid reflex
corneosclera
corneoscleral
  c. border
  c. button
  c. forceps
  c. groove
  c. incision
  c. junction
  c. laceration
  c. lamellae
  c. melt
  c. punch
  c. right/left-hand scissors
  c. scissors
  c. sulcus
  c. trabeculum
corneoscleralis
  pars c.
corneoscope
  IDI c.
cornpicker's pupil
corona
  c. ciliaris
  Zinn's c.
coronal
coronaria
  cataracta c.
coronary cataract
coroparelcysis
coroplasty
coroscopy
Cor-Oticin

corotomy
corpus
    c. adiposum orbitae
    c. callosum
    c. ciliare
    c. ciliaris
    vitreum c.
    c. vitreum
corpuscle
    corneal c.
    hyaloid c.
    Toynbee's c.
    Virchow's c.
correctable
corrected
    c. lens
    c. spectacle lens
correction
    aphakic c.
    astigmatism c.
    Byron Smith's lazy T c.
    dioptric c.
    epicanthal c.
    optical c.
    spectacle c.
    with c. (cc)
    without c. (sc)
corrective movement
correlation coefficient
correspondence
    abnormal c.
    abnormal harmonious
      retinal c.
    abnormal retinal c. (ARC)
    abnormal unharmonious
      retinal c.
    anomalous c.
    anomalous retinal c. (ARC)
    dysharmonious c.
    harmonious c.
    harmonious abnormal
      retinal c.
    harmonious retinal c.
    Herring's law of motor c.
    normal c.
    normal retinal c. (NRC)
    c. points
    retinal c.
    sensory c.
corresponding
    c. point
    c. retinal points
corridor incision

corrugans
    fibrosis choroideae c.
corrugator
Cort-Dome
Cortef
    Delta C.
    Neo-C.
cortex
    aspiration of c.
    brain c.
    calcarine c.
    cerebellar c.
    cerebral c.
    c. lens
    c. lentis
    occipital c.
    parastriate visual c.
    peristriate visual c.
    primary visual c.
    residual c.
    striate c.
    striate visual c.
    visual c.
cortical
    c. blindness
    c. cataract
    c. change
    c. cleanup
    c. cleft
    c. clefting
    c. opacification
    c. psychic blindness
    c. spokes
    c. spokes cataract
    c. stripping
    c. substance of lens
    c. vacuole
    c. visual impairment
    c. visual insufficiency
cortices
corticolysis
corticonuclear fiber
corticopupillary reflex
corticose vein
corticosteroid-induced
    c.-i. cataract
    c.-i. glaucoma
corticosteroid therapy
corticotropin
cortisol
cortisone
    c. acetate
Cortisporin

Cortone
coruscation
Corynebacterium diphtheriae
coryza
cosmesis
cosmetic
    c. contact lens
    c. contact shell implant
    c. defect
    c. iris
    c. shell contact lens
Costenbader incision spreader
Coston-Trent iris retractor
cottonoid
Cotton's effect
cotton-wool
    c.-w. exudate
    c.-w. patches
    c.-w. spot
couching
    cataract c.
    c. of cataract
    c. needle
cough headache
Coumadin
coumarin derivative
counseling
    genetic c.
count
    complete blood c. (CBC)
    endothelial cell c.
    finger c.
    Kestenbaum's capillary c.
counterpressor
    Amenabar c.
    angled c.
    Gill c.
counting
    finger c.
    c. fingers (CF)
coup injury
course
    arcuate c.
    extramedullary c.
cover
    Expo Bubble eye c.
    Eye-Pak II c.
    c. test (CT)
cover-uncover test
Cowen's sign
cow face
COWS
    cold-opposite, warm-same

Coxiella burnetii
Cozen-McPherson tying forceps
CPC
    central posterior curve
CPEO
    chronic progressive external
    ophthalmoplegia
CPI90-100
    insulin pump CPI90-100
C/R
    chorioretinal
CR-39 lens
CRA
    central retinal artery
crack
    lacquer c.
cranial
    c. arteritis
    c. foramen
    c. foramina
    c. nerve (CN)
    c. nerve palsy
    c. stenosis syndrome
cranii
    frons c.
craniofacial
    c. anomaly
    c. dysostosis
    c. fibro-osseous tumor
    c. syndrome
craniometaphyseal dysplasia
cranio-orbital surgery
craniopharyngioma
craniostenosis, pl. **craniostenoses**
craniosynostosis
craniotabes
craniotomy
    frontal c.
cranium
    frons of c.
CRAO
    central retinal artery occlusion
crapulosa
    amblyopia c.
crassus, pl. **panni**
    pannus c.
Crawford
    C. fascial stripper
    C. forceps
    C. lacrimal set
    C. needle
    C. stripper
    C. tube

Crawford's
C. fascia
C. method
C. sling operation
C. technique
C-reactive protein
cream
Drysol c.
crease
eyelid c.
lid c.
superior eyelid c.
creatine
creatinine clearance test
Credé's
C. method
C. prophylaxis
creep
crenated
crepe bandage dressing
crepitance
crepitation
crepitus
crescent
c. choroid
congenital c.'s
c. corneal graft
c. graft
homonymous c.
monocular temporal c.
c. myopia
myopic c.
c. operation
scleral c.
temporal c.
c. tonofilms
crescentic
CREST
calcinosis, Raynaud's
phenomenon, esophageal
motility disorder, sclerodactyly,
and telangiectasia
CREST syndrome
crest
lacrimal c.
lacrimal anterior c.
lacrimal posterior c.
neural c.
orbital c.
cretinism
Creutzfeldt-Jakob disease

cribra
c. orbitalia
c. orbitalis of Welcker
cribral
cribrate
cribriform
c. field
c. ligament
c. plate
c. spot
cribrosa
area c.
lamina c.
scleral lamina c.
cribrum
cri du chat syndrome
Crile needle holder
crisis, pl. **crises**
glaucomatocyclitic c.
ocular c.
oculogyric c.
Pel's c.
cristallinus
humor c.
Critchett's operation
criterion-free measurement
critical
c. angle
c. corresponding frequency
(CCF)
c. flicker fusion frequency
c. illumination
Crock's
C. encircling operation
C. operation
crocodile
c. lens
c. shagreen
c. tears
crofilcon A
Crohn's disease
cromoglycate
sodium c.
cromolyn
c. sodium
c. sodium 46
Cronassial
Crookes
C. glass
C. lens
Cross
Lancaster C.

cross
  c. cover test
  c. cylinder
  c. eyes
  optical c.
cross-action
  c.-a. capsule forceps
  c.-a. clamp
  c.-a. towel clamp
crossed
  c. amblyopia
  c. cylinders
  c. diplopia
  c. eyes
  c. fixation
  c. hemianopsia
  c. lens
  c. parallax
  c. reflex
cross-eye
cross-eyes
  alternating c.-e.
cross-fixation
crossing
  arteriolovenous c.'s
cross-polarization photography
cross-vector A-scan
croup
croupous
  c. conjunctivitis
  c. rhinitis
Crouzon's
  C. craniofacial dysostosis
  C. disease
  C. syndrome
crowding phenomenon
crow-foot closure
crown
  borosilicate c.
  ciliary c.
  c. glass
  c. glass lens
  spectacle c.
CRT
  cathode ray tube
cruciata
  amblyopia c.
crusher
  Lieberman phaco c.
crusting
  eyelid c.
  lid c.
  c. lids

crutch glasses
CRV
  central retinal vein
CRVO
  central retinal vein occlusion
cryoablation
cryoapplication
Cryo-Barrages vitreous implant
cryocoagulation
cryoedema
cryoenucleator
  Gallie c.
cryoextraction
  open-sky c.
  c. operation
cryoextractor
  Alcon c.
  Amoils c.
  Beaver c.
  Beaver cataract c.
  Bellows c.
  Keeler c.
  Kelman c.
  Rubinstein c.
  Thomas c.
cryofreeze
cryogenic
cryoglobulin
cryoglobulinemia
cryolathe
  Barraquer c.
cryopencil
  Amoils c.
  Mira endovitreal c.
cryopexy
  double c.
  double freeze-stalk c.
  double freeze-thaw c.
  c. probe
cryophake
  Alcon c.
  Amoils c.
  Bellows c.
  Keeler c.
  Kelman c.
  Rubinstein c.
cryopreservation
cryoprobe
  Amoils c.
  cryoptor c.
  Rubinstein c.
  Thomas c.

cryoptor
    c. cryoprobe
    Thomas c.
cryoretinopexy
cryoretractor
    Thomas c.
cryostat
Cryostylet 2000
cryostylet, cryostylette
cryosurgery
cryosurgical
    c. unit
Cryosystem
    Keeler-Amoils
      Ophthalmic C.
cryotherapy
    freeze-thaw c.
    c. operation
    c. probe
cryounit
crypt
    Fuchs' c.
    iris c.
cryptococcosis
Cryptococcus
    C. neoformans
cryptoglioma
cryptophthalmus, cryptophthalmia
cryptosporidiosis
crystal
    conjunctival c.'s
    corneal c.'s
    cystine c.
    refractile c.
    uric acid c.'s
crystallin
    gamma c.
crystallina
    lens c.
crystalline
    c. capsule
    c. cataract
    c. corneal dystrophy
    c. deposits
    c. dystrophy
    c. humor
    c. infiltrate
    c. keratopathy
    c. lens
    c. lens equator
    c. retinopathy
crystallitis
Csapody's orbital repair operation

CSF
    cerebrospinal fluid
CSR
    central serous retinopathy
CT
    computed tomography
    cover test
      CT scan
CTM
    Carlo Traverso maneuver
CU-8 needle
CUA needle
cuboidal
cuff
    blood pressure c.
    Honan c.
    opacified c.
    Watzke c.
Cuignet's
    C. method
    C. test
cul-de-sac
    conjunctival c.-d.-s.
    glaucomatous c.-d.-s.
    c.-d.-s. irrigating vectis
    c.-d.-s. irrigation T-tube
    c.-d.-s. irrigator
    ocular c.-d.-s.
    ophthalmic c.-d.-s.
    optic c.-d.-s.
Culler
    C. fixation forceps
    C. iris spatula
    C. lens spoon
    C. muscle hook
    C. speculum
culture
    bacterial c.
    c. media
cuneate-shaped scotoma
cuneiform cataract
cup
    bleb c.
    eye c.
    flat c.
    Galin bleb c.
    glaucomatous c.
    large physiologic c.
    ocular c.
    ophthalmic c.
    optic c.
    perilimbal suction c.
    physiologic c.

cupped disk
Cupper-Faden operation
Cüppers
  C. method of pleoptic
  C. Visuscope
cupping
  c. of disk
  glaucomatous c.
  optic c.
  c. of optic disk
  optic disk c.
  c. of optic nerve
  pathologic c.
cup-to-disk ratio (C/D)
cupuliform cataract
cupulolithiasis
curb tenotomy
Curdy
  C. blade
  C. sclerotome
Curdy-Hebra blade
curettage
curette, curet
  Alvis c.
  chalazion c.
  corneal c.
  Fink c.
  Gifford c.
  Gifford corneal c.
  Gills-Welsh c.
  Green c.
  Heath c.
  Heath chalazion c.
  Hebra c.
  Heyner c.
  Kraff capsule polisher c.
  Meyhoeffer c.
  Meyhoeffer chalazion c.
  Skeele c.
  Spratt mastoid c.
  Visitec capsule polisher c.
curetted
curl
  c. backshell implant
  c. temple
curling of capsule
Curran knife needle
Curschmann-Steinert disease
curvature
  c. aberration
  c. ametropia
  anterior corneal c.
  corneal c.

  c. hyperopia
  c. of lens
  c. myopia
curve
  anterior central c. (ACC)
  anterior peripheral c. (APC)
  base c.
  bell-shaped c.
  central posterior c. (CPC)
  contact lens c.
  intermediate posterior c.
    (IPC)
  luminosity c.
  peripheral c.
  peripheral posterior c.
    (PPC)
  posterior central c. (PCC)
  posterior intermediate c.
    (PIC)
  posterior peripheral c.
    (PPC)
  c. response
  Steiger's c.'s
  Stromberg's c.'s
  visibility c.
  c. width
curved
  c. needle eye spud
  c. reflecting surface
  c. scleral-limbal incision of
    Flieringa
  c. tying forceps
curved-top bifocal
curves of spectacle lens
curvilinear
cushingoid
Cushing's
  C. disease
  C. syndrome
Cusick goniotomy knife
Cusick-Sarrail ptosis operation
Cusick's operation
Custodis
  C. sponge
  C. suture
Custodis'
  C. nondraining procedure
  C. operation
  C. procedure
  C. scleral buckling
cut
  sector c.'s
cutaneomucouveal syndrome

cutaneous
c. horn
c. melanoma
c. myiasis
c. pupillary reflex
c. tissue
cutdown incision
Cuterebra
cuticular
c. layer
c. stitch
cutis hyperelastica
Cutler
C. implant
C. lens spoon
Cutler-Beard
C.-B. bridge flap
C.-B. operation
Cutler's operation
cutter
Buettner-Parel c.
Buettner-Parel vitreous c.
Douvas c.
Douvas vitreous c.
guillotine-type c.
infusion suction cutter
vitreous c.
Kloti c.
Kloti vitreous c.
Machemer c.
Machemer vitreous c.
Maguire-Harvey c.
Maguire-Harvey vitreous c.
O'Malley-Heintz c.
O'Malley-Heintz vitreous c.
Parel-Crock c.
Parel-Crock vitreous c.
rotating-type c.
Tolentino c.
Tolentino vitreous c.
VISC vitreous c.
vitreoretinal infusion c.
vitreous c.
vitreous infusion suction c.
(VISC)
cutting
c. board
c. bur
lathe c.
CVA
cerebrovascular accident
C value
C-valve

cyanoacrylate
c. adhesive
butyl c.
ethyl c.
c. retinopexy
c. tissue adhesive
cyanocobalamin
cyanographic contrast material
cyanographin contrast material
cyanolabe
cyanopia
cyanopsia
c. retinae
cyanopsin
cyanosis
bulbar c.
c. bulbi
compression c.
retina c.
c. retinae
cyanotic heart disease
cyclectomy
cyclic
c. adenosine monophosphate
(cAMP)
c. esotropia
c. guanosine monophosphate
c. nucleotide
c. ocular motor spasm
c. strabismus
cyclicotomy
cyclitic membrane
cyclitis
chronic c.
Fuchs' c.
Fuchs' heterochromic c.
heterochromia c.
heterochromic c.
heterochromic Fuchs' c.
c. in pars planitis
plastic c.
pure c.
purulent c.
serous c.
cycloanemization
cycloceratitis
cyclochoroiditis
cyclocoagulation
cyclocongestive glaucoma
cyclocryopexy
cyclocryotherapy
YAG c.
cyclodamia

cyclodestructive procedure
cyclodeviation
cyclodialysis
    Allen c.
    c. cannula
    c. clefts
    Heine's c.
    c. spatula
cyclodiathermy
    Castroviejo-Scheie c.
    c. electrode
    c. operation
cyclodiplopia
cycloduction
cycloelectrolysis
cyclofilcon A
cyclofusion
cyclogram
Cyclogyl
cyclokeratitis
Cyclomydril
cyclopea
cyclopean eye
cyclopentolate
    c. hydrochloride
cyclophoria
    accommodative c.
    minus c.
    c. minus
    c. negative
    plus c.
    c. plus
    position c.
    c. positive
cyclophorometer
cyclophosphamide
cyclophotocoagulation
    Nd:YAG c.
    transpupillary c.
cyclopia
cycloplegia
cycloplegic refraction
cyclops
cycloscope
cycloscopy
cycloserine
cyclospasm
cyclosporine
cyclotherapy
    laser c.
cyclotome
cyclotomy

cyclotropia
    minus c.
    c. minus
    c. negative
    c. plus
    c. positive
cyclovergence
cycloversion
cyclovertical muscle
Cyl, cyl.
    cylinder
cylicotomy
cylinder (C, Cyl, cyl.)
    anterior c.
    c. axis
    concave c.
    cross c.
    crossed c.'s
    Jackson cross c.
    c. lens
    c. lenses
    minus c.
    c. retinoscopy
    c. spectacle lens
cylindric, cylindrical
    c. refraction
cylindroma
cyst
    aneurysmal bone c.
    arachnoidal c.
    bilateral c.
    Blessig-Iwanoff c.
    Blessig's c.
    blood c.
    bone c.
    chocolate c.
    colloid c.
    colobomatous c.
    conjunctival c.
    corneal c.
    Dandy-Walker c.
    c. degeneration
    dermoid c.
    echinococcus c.
    epibulbar dermoid c.
    epidermal inclusion c.
    epidermoid c.
    epithelial c.
    epithelial implantation c.
    epithelial inclusion c.
    c. fibrosis
    foveal c.
    hematic c.

inclusion c.
infundibular c.
intraepithelial c.
iris c.
Iwanoff's c.'s
lacrimal ductal c.
meibomian c.
orbital c.
pearl c.
proteinaceous c.
pupillary c.
pupillary iris c.
renal medullary c.
retinal c.
scleral c.
sebaceous c.
spontaneous congenital
  iris c.
subconjunctival c.
sudoriferous c.
tarsal c.
traumatic corneal c.
traumatic scleral c.
cystadenoma
cystic
  c. cataract
  c. eye
  c. fibrosis
  c. hydrocystoma tumor
  c. microphthalmia
cysticerci
cysticercoid
cysticercosis
cysticercus, pl. cysticerci
  intraocular c.
cysticum
  epithelioma adenoides c.
cystine crystal
cystinosis
  nephropathic c.
cystitome, cystotome
  air c.
  Atkinson 25-G short
    curved c.
  Azar curved c.
  Beaver Ocu-1 curved c.
  Blumenthal irrigating c.
  double-cutting sharp c.
  Drews angled c.
  Graefe c.
  irrigating c.
  Kelman c.
  Kelman air c.

Knolle-Kelman cannulated c.
Kratz angled c.
Lewicky formed c.
Lieppman c.
Look c.
McIntyre reverse c.
Mendez c.
Nevyas double sharp c.
Visitec c.
Visitec double-cutting c.
von Graefe c.
Wheeler c.
Wilder c.
cystitomy
cystoid
  c. body
  c. cicatrix
  c. cicatrix of limbus
  c. degeneration
  c. macular degeneration
    (CMD)
  c. macular dystrophy
  c. macular edema (CME)
  c. macular hole
  c. maculopathy
  c. retinal degeneration
cystotome (*var. of* cystitome)
cytidine (C)
cytochalasin
cytogenetics
cytoid body
cytologic examination
cytology
  conjunctival impression c.
  impression c.
cytomegalic
  c. inclusion disease
  c. inclusion virus
cytomegalovirus
  c. retinitis
cytopathy
  mitochondrial c.
cytoplasm
  foam-appearing c.
cytoplasmic
  c. filament
  c. organelles
cytosegrosome
cytosine arabinoside (ara-C)
cytosome
cytotoxic antibody
Cytovene
Czapski microscope

Czermak
accommodation phosphene
of C.
C. keratome
Czermak's pterygium operation

D
- deciduous
- deuterium
- dexter
- diopter
- duration

Dacriose
Dacron suture
dacryadenalgia
dacryadenitis
dacryadenoscirrhus
dacryagogatresia
dacryagogic
dacryagogue
dacrycystalgia
dacrycystitis
dacryelcosis
dacryoadenalgia
dacryoadenectomy operation
dacryoadenitis
- infectious d.

dacryoblennorrhea
dacryocanaliculitis
dacryocele
- congenital d.

dacryocyst
dacryocystalgia
dacryocystectasia
dacryocystectomy operation
dacryocystis
- phlegmonous d.
- syphilitic d.
- trachomatous d.
- tuberculous d.

dacryocystitis
- acute d.
- chronic d.
- congenital d.
- phlegmonous d.
- syphilitic d.
- trachomatous d.
- tuberculous d.

dacryocystoblennorrhea
dacryocystocele
dacryocystoethmoidostomy
dacryocystogram
dacryocystography
dacryocystoptosis, dacryocystoptosia
dacryocystorhinostenosis
dacryocystorhinostomy (DCR)

dacryocystorhinotomy operation
dacryocystostenosis
dacryocystostomy operation
dacryocystotome
dacryocystotomy operation
dacryogenic
dacryogram
dacryohelcosis
dacryohemorrhea
dacryolin
dacryolith
- Desmarres' d.

dacryolithiasis
dacryoma
dacryon
dacryops
dacryopyorrhea
dacryopyosis
dacryorhinocystotomy
dacryorrhea
dacryoscintigraphy
dacryosinusitis
dacryosolenitis
dacryostenosis
dacryostomy
- Arroyo's d.
- Arruga's d.
- Dupuy-Dutemps d.
- Kuhnt's d.

dacryosyrinx
DAF syndrome
Dailey cataract needle
Dailey's operation
daily-wear lenses
Daisy irrigation-aspiration instrument
Dakrina
Dalcaine
Dalen-Fuchs nodule
Dalgleish's operation
Dallas lens-inserting forceps
Dalma's sentinel
Dalrymple's
- D. disease
- D. sign

daltonian
daltonism
dam
- rubber d.

damage
    brain d.
    glaucomatous optic nerve d.
    (GOND)
    solar d.
dammini
    Ixodes d.
danazol
Danberg
    D. forceps
    D. iris forceps
Dan chalazion forceps
Dandy-Walker cyst
Dan-Gradle cilia forceps
Dannheim
    D. eye implant
    D. implant
dantrolene sodium
dapiprazole HCl
dapsone
Daranide
Daraprim
Darin lens
dark
    d. adaptation
    d. adaptometry
    d. disk
dark-adapted eye
dark-field
    d.-f. examination
    d.-f. illumination
dark-ground illumination
dark-room
    d.-r. test
    d.-r. testing
Darling capsulotome
Darling's capsulotomy
Dartmouth Eye Institute
DaSilva dermatome
Daubenton's plane
Daviel
    D. lens spoon
    D. scoop
Daviel's operation
Davis
    D. forceps
    D. knife needle
    D. spud
    D. trephine
Davis-Geck
    D.-G. blepharoplasty
    D.-G. suture

day
    d. blindness
    d. sight
    d. vision
Dazamide
dazzle reflex
dazzling glare
DBC
    distance between centers
DBL
    distance between nasal lines
D chromosome ring syndrome
DCR
    dacryocystorhinostomy
DDH
    dissociated double hypertropia
DDT
    dye disappearance test
Dean
    D. blade
    D. iris knife
    D. knife holder
    D. knife needle
    D. needle
debridement
    epithelial d.
debrider
    corneal d.
    Sauer d.
    Sauer corneal d.
debris
    capsular d.
    cellular d.
    desquamated epithelial d.
    phagocytosed cellular d.
debris-laden tear film
Decadron Phosphate
decalvans
    keratosis follicularis
    spinulosa d.
decarboxylation
    ornithine d.
decenter
decentered
    d. lens
    d. spectacles
decentration
    d. of contact lens
    d. of lens
deciduous (D)
decimate

declination
decompensation
corneal d.
decompression
Dickson-Wright orbit d.
lateral orbital d.
orbital d.
d. of orbit operation
transantral d.
decompressive surgery
decreased corneal sensation
decreasing vision
decussate
decussation
oculomotor d.
optic d.
deep
d. blunt rake retractor
d. congestion
d. corneal stromal opacities
d. filiform dystrophy
d. keratitis
d. parenchymatous
dystrophy
d. punctate keratitis
d. pustular keratitis
d. scleritis
defect
acquired color d.
afferent d.
afferent pupillary d. (APD)
altitudinal d.
altitudinal field d.
arcuate d.
arcuate field d.'s
arteriovenous crossing d.
AV crossing d.
bilateral homonymous
altitudinal d.
binasal field d.
bitemporal field d.
chiasmatic field d.'s
color d.
compressive d.
compressive optic nerve d.
congruous field d.
corkscrew visual field d.
cosmetic d.
field d.
functional d.
glaucoma field d.
gun-barrel field d.
homonymous field d.

incongruous field d.
inferior altitudinal d.
Marcus Gunn afferent d.
Marcus Gunn relative
afferent d.
monocular field d.
nasal step d.
nerve fiber bundle d.
paracentral d.
parietal lobe field d.
patchy window d.'s
"pie on the floor" d.
"pie in the sky" d.
quadrantic d.
relative afferent pupillary d.
(RAPD)
sector d.
sector-shaped d.
superior homonymous
quadrantic d.
temporal lobe field d.
vascular filling d.
visual d.
visual corkscrew d.'s
window d.
deferoxamine
deficiency
aqueous tear d. (ATD)
familial lecithin:cholesterol
acyl transferase d.
familial lipoprotein d.
folic acid d.
growth hormone d.
vitamin A d.
definition
area of critical d.
deflection
deformans
osteitis d.
deformity angle
degeneratio
d. hyaloidea granuliformis
d. hyaloideoretinas
hereditaria
d. spherularis elaioides
degeneration
aberrant d. of third nerve
age-related macular d.
(AMD, ARMD)
amyloid corneal d.
atrophic age-related
macular d. (AAMD)
atrophic macular d.

degeneration *(continued)*
    Best's d.
    Biber-Haab-Dimmer d.
    Bietti's tapetoretinal d.
    calcareous d.
    central retinal d.
    chorioretinal d.
    cobblestone d.
    cobblestone retinal d.
    cone d.
    cone-rod d.
    congenital macular d.
    d. of cornea
    corneal d.
    corneal furrow d.
    cyst d.
    cystoid d.
    cystoid macular d. (CMD)
    cystoid retinal d.
    diabetic macular d.
    disciform d.
    disciform macular d.
    Doyne's familial colloid d.
    Doyne's honeycombed d.
    dry senile macular d.
    ectatic marginal d. of
      cornea
    equatorial d.
    familial colloid d.
    familial pseudoinflammatory
      macular d.
    furrow d.
    hepatolenticular d.
    hereditary d.
    heredomacular d.
    hyaline d.
    hyaloideoretinal d.
    hydropic d.
    Kozlowski's d.
    Kuhnt-Junius d.
    Kuhnt-Junius macular d.
    lattice d.
    lattice retinal d.
    lenticular d.
    lipid d.
    macular d.
    macular disciform d.
    marginal d.
    marginal corneal d.
    marginal furrow d.
    myopic d.
    nodular d.
    paving-stone d.

    pellucid d.
    pellucid marginal d.
    pellucid marginal corneal d.
    pellucid marginal retinal d.
    peripheral cystoid d.
    peripheral tapetochoroidal d.
    pigmentary perivenous
      chorioretinal d.
    primary pigmentary d. of
      retina
    progressive cone d.
    progressive myopic d.
    reticular cystoid d.
    retinal d.
    retinal lattice d.
    rod-cone d.
    Salzmann's d.
    Salzmann's nodular d.
    Salzmann's nodular
      corneal d.
    scleral d.
    senescent disciform
      macular d.
    senescent macular d.
    senile disciform d.
    senile disciform macular d.
    senile exudative macular d.
    senile macular d. (SMD)
    Sorsby's macular d.
    Sorsby's pseudoinflammatory
      macular d.
    spheroid d.
    spinocerebellar d.
    striatal nigral d.
    superficial reticular d. of
      Koby
    tapetochoroidal d.
    tapetoretinal d.
    Terrien's d.
    Terrien's marginal d.
    tractional retinal d.
    trophic retinal d.
    vitelliform d.
    vitelliform macular d.
    vitelline macular d.
    vitelliruptive d.
    vitreoretinal d.
    Vogt's d.
    Wagner's hereditary
      vitreoretinal d.
    Wagner's hyaloid retinal d.
    Wilson's d.
    xerotic d.

degenerative
d. myopia
d. ocular disease
d. pannus
d. retinal disease
degenerativus
pannus d.
Degest
Degest-2
Degos' syndrome
degradation
image d.
de Grandmont's operation
degree
prism d.
DeGrouchy's syndrome
dehisced
dehiscence
iris d.
Zuckerkandl's d.
dehiscent
dehiscing
dehydration
corneal d.
Dehydrex
dehydrogenase
glucose 6-phosphate d.
dehydroretinal
deinsertion
Deiter's operation
DeJean's syndrome
De Klair's operation
Deknatel silk suture
delacrimation
de Lange's syndrome
de Lapersonne's operation
De LaVega lens pusher
De LaVega vitreous aspirating cannula
delayed
d. hypersensitivity
d. rectifier
d. visual maturation
delayed-type hypersensitivity
deletion
chromosome d.
d. mapping
delicate serrated straight dressing forceps
delimiting keratotomy
deliver
delivery system

dellen
corneal d.
d. of Fuchs
Deller's modification
Delta Cortef
Deltasone
Del Toro's operation
demacurium
demarcation line of retina
demecarium
d. bromide
demecariumdemecarium bromide
demeclocycline
Demerol
demodectic blepharitis
Demodex folliculorum
demonstration
d. eyepiece
d. ophthalmoscope
demonstrator
halo d.
DeMosier's syndrome
Demours' membrane
demyelinate
demyelinating
d. disease
d. plaque
demyelination
autoimmune d.
demyelinative disease
demyelinization
demyelinizing
Dendrid
dendriform
d. keratitis
d. ulcer
dendrite
corneal d.
dendritic
d. cataract
d. corneal ulcer
d. ghosts
d. herpes simplex corneal ulcer
d. herpes zoster keratitis
d. keratitis
d. keratopathy
d. lesion
d. ulcer
denervate
denervated
denervation supersensitivity

dense
 d. brunescent nucleus
 d. core granules
 d. opacities
denser
densitometer
density
 arciform d.
 conjunctival goblet cell d.'s
 corneal optical d.
dental infection
dentate
dentation
denudation
denude
denuding
deorsumduction
deorsumvergence
 left d.
 right d.
deorsumversion
deoxyribonucleic acid (DNA)
depigmented spot
Depo-Medrol
deposit
 calcareous d.
 colloid d.'s
 conjunctival d.'s
 corneal d.'s
 crystalline d.'s
 iron d.
 refractile d.
deposition
 calcium d.
 copper d.
 iron d.
 pigment d.
depressed fracture
depression
 chin d.
 d. of orbital floor
 posterior corneal d.
depressor
 muscle d.
 O'Connor d.
 orbital d.
 Schepens d.
 Schepens scleral d.
 Schepens thimble d.
 Schocket scleral d.
 scleral d.
 Wilder scleral d.
deprimens oculi

deprivation
 d. amblyopia
 stimulus d.
depth
 d. of chamber
 d. of field
 focal d., d. of focus
 d. gauge
 d. perception
 sagittal d.
derangement
 pigment d.
Derby's operation
Derf needle holder
derivative
 coumarin d.
 ergot d.
 phenothiazine d.
dermabrasion
dermal nevus
Dermalon suture
dermatan sulfate
dermatitidis
 Blastomyces d.
dermatitis
 atopic d.
 contact d.
 d. herpetiformis
 infectious eczematoid d.
dermatochalasis
 eyelid d.
dermatoconjunctivitis
 contact d.
dermatogenic cataract
dermatolysis
 d. palpebrarum
dermatome
 DaSilva d.
 Hall d.
dermatomyositis
dermato-ophthalmitis
dermatosis
dermis-fat graft
dermis patch graft
dermochondral corneal dystrophy of François
dermoid
 congenital d.
 congenital limbal corneal d.
 conjunctival d.'s
 d. cyst
 d. of orbit

orbital d.
d. tumor
dermolipoma
Dermostat implant
desaturation
red d.
Descartes' law
Descemet
D. membrane punch
D. punch
descemetitis
descemetocele
Descemet's
D. folds
D. membrane
D. membrane detachment
desensitization immunotherapy
desferrioxamine
desiccant
desiccate
desiccation keratitis
Desmarres
D. chalazion forceps
D. corneal dissector
D. fixation pick
D. forceps
D. knife
D. lid clamp
D. lid elevator
D. lid retractor
D. marker
D. refractor
D. retractor
D. scarifier
Desmarres'
D. chalazion
D. dacryolith
D. law
D. operation
desmosomal cellular attachment
desmosome
desquamated epithelial debris
desquamation
dessicated
de-STAT
detached
d. iris
d. retina
d. vitreous
detachment
aphakic d.
bullous d.
choroidal d.

ciliochoroidal d.
Descemet's membrane d.
disciform d. of retina
exudative retinal d.
funnel-shaped retinal d.
macular d.
morning glory retinal d.
nonrhegmatogenous d.
nonrhegmatogenous
retinal d.
open-funnel d.
pigment epithelial d. (PED)
posterior vitreal d. (PVD)
pseudophakic d.
retinal d., d. of retina (RD)
rhegmatogenous d.
rhegmatogenous retinal d.
serous d.
serous macular d.
tear-induced retinal d.
traction d.
tractional retinal d.
vitreal d.
vitreous d.
detamide
detectable foci
deterenol
deterenol HCl
deturgescence
d. of cornea
corneal d.
deturgescent state
deutan
deuteranoma
deuteranomalopia
deuteranomalous
deuteranomaly
deuteranope
deuteranopia
deuteranopic
deuterium (D)
deuton color blindness
Deutschman cataract knife
devascularization
development
fetal d.
visual d.
developmental
d. anomaly
d. cataract
deviant color
deviating eye

deviation
    commitant vertical d.
    conjugate d.
    conjugate d. of eyes
    convergent d.
    dissociated vertical d.
        (DVD)
    Hering-Hellebrand d.
    heterotropic d.
    horizontal d.
    incomitant vertical d.
    latent d.
    manifest d.
    minimum d.
    primary d.
    Roth-Bielschowsky d.
    secondary d.
    skew d.
    d. squint
    squint d.
    standard d.
    strabismic d.
    supranuclear d.
    torsional d.
    tropia d.
    tropic d.
    vertical d.
    vertical comitant d.
deviational nystagmus
device
    doubling d.
    Joseph d.
    Keratolux fixation d.
    laser-argon d.
    laser-ruby d.
    oblique prism d.
    Ocusert d.
    Putterman-Chaflin ocular d.
    Putterman-Chaflin ocular
        asymmetry d.
    retrieval d.
    Welch four-drop d.
Devic's disease
DeVilbiss
    D. irrigating/aspirating unit
de Vincentiis operation
deviometer
devitalized
DeWecker
    D. iris scissors
    D. scissors
DeWecker-Pritikin scissors
DeWecker's anterior sclerotomy

de Wecker's operation
Dexacidin
Dexair
    Neo D.
dexamethasone
    neomycin and d.
    neomycin, polymixin B,
        and d.
    d. phosphate
    d. sodium phosphate
    d. solution
Dexasporin
Dexedrine
Dexon suture
Dexsone
dexter (D)
dextra
    visio oculus d.
dextran
dextroclination
dextrocular
dextrocularity
dextrocycloduction
dextrocycloversion
dextrodepression
dextroduction
dextrogyration
dextrose
dextrotorsion
dextroversion
dextroverted
DFP
    diisopropyl fluorophosphate
diabetes
    adult-onset d.
    d. albuminurinicus
    alloxan d.
    artificial d.
    brittle d.
    bronze d.
    chemical d.
    experimental d.
    gestational d.
    gouty d.
    growth-onset d.
    d. innocens
    d. inositus
    d. insipidus
    insulin-deficient d.
    insulin-dependent d. mellitus
        (IDDM)
    juvenile d.
    ketosis-prone d.

ketosis-resistant d.
Lancereaux's d.
latent d.
lipoatrophic d.
lipoplethoric d.
lipuric d.
masked d.
maturity-onset d.
d. mellitus
Mosler's d.
nephrogenic d. insipidus
non-insulin-dependent d. mellitus (NIDDM)
overflow d.
overt d.
pancreatic d.
phlorhizin d.
phosphate d.
piqûre d.
puncture d.
renal d.
skin d.
steroid d.
steroidogenic d.
subclinical d.
temporary d.
toxic d.
type I d.
type II d.

diabetic
d. acidosis
d. amaurosis
d. Argyll-Robertson pupil
d. cataract
d. iritis
d. macular degeneration
d. maculopathy
d. melanosis
d. optic atrophy
d. retinitis
d. retinopathy
d. traction

diabetic-osmotic cataract

diagnosis
laboratory d.
neuro-ophthalmologic d.

diagnostic
d. contact lens
d. fiberoptic lens
d. fitting set
d. positions of gaze
d. program

dial
astigmatic d.
clock d.
Mendez astigmatism d.
Regan-Lancaster d.
sunburst d.

dialer
angled iris hook and IOL d.
intraocular lens d.
Visitec intraocular lens d.

dialing

dialysis
d. retinae
retinal d.

diameter
chord d.
contact lens d.
contact lens chord d.
d. of cornea
corneal d.
effective d.
iris d.
minimal effective d. (MED)
visible iris d. (VID)

diamond
d. blade
d. blade knife
d. bur
d. dye
d. knife

diamond-dusted
d.-d. knife
d.-d. knife blade

Diamox Sequels

Dianoux's operation

diaphanoscopy

diaphanous

diaphoresis

diaphragm
Potter-Bucky d.

diaschisis

diastase stain

diastasis
iris d.

diathermocoagulator

diathermy
d. applications
d. electrode
Mira d.
d. operation
d. points
d. puncture

diathermy *(continued)*
    d. tip
    d. unit
diathesis
    albinism-hemorrhagic d.
diazepam
dichlorphenamide
dichroic
dichroism
    circular d.
dichromasy
dichromat
dichromatic
    d. light
    d. vision
dichromatism
    congenital d.
dichromatopsia
dichromic
Dickey-Fox operation
Dickey's operation
Dickson-Wright
    D.-W. operation
    D.-W. orbit decompression
diclofenac sodium
dicoria
Dicumarol
Dieffenbach serrefine
Dieffenbach's operation
diencephalic syndrome
diet
    arginine-reduced d.
diethylamide
    lysergic acid d. (LSD)
diethylcarbamazine
Difei glasses
difference
    light d.
difficulty
    separation d.
diffraction
    Fraunhofer's d.
diffuse
    d. angiokeratoma
    d. anterior scleritis
    d. cataract
    d. choroidal sclerosis
    d. choroiditis
    d. deep keratitis
    d. drusen
    d. inflammatory eyelid
    atrophy
    d. unilateral neuroretinitis

    d. unilateral subacute
    neuroretinitis (DUSN)
diffusion
    circle d.
    d. factor
diffusum
    angiokeratoma corporis d.
Digilab
    D. perimeter
    D. tonometer
Digital
    D. B System
    D. B System ultrascan
digital
    d. pressure
    d. subtraction angiography
    d. tonometry
Digitalis
    D. purpurea
digitalis
    d. glycoside
    d. toxicity
digitizer
digoxin
dihematoporphyrin ether
diisopropyl fluorophosphate (DFP)
diktyoma, dictyoma
dilacerated cataract
dilaceration
Dilantin
Dilatair
dilatation
    homatropine d.
dilate
dilated pupil
dilation
    ectatic d.
    lag d.
    d. lag
    d. of punctum
    d. of punctum operation
    pupil d.
dilator
    Berens d.
    Castroviejo-Galezowski d.
    Castroviejo lacrimal d.
    French lacrimal d.
    Galezowski lacrimal d.
    Heath d.
    Heyner d.
    Hosford lacrimal d.
    House lacrimal d.
    iris d.

Jones d.
Jones punctum d.
lacrimal d.
Muldoon lacrimal d.
muscle d.
d. muscle
d. muscle of pupil
Nettleship-Wilder d.
punctal d.
punctum d.
pupil d.
Rolf d.
Ruedemann lacrimal d.
Weiss gold d.
Wilder d.
Wilder lacrimal d.
Ziegler d.
Ziegler lacrimal d.
dilution
pigmentary d.
dimefilcon A
dimercaprol
dimethylpolysiloxane
dimethyl sulfate
Dimitry
D. chalazion trephine
D. erysiphake
Dimitry-Bell erysiphake
Dimitry-Thomas erysiphake
Dimmer's
D. keratitis
D. nummular keratitis
dimness of vision
dimple
Fuchs' d.
d. veil
dimpling of eyeball
dinitrochlorobenzene (DNCB)
dinitrofluorobenzene
2,4-dinitrophenol
diode
d. endolaser
d. laser
Diodoquin
diopsimeter
diopter (D)
prism d. (PD)
d. prism
Dioptimum System
dioptometer
dioptometry
dioptoscope
dioptoscopy

dioptre
dioptric
d. aberration
d. apparatus
d. correction
d. media
d. power
d. system
dioptrometer
dioptrometry
Dioptron
D. Nova
D. Ultima
dioptroscope
dioptroscopy
dioptry
dioxide
carbon d.
sulfur d.
diphenhydramine
d. hydrochloride
diphenylhydantoin
diphtheria
diphtheriae
Corynebacterium d.
diphtheritic conjunctivitis
diphtheroid
dipivalyl epinephrine
dipivefrin
d. HCl
diplegia
congenital facial d.
diplexia
diplobacillary
d. blepharitis
d. conjunctivitis
diplobacillus of Petit
diplocoria
diplopia
binocular d.
cerebral d.
crossed d.
direct d.
heteronymous d.
homonymous d.
horizontal d.
monocular d.
paradoxical d.
simple d.
stereoscopic d.
torsional d.
uncrossed d.
vertical d.

diplopiometer
diploscope
dipping
    ocular d.
diprivan
dipstick
direct
    d. astigmatism
    d. diplopia
    d. glare
    d. gonioscopic lens
    d. illumination
    d. image
    d. method
    d. ophthalmoscope
    d. ophthalmoscopy
    d. parallax
    d. pupillary response
    d. reflex
    d. vision
direction
    angle of d.
    line of d.
    principal line of d.
    principal visual d.
    visual d.
direct-light
    d.-l. reflex
    d.-l. refraction
    d.-l. response
director
    grooved d.
dirofilariasis
Disabilities
    Association for Children
    and Adults with
    Learning D. (ACLD)
disability
    auditory perceptual d.
    motor-output d.
disappearance
    fluorescein dye d.
disc (*var. of* disk)
discharge
    conjunctival d.
    mucous d.
    socket d.
disci
    excavatio d.
disciform
    d. chorioretinopathy
    d. degeneration
    d. degeneration of retina

    d. detachment of retina
    d. herpes simplex keratitis
    d. keratitis
    d. macular degeneration
    d. opacity
disciformans
    retinitis d.
discission
    d. hook
    d. knife
    d. of lens operation
    Moncrieff's d.
    d. needle
    posterior d.
discitis
disclination
discoid lupus erythematosus
discoloration
disconjugate gaze
discontinuity
    zone of d.
discoria
discrete
    d. colliquation
    d. colliquative
discrimination
    color d.
    contrast d.
    light d.
    spatial d.
    two-light d.
    visual d.
discus, pl. **disci**
    d. nervi optici
    d. opticus
disease
    acyanotic heart d.
    Addison's d.
    Albers-Schönberg d.
    Albright's d.
    Alström's d.
    Alzheimer's d.
    Anderson-Fabry d.
    Apert's d.
    Apollo's d.
    Arlt's d.
    arteriolar occlusive d.
    autoimmune d.
    autosomal dominant d.
    autosomal recessive d.
    bacterial d.
    Ballet's d.
    Basedow's d.

Batten-Mayou d.
Batten's d.
Bechterew's d.
Behçet's d.
Behr's d.
Benson's d.
Berlin's d.
Best's d.
Bielschowsky-Jansky d.
Bielschowsky's d.
blinding d.
Bourneville's d.
Bowen's d.
Bower's d.
Bright's d.
brittle-bone d.
broad-beta d.
Buerger's d.
Caffey's d.
caisson's d.
cardiac valvular d.
cardiovascular d.
carotid occlusive d.
cat-scratch d.
cerebellar d.
cervical vascular d.
Charcot-Marie-Tooth d.
Chédiak-Higashi d.
chiasmal d.
chlamydial d.
chronic granulomatous d.
Coats' d.
Cogan's d.
collagen d.
collagen and rheumatoid-
  related d.
collagen vascular d.
congenital heart d.
Creutzfeldt-Jakob d.
Crohn's d.
Crouzon's d.
Curschmann-Steinert d.
Cushing's d.
cyanotic heart d.
cytomegalic inclusion d.
Dalrymple's d.
degenerative ocular d.
degenerative retinal d.
demyelinating d.
demyelinative d.
Devic's d.
disseminated lupus
  erythematosus d.

Dyggve's d.
Eales' d.
endogenous d.
Englemann's d.
epithelial herpetic d.
Erdheim-Chester d.
exogenous d.
extraorbital d.
Faber's d.
Fabry's d.
Farber's d.
Favre's d.
fibrocystic d.
Flajani's d.
Flatau-Schilder d.
flecked retina d.
Föerster's d.
Franceschetti's d.
Francis' d.
Gaucher's d.
genetic d.
Gierke's d.
Gilchrist's d.
glycogen storage d.
Goldmann-Favre d.
gonococcal d.
gouty episcleritis d.
Graefe's d.
graft-versus-host d.
Graves' d.
Hand-Schüller-Christian d.
Hansen's d.
Harada's d.
Heerfordt's d.
helminthic d.
Hippel's d.
Hodgkin's d.
Hunter's d.
Huntington's d.
Hurler's d.
Hutchinson's d.
hydatid d.
I-cell d.
immune complex d.
inclusion d.
infantile Refsum d.
infectious d.
inflammatory bowel d.
Jansky-Bielschowsky d.
Jensen's d.
Kawasaki's d.
Kimmelstiel-Wilson d.
Kimura's d.

disease *(continued)*
 Koeppe's d.
 Krabbe's d.
 Krill's d.
 Kufs' d.
 Kuhnt-Junius d.
 Kyrle's d.
 Lauber's d.
 Leber's d.
 Letterer-Siwe d.
 Lindau's d.
 Lindau-von Hippel d.
 Lyell's d.
 Lyme d.
 lysosomal storage d.
 macular d.
 marble bone d.
 Marfan's d.
 Marie-Strümpell d.
 Masuda-Kitahara d.
 medullary cystic d.
 medullary optic d.
 metabolic storage d.
 Mikulicz's d.
 Milroy's d.
 miner's d.
 Möbius' d.
 multifactorial d.
 multifocal chorioretinal d.
 mycobacterial d.
 nephropathic cystine
  storage d.
 Newcastle d.
 Nicolas-Favre d.
 Niemann-Pick d.
 Niemann-Pick type C d.
 Norrie's d.
 occlusive d.
 occlusive vascular d.
 ocular d.
 ocular syphilitic d.
 oculoglandular d.
 Oguchi's d.
 optic nerve d.
 Paget's d.
 pancreatic d.
 Parry's d.
 pauciarticular d.
 phytanic acid storage d.
 plus d.
 Pompe's d.
 protozoan d.
 pulseless d.

Purtscher's d.
Recklinghausen's d.
Refsum's d.
Reis-Bücklers d.
Reiter's d.
Rendu-Osler-Weber d.
rheumatic valvular d.
rheumatoid-related d.
rickettsial d.
Ritter's d.
Robles' d.
Sachs' d.
Sanders' d.
Sandhoff's d.
Sanfilippo's d.
sarcoid granulomatous d.
Schilder's d.
sex-linked d.
shipyard d.
Sichel's d.
sickle cell hemoglobin C d.
sickle cell hemoglobin D d.
sickle cell thalassemia d.
Simmonds' d.
Sjögren's d.
Spielmeyer-Sjögren d.
Spielmeyer-Stock d.
Spielmeyer-Vogt d.
spirochetal d.
Stargardt's d.
Steele-Richardson-
 Olszewski d.
Still's d.
stromal d.
Sturge-Weber d.
syphilitic ocular d.
systemic d.
Takayasu's d.
Tangier's d.
Tay's d.
Tay-Sachs d.
Thygeson's d.
thyroid d.
thyroid eye d.
Urbach-Wiethe d.
van der Hoeve's d.
vascular occlusive d.
venereal d.
venous occlusive d.
viral ocular d.
Vogt-Koyanagi-Harada d.
Vogt's d.
Vogt-Spielmeyer d.

von Gierke's d.
von Hippel-Lindau d.
von Hippel's d.
von Recklinghausen's d.
Wagner's d.
Weil's d.
Westphal-Strümpell d.
Whipple's d.
Wilson's d.
X-linked d.
X-linked recessive d.
disequilibrium
disinfecting solution
disinfection
thermal d.
disinserted
d. muscle
d. retina
disinsertion
levator aponeurosis d.
d. of retina
disjugate
d. movement
d. movement of eyes
disjunctive
d. movement
d. nystagmus
disk, disc
Airy d.
anagioid d.
anomalous d.'s
aperture d.
choked d.
ciliary d.
color d.
conus of optic d.
cupped d.
cupping of d.
dark d.
dragged d.
d. drusen
d. drusen hemorrhage
excavation of optic d.
d. forceps
gelatin d.
hypoplastic d.
ischemic d.
Krill's d.
micrometer d.
morning glory d.
nasal border of optic d.
d. neovascularization
neovascularization of d.

d. neurovascular vessels
Newton's d.
new vessels d.
d. new vessels
optic d.
d. pallor
pallor of d., pallor of d.
pinhole d.
pinkeye d.
Placido's d.
Rekoss' d.
stenopeic d., stenopaic d.
stroboscopic d.
swelling of d.
tilted d.
Whipple's d.
disk-shaped cataract
dislocated lens
dislocation
congenital lens d.
intraocular lens d.
d. of lens
lens d.
posterior d.
dislocator
Kirby d.
Kirby lens d.
dismutase
human superoxide d. (hSOD)
disodium
d. ethylenediaminetetraacetic acid
d. hydrogen phosphate
disorder
adrenal d.
amino acid metabolism d.
attention deficit d.
autosomal d.
bullous d.
canalicular d.
congenital d.
connective tissue d.
d. of eye
eye movement d.
hemorrhagic d.
histiocytic d.
hyperkeratotic d.
infranuclear d.
intestinal d.
lymphoproliferative d.
mendelian d.
metabolic d.

disorder *(continued)*
    myelin d.
    oculodermal d.
    ophthalmic d.
    outflow d.
    parathyroid d.
    peroxisomal d.
    prechiasmal d.
    retinal d.
    Sanders' d.
    Sanfilippo's d.
    skeletal d.
    skin d.
    supranuclear d.
    thyroid d.
    vitreoretinal d.
    X-linked dominant d.
    X-linked recessive d.
disorganized globe
disparate
    d. point
    d. retinal points
disparity, pl. disparities
    d. angle
    binocular disparities
    bitemporal d.
    conjugate d.
    fixation d.
    retinal d.
dispersing lens
dispersion
    chromatic d.
    circle of d.
    corneal endothelial
      pigmentary d.
    pigment d.
    point of d.
    d. prism
    d. syndrome
displacement
    image d.
    macular d.
    object d.
    d. threshold
disposable
    d. cautery
    d. contact lens
    d. ocutome
    d. trephine
disruption
    posterior capsular
      zonular d.
dissected half-thickness

dissecting scissors
dissection
dissector
    Barraquer corneal d.
    Berens corneal d.
    Castroviejo corneal d.
    corneal d.
    corneal knife d.
    Desmarres corneal d.
    Green d.
    Green corneal d.
    d. knife
    Martinez d.
    Troutman corneal d.
    Troutman lamellar d.
disseminated
    d. asymptomatic unilateral
      neovascularization
    d. choroiditis
    d. intravascular coagulation
    d. lupus erythematosus
      disease
    d. nonosteolytic
      myelomatosis
dissimilar
    d. image test
    d. segment
    d. target test
dissipation
    circle d.
dissociated
    d. alkaloid
    d. double hypertropia
      (DDH)
    d. hyperdeviation
    d. hypertropia
    d. nystagmus
    d. position
    d. vertical deviation (DVD)
    d. vertical divergence
      (DVD)
dissociation
    light-near d.
dissociative state
distance
    d. acuity
    angular d.
    d. between centers (DBC)
    center of rotation d.
    equivalent d.
    focal d.
    infinite d.
    intercanthal d. (ICD)

interpupillary d. (IPD)
intraocular d.
d. and near (D&N)
object d.
prism diopters or
  pupillary d.
pupillary d. (PD)
vertex of d.
d. visual acuity (DVA)
**distance between nasal lines
  (DBL)**
distant gaze
distantial aberration
distichia, distichiasis
acquired d.
distometer
distortion
d. aberration
barred d.
barrel d.
corneal d.
d. of lens
pin-cushion d.
d. of vision
distraction
conus d.
d. conus
distribution
Gaussian's d.
normal d.
districhiasis
disturbance
visual d.
diuretic
diurnal
d. intraocular pressure
  measurement
variation d.
d. variation
DIVA test
divergence
d. amplitudes
dissociated vertical d.
  (DVD)
excess d.
d. excess
d. excess exotropia
fusional d.
d. insufficiency
d. insufficiency exotropia
negative vertical d.
d. paralysis
point of d.

positive vertical d.
relative d.
d. reserves
strabismus d.
vertical d.
divergent
d. beams
d. light
d. ray
d. squint
d. strabismus
diverging
d. lens
d. meniscus
d. meniscus lens
divers' spectacles
diverticula of lacrimal sac
divided spectacles
Dix
D. foreign body spud
D. spud
Dix-Hallpike test
**Dixon-Thorpe vitreous foreign body
  forceps**
dizziness
DK
DK value
DMV II contact lens remover
D&N
distance and near
DNA
deoxyribonucleic acid
recombinant DNA (rDNA)
DNCB
dinitrochlorobenzene
Docustar fundus camera
Dodick lens-holding forceps
Doherty
D. implant
D. sphere
D. sphere implant
Dohlman plug
do-it-yourself
dolichocephaly
dolichoectasia
dolichomorphism
Dollinger's tendinous ring
doll's
d. eye
d. eye maneuver
d. eye reflex
d. eye sign

doll's *(continued)*
>d. head maneuver
>d. head phenomenon

dolorosa
>atrophia d.

D'ombrain's operation
dominance
>ocular d.

dominant
>d. cystoid macular dystrophy
>d. eye
>d. gene
>d. inheritance
>d. progressive foveal dystrophy
>d. slowly progressive macular dystrophy

Donaldson eye patch
Donaldson-Fitzpatrick oculocutaneous albinism
Donders'
>D. chart
>D. glaucoma
>D. law
>D. line
>D. procedure
>D. rings

donor
>d. cornea
>d. eye
>d. graft
>d. material
>d. tissue

dopamine
Dopastat
Doppler
>D. ultrasonogram
>D. ultrasonography

Dorello's canal
Dorsacaine
dorsalis
>tabes d.

dorsal midbrain syndrome
dorsolateral
Doryl
dot
>Gunn's d.
>d. hemorrhage
>Horner-Trantas d.'s
>lamina d.'s
>Marcus Gunn d.
>Mittendorf d.

Morgan's d.
Trantas' d.
white d.'s

dot-and-blot hemorrhage
dot-like lens
double
>d. arcuate scotoma
>d. concave lens
>d. convex lens
>d. cryopexy
>d. dissociated hypertropia
>d. elevator palsy
>d. freeze-stalk cryopexy
>d. freeze-thaw cryopexy
>d. homonymous hemianopsia
>d. hypertropia
>d. irrigating/aspirating cannula
>d. Maddox rod test
>d. refraction
>d. slab-off contact lens
>d. slab-off lens
>d. spatula
>d. tantalum clip
>d. vision

double-armed suture
double-blind study
double-contrast visualization
double-cutting sharp cystitome
double-pronged forceps
double-row diathermy barrage
doublet
>achromatic d.
>Wollaston's d.

doubling device
Doubra lens
Dougherty irrigating/aspirating unit
Douglas cilia forceps
douloureux
>tic d.

Douvas
>D. cutter
>D. rotoextractor
>D. vitreous cutter

Douvas-Barraquer speculum
Douvas' honeycombed choroiditis
down
>endothelial cell side d.
>d. to finger-counting

downbeat nystagmus
down-gaze

downgrowth
    epithelial d.
Down syndrome
downward
    d. gaze
    d. squint
doxorubicin
doxycycline
Doyne's
    D. choroiditis
    D. familial colloid
      degeneration
    D. familial honeycombed
      choroiditis
    D. guttate iritis
    D. honeycombed choroiditis
    D. honeycombed
      choroidopathy
    D. honeycombed
      degeneration
    D. honeycombed dystrophy
    D. iritis
    D. syndrome
Draeger
    D. forceps
    D. high vacuum erysiphake
    D. tonometer
dragged
    d. disk
    d. macula
    d. retina
drain
    Mentor pre-cut d.
    Penrose d.
drainage
    d. angle
    lacrimal d.
    d. of lacrimal gland
    d. of lacrimal gland
      operation
    d. of lacrimal sac
    d. of lacrimal sac operation
    lymphatic d.
    sclerotomy with d.
    subretinal fluid d.
    uveovertex d.
drape
    1021 d.
    Alcon disposable d.
    Barrier d.
    Blair head d.
    Eye-Pak d.
    Eye-Pak II d.

    Hough d.
    mini ophthalmic d.
    3M Steri-Drape d.
    Opraflex d.
    Pro-Ophtha d.
    Steri-Drape d.
    Surgikos d.
    Surgikos disposable d.
    VISIFLEX d.
dressing
    binocle d.
    binocular d.
    Blenderm tape d.
    bolus d.
    Borsch d.
    collodion d.
    compression d.
    crepe bandage d.
    Elastoplast d.
    Expo Bubble d.
    eye pad d.
    fluff d.
    fluffed gauze d.
    d. forceps
    Harman eye d.
    lens d.
    moistened fine mesh
      gauze d.
    monocular d.
    nasal-tip d.
    pressure d.
    pressure patch d.
    Pro-Ophtha d.
    ribbon gauze d.
    saline saturated wool d.
    sterile adhesive bubble d.
    Telfa d.
    Telfa plastic film d.
    tie-over d.
    tie-over Sellotape d.
    tulle gras d.
    wet d.
    wool saturated in saline d.
Drews
    D. angled cystitome
    D. cannula
    D. capsule polisher
    D. cataract needle
    D. cilia forceps
    D. inclined prism
    D. irrigating/aspirating unit
    D. irrigating cannula

Drews *(continued)*
    D. lens
    D. syndrome
Drews-Knolle reverse irrigating vectis
Drews-Rosenbaum
    D.-R. iris retractor
    D.-R. irrigating/aspirating unit
Drews-Sato
    D.-S. suture pickup hook
    D.-S. suture pickup spatula
    D.-S. tying forceps
drift movements
drippings
    candle wax d.
droop
    lid d.
drooping
    d. of eyelid
    d. upper eyelid
droperidol
dropout
    nerve fiber layer d.
    pigmentary d.
dropped-socket appearance
dropper
    eye d.
    Undine d.
drops
    AC eye d.
    Boston reconditioning d.
    Boston Advance reconditioning d.
    Collyrium eye d.
    Comfort d.
    eye d.
    Lens Plus rewetting d.
    Mallazine d.
    Moisture d.
    Sensitive Eyes d.
    Twenty/Twenty d.
droxifilcon A
Drualt
    bundle of D.
Drualt's bundle
drug
    d. abuse retinopathy
    anticataract d.
    cataractogenic d.
    d. fever
    d. idiosyncrasy
    immunosuppressive d.

    d. interaction
    nonsteroidal anti-inflammatory d. (NSAID)
    ophthalmic d.
    sulfa d.
    systemic d.
    topical d.
drug-induced
    d.-i. cataract
    d.-i. glaucoma
    d.-i. nystagmus
drum
    optokinetic d.
drusen
    basal laminar d.
    buried d.
    diffuse d.
    disk d.
    equatorial d.
    familial d.
    giant d.
    hard d.
    intrapapillary d.
    macular d.
    nerve head d.
    d. of optic disk, optic disk d.
    optic nerve d.
    d. of optic papilla
    soft d.
Dry
    D. Eyes
    D. Eye Therapy
dry
    d. eye
    d. eye syndrome
    d. senile degenerative maculopathy
    d. senile macular degeneration
    d. spot
dry-shelled cataract
Drysol cream
DS-9 needle
D-15 test
D_1 trisomy
D trisomy syndrome
dual lens
Dualoop
Dual-Wet
Duane retractor
Duane's
    D. accommodation chart

D. classification
D. classification of squint
D. retraction syndrome
D. syndrome
duboisii
    Histoplasma d.
Duchenne's dystrophy
duct
    ampulla of lacrimal d.
    canalicular d.
    catheterization of
      lacrimal d.
    catheterization of
      lacrimonasal d.
    excretory d.
    lacrimal d.
    lacrimonasal d.
    meibomian d.
    nasal d.
    nasolacrimal d.
    probing lacrimonasal d.
    tear d.
    d. T-tube lacrimal
duction
    forced d.
    full versions and d.'s
    passive d.
    d. test
    d.'s and versions (D&V)
    versions and d.'s
    vertical d.'s
ductional
ductule
ductulus
ductus
    d. lacrimales
    d. nasolacrimalis
Duddell's membrane
Duke-Elder
    D.-E. lamp
    D.-E. operation
Dulaney lens
Dunnington's operation
duochrome test
Duo-Flow
Duolube
duplication
    chromosomal d.
duplicity theory of vision
Dupuy-Dutemps
    D.-D. dacryocystorhinostomy
    dye test

    D.-D. dacryostomy
    D.-D. operation
dura
DURAcare
DURAcare II
dural
    d. arteriovenous
      malformation
    d. cavernous sinus fistula
    d. sheath
    d. shunt
    d. shunt syndrome
Duralone
Duranest
    D. HCl
    D. HCl with epinephrine
Duratears Naturale
duration (D)
Dura-T lens
Durazyme
Duredge knife
Durham tonometer
Duricef
Durr's operation
DUSN
    diffuse unilateral subacute
      neuroretinitis
dusting
    fibrin d.
dust-like opacities
Dutcher bodies
Duverger-Velter operation
D&V
    ductions and versions
DVA
    distance visual acuity
DVD
    dissociated vertical deviation
    dissociated vertical divergence
dwarfism
    pituitary d.
    polydystrophic d.
Dwelle
dyclonine
dye
    diamond d.
    d. disappearance test (DDT)
    fluorescein d.
    Haag-Streit fluorescein d.
    d. laser
    materials primary d.
    d. test

Dyer
    D. nomogram system of lens ordering
    D. nomogram system of ordering contact lens
dyflos
Dyggve's disease
dynamic
    d. refraction
    d. strabismus
dynamics
dynopter
Dynosol
Dyonics syringe injector
dyostosis
    mandibulofacial d.
dysadaptation
dysaptation
dysautonomia
    familial d.
    familial autonomic d.
dysautonomic
dyscephalic
    d. syndrome
    d. syndrome of François
dyscephaly
    mandibulo-oculofacial dysmorphia and d.
    oculomandibulofacial d.
dyschromasia
dyschromatopsia
    cerebral d.
dysconjugate gaze
dyscoria
dyscrasia
    blood d.
dyscrinic rhinitis
dysfunction
    brain d.
    brainstem d.
    cerebellar d.
    cone d.
    familial autonomic d.
    intraorbital nerve d.
    minimal brain d.
    oculosympathetic d.
    phagocytic d.
    pontomesencephalic d.
dysgenesis
    corneal d.
    iridocorneal d.
    iridocorneal mesodermal d.
    mesodermal d.

dysgerminoma
dysharmonious correspondence
dyskeratosis
    benign d.
    d. congenita
    hereditary benign intraepithelial d.
    intraepithelial d.
    malignant d.
    d. palmoplantaris
dyslexia
    endogenous d.
dyslipoproteinemia
dysmegalopsia
dysmetria
    ocular d.
dysmetropsia
dysmorphic
dysmorphopsia
dysopsia algera, dysopia algera
dysoric retinopathy
dysostosis, pl. dysostoses
    acrofacial d.
    craniofacial d.
    Crouzon's craniofacial d.
    Franceschetti's mandibulofacial d.
    mandibular d.
    mandibulofacial d.
    otomandibular d.
dysphoric
dysplasia
    anhidrotic ectodermal d.
    arteriohepatic d.
    chiasmal d.
    conjunctival d.
    corneal d.
    craniometaphyseal d.
    ectodermal d.
    encephalo-ophthalmic d.
    facial d.
    fibrous d.
    forebrain d.
    hereditary mucoepithelial d.
    hereditary renal-retinal d.
    oculoauricular d.
    oculoauriculovertebral d.
    oculodentodigital d.
    oculovertebral d.
    ophthalmomandibulo-melic d., OMM d.
    optic nerve d.
    orodigitofacial d.

polyostotic fibrous d.
retinal d.
septo-optic d.
vitreoretinal d.
dysplastic coloboma
Dysport
dysproteinemia
dysproteinemic retinopathy
dysthyroidism
dysthyroid optic neuropathy
dystonia
blepharospasm-
oromandibular d.
dystopia
d. canthorum
foveal d.
orbital d.
dystrophia
d. adiposa corneae
d. endothelialis corneae
d. epithelialis corneae
dystrophica
myotonia d.
dystrophy
amorphous d.
amorphous corneal d.
annular macular d.
anterior membrane d.
basement membrane d.
benign concentric annular
macular d.
Best's vitelliform d.
Best's vitelliform macular d.
Biber-Haab-Dimmer d.
Biber-Haab-Dimmer
corneal d.
Bietti's d.
Bietti's crystalline
corneoretinal d.
Bückler's I d.
Bückler's II d.
Bückler's III d.
butterfly d.
butterfly macular d.
butterfly-shaped pigment
epithelial d.
central areolar choroidal d.
central areolar pigment
epithelial d.
central cloudy d.
central cloudy corneal d.
central cloudy
parenchymatous d.

central pigmentary retinal d.
central speckled d.
central speckled corneal d.
choroidal d.
choroidoretinal d.
Cogan's d.
Cogan's corneal d.
Cogan's microcystic d.
Cogan's microcystic corneal
epithelial d.
Cogan's microcystic
epithelial corneal d.
cone d.
cone-rod d.
congenital d.
congenital endothelial d.
congenital hereditary
corneal d.
congenital hereditary
endothelial d.
congenital hereditary
endothelial corneal d.
d. of cornea
corneal d.
corneal endothelial d.
corneal endothelial
guttate d.
corneal guttate d.
corneal stromal d.
corneal vortex d.
crystalline d.
crystalline corneal d.
cystoid macular d.
deep filiform d.
deep parenchymatous d.
dominant cystoid
macular d.
dominant progressive
foveal d.
dominant slowly progressive
macular d.
Doyne's honeycombed d.
Duchenne's d.
ectatic d.
ectatic corneal d.
elastodystrophy d.
endothelial d.
endothelial cell d.
endothelial d. of cornea
epithelial d.
epithelial basement
membrane d.
Favre's d.

dystrophy *(continued)*
    Fehr's macular d.
    fenestrated sheen macular d.
    filiform d.
    fingerprint d.
    fingerprint corneal d.
    flecked d.
    flecked d. of cornea
    flecked corneal d.
    Fleischer's d.
    foveomacular vitelliform d.
    Franceschetti's d.
    François d.
    Fuchs' d.
    Fuchs' combined corneal d.
    Fuchs' endothelial d.
    Fuchs' endothelial
      corneal d.
    Fuchs' endothelial-
      epithelial d.
    Fuchs' epithelial d.
    Fuchs' epithelial corneal d.
    Fuchs' epithelial-
      endothelial d.
    furrow d.
    Goldmann-Favre d.
    granular d.
    granular corneal d.
    Grayson-Wilbrandt d.
    Grayson-Wilbrandt anterior
      corneal d.
    Grayson-Wilbrandt
      corneal d.
    Groenouw's d.
    Groenouw's corneal d.
    Groenouw's type I d.
    Groenouw's type II d.
    gutter d. of cornea
    hereditary anterior
      membrane d.
    hereditary endothelial d.
    hereditary epithelial d.
    hereditary epithelial
      corneal d.
    hereditary hemorrhagic
      macular d.
    hereditary macular d.
    hereditary vitelliform d.
    honeycomb d.
    juvenile corneal epithelial d.
    juvenile epithelial d.
    keratoconus d.
    lattice d.

    lattice corneal d.
    Lefler-Wadsworth-Sidbury
      foveal d.
    leukodystrophy d.
    macroreticular d.
    macular d.
    macular corneal d.
    Maeder-Danis d.
    mandibulofacial d.
    map-dot d.
    map-dot corneal d.
    map-dot-fingerprint d.
    map-dot-fingerprint corneal
      epithelial d.
    marginal d.
    marginal crystalline d.
    Meesman's d.
    Meesman's epithelial d.
    Meesman's epithelial
      corneal d.
    Meesman's juvenile
      epithelial d.
    Melsman's d.
    Melsman's corneal d.
    microcystic d.
    microcystic corneal d.
    microcystic epithelial d.
    muscular d.
    myotonic d.
    neonatal
      adrenoleukodystrophy d.
    oculocerebrorenal d.
    oculopharyngeal d.
    ophthalmoplegic muscular d.
    parenchymatous d.
    parenchymatous corneal d.
    pattern d.
    pattern d. of pigment
      epithelium of Byers and
      Marmor
    pericentral rod-cone d.
    pigment epithelial d.
    Pillat's d.
    polymorphous d.
    posterior polymorphic d.
      (PPMD)
    posterior polymorphous d.
    posterior polymorphous
      corneal d.
    progressive cone d.
    progressive cone-rod d.
    progressive foveal d.
    progressive macular d.

progressive
  tapetochoroidal d.
pseudoinflammatory
  macular d.
Reis-Bücklers d.
Reis-Bücklers corneal d.
Reis-Bücklers ring-shaped d.
Reis-Bücklers superficial
  corneal d.
reticular d. of cornea
retinal d.
retinal pigmentary d.
ring-like corneal d.
ring-shaped d.
rod and cone d.
rod-cone d.
Salzmann's d.
Salzmann's corneal d.
Salzmann's nodular
  corneal d.
Schlichting's d.
Schnyder's crystalline d.

Schnyder's crystalline
  corneal d.
Sjögren's reticular d.
Sorsby's
  pseudoinflammatory d.
Sorsby's pseudoinflammatory
  macular d.
speckled corneal d.
Stocker-Holt d.
Stocker-Holt-Schneider d.
stromal d.
stromal corneal d.
tapetochoroidal d.
vitelliform d.
vitelliruptive macular d.
vitreo-tapetoretinal d.
vortex d.
vortex corneal d.
d. of Waardenburg-Jonkers
Wagner's vitreoretinal d.
dysversion
  congenital d.

E
esophoria
EA-290
Toctron EA-290
EACA
ε-aminocaproic acid
Eagle Vision-Freeman punctum plug
Eales' disease
early
e. antigen
e. lens opacities
e. mature cataract
e. receptor potential (ERP)
e. receptor potential mottling (ERPM)
Early Treatment Diabetic Retinopathy Study (ETDRS)
Easterman's visual function
EasyClean/GP
Easy Eyes
Eaton-Lambert syndrome
Eber needle-holder forceps
EBV
Epstein-Barr virus
EBV nuclear antigen
EBV-associated antigen
E Carpine
ECCE
extracapsular cataract extraction
eccentric
e. fixation
e. gaze
e. limitation
e. viewing
e. vision
eccentrically
ecchymosis, pl. ecchymoses
e. of eyelid
ecchymotic
eccrine acrospermia
E chart
echinococcosis
echinococcus cyst
Echinococcus granulosa
echinophthalmia
echo
linear e.'s
reflectance e.
reflected e.

Echodide
echogram
echography
kinetic e.
orbital e.
quantitative e.
topographic e.
echo-ophthalmogram
echo-ophthalmography
EchoScan by Nidek
echothiophate
e. iodide
e. phospholine
eclamptic retinopathy
eclipse
e. amblyopia
e. blindness
e. retinopathy
e. scotoma
Econochlor
Econopred Plus
ecothiopate
ectasia, ectasis
corneal e.
iris e.
nasal fundus e.
e. of sclera
scleral e.
ectatic
e. corneal dystrophy
e. dilation
e. dystrophy
e. marginal degeneration of cornea
ecthyma
e. contagiosum
e. gangrenosum
ectiris
ectochoroidea
ectocornea
ectoderm
surface e.
ectodermal dysplasia
ectodermatosis
ectodermosis
ectopia
cilia e.
e. iridis
e. lentis
e. maculae

ectopia *(continued)*
    macular e.
    posterior pituitary e.
    e. pupillae congenita
ectopic
    e. eyelash
    e. tissue
ectropion, ectropium
    Adams' e.
    atonic e.
    Cibis' e.
    e. cicatriceum
    cicatricial e.
    complex e.
    congenital e.
    e. of eyelid
    eyelid e.
    flaccid e.
    inflammatory e.
    involutional e.
    involutional senile e.
    e. luxurians
    mechanical e.
    medial e.
    paralytic e.
    e. paralyticum
    pigment layer e.
    e. sarcomatosum
    senescent e.
    senile e.
    e. senilis
    spastic e.
    e. spasticum
    tarsal e.
    e. uveae
ectropionize
eczema
    atopic e.
eczematoid blepharitis
eczematosus
    pannus e.
eczematous
    e. conjunctivitis
    e. pannus
edema
    aphakic cystoid macular e.
    aphakic macular e.
    Berlin's e.
    boggy e.
    brawny e.
    central e.
    choroidal e.
    conjunctival e.

    e. of cornea
    corneal e.
    cystoid macular e. (CME)
    endothelial cell e.
    epithelial e.
    e. of eyelid
    eyelid e.
    Iwanoff's retinal e.
    macular e.
    microcystic e.
    e. of optic disk
    periorbital e.
    periretinal e.
    phakic cystoid macular e.
    phakic macular e.
    e. residue
    retinal e.
    Stellwag's brawny e.
    stromal e.
    subconjunctival e.
edematous
edge
    e. coating
    e. contour
    epithelial rolled e.'s
    fimbriated e.
    e. stand-off
edging
    e. of lens
    e. of spectacle lens
Edinger's fibers
Edinger-Westphal (EW)
    E.-W. nucleus
edipism
edrophonium
    e. chloride
    e. chloride test
    e. test
EDTA
    ethylenediaminetetraacetic acid
Edwards' syndrome
EEG
    electroencephalogram
effect
    Abney's e.
    autokinetic e.
    Bracken's e.
    braid e.
    Braid's e.
    cat's eye e.
    copper-wire e.
    Cotton's e.
    ocular e.

pantoscopic e.
prismatic e.
Purkinje's e.
radiation e.
Raman's e.
Stiles-Crawford e.
sunburst e.
telephoto e.
Tyndall's e.
Zeeman's e.
effective diameter
efferent
e. fibers
e. nerve
efficacy
efficiency
visual e.
effusion
ciliochoroidal e.
uveal e.
Efricel
E game
EGF
epidermal growth factor
Egger's line
egilops
egress
egressed
EGTA
ethyleneglycoltetraacetate
Egyptian
E. conjunctivitis
E. ophthalmia
Ehlers-Danlos syndrome
Ehrhardt lid forceps
Ehrlich-Türck line
Ehrmann's test
eidoptometry
eight-ball
e.-b. hemorrhage
e.-b. hyphema
eighth cranial nerve
eikonometer, eiconometer
EKC
epidemic keratoconjunctivitis
elastica
tela e.
elasticity
elastic pseudoxanthoma
elasticum
pseudoxanthoma e. (PXE)
xanthoma e.
elastodysplasia

elastodystrophy
e. dystrophy
Elastoplast
E. bandage
E. dressing
E. eye occlusor
elastorrhexis
elastosis
e. dystrophica
senescent e.
senile e.
Elavil
Eldridge-Green lamp
electric
e. cataract
e. light blindness
e. ophthalmia
e. retinopathy
e. shock cataract
electrica
ophthalmia e.
electrocauterizer
electrocautery
Fine micropoint e.
Geiger e.
Hildreth e.
Mentor wet-field e.
Mira e.
Mueller e.
ophthalmic e.
Op-Temp disposable e.
Parker-Heath e.
Prince e.
Rommel e.
Rommel-Hildreth e.
Scheie e.
Todd e.
Valilab e.
von Graefe e.
Wadsworth-Todd e.
wet-field e.
Ziegler e.
electrocoagulation
electrode
Berens e.
Cibis e.
coagulating e.
cyclodiathermy e.
diathermy e.
Gradle e.
Guyton e.
Kronfeld e.
Pischel e.

electrode *(continued)*
    Schepens e.
    Walker e.
    Weve e.
electrodiaphake
electroencephalogram (EEG)
electroencephalograph
electroencephalography
electroepilation
electrokeratotome
    Castroviejo e.
electrolysis
electromagnetic
    e. energy
    e. radiation
    e. removal of foreign body
    e. scleral search coil
    e. spectrum
electromucotome
    Steinhauser e.
electromyogram (EMG)
electromyography
electron
    e. interferometer
    e. interferometry
    e. microscope
    e. microscopy
    e. volt
electronic tonometer
electronystagmogram (ENG)
electronystagmograph
electronystagmography (ENG)
electro-oculogram (EOG)
electro-oculograph
electro-oculography (EOG)
electro-olfactogram (EOG)
electroparacentesis
electroperimeter
electrophoresis
    hemoglobin e.
    protein e.
    serum protein e.
electrophysiological
    e. test
    e. testing
electrophysiology
electroretinogram (ERG)
    flash e.
    pattern e.
    pattern-evoked e. (PERG)
electroretinograph
    Ganzfeld e.
electroretinography (ERG)

electrospinogram
element
    encircling e.
    Kollmorgen's e.'s
    retinal e.
elephantiasis
    e. neuromatosis
    e. nostras
    e. oculi
elevation
    e. angle
    chin e.
elevator
    Desmarres lid e.
    Freer e.
    Freer periosteal e.
    Joseph e.
    e. muscle
    e. palsy
    Tenzel e.
Eliasoph lid retractor
ELISA
    enzyme-linked immunosorbent
    assay
Ellingson's syndrome
Elliot
    E. corneal trephine
    E. trephine
    E. trephine handle
Elliot's
    E. operation
    E. sign
ellipse
ellipsoid
ellipsoidal back surface
elliptical nystagmus
elliptic nystagmus
Ellis
    E. foreign body needle
    E. foreign body spud
    E. foreign body spud
      needle probe
    E. needle holder
    E. needle probe
    E. spud
Elschnig
    E. body
    E. capsule forceps
    E. cataract knife
    E. corneal knife
    E. cyclodialysis spatula
    E. extrusion needle
    E. fixation forceps

E. forceps
E. knife
E. pterygium knife
E. refractor
E. retractor
E. spatula
E. spoon
E. trephine
Elschnig-O'Brien forceps
Elschnig-O'Connor
E.-O. fixation forceps
E.-O. forceps
Elschnig's
E. blepharorrhaphy
E. canthorrhaphy
E. canthorrhaphy operation
E. central iridectomy
E. conjunctivitis
E. iridectomy
E. keratoplasty
E. operation
E. pearl
E. spot
E. syndrome
Elschnig-Weber loupe
Ely's operation
embedded
embolism
retinal e.
embolus, pl. emboli
calcium e.
carotid e.
cholesterol e.
fat e.
fibrin-platelet e.
platelet-fibrin e.
embryogenesis
embryology
embryonal
e. carcinoma
e. cataract
e. epithelial cyst of iris
e. medulloepithelioma
e. medulloepithelioma of ciliary body
e. nuclear cataract
e. tumor of ciliary body
embryonic
e. cataract
e. fixation syndrome
e. plate
embryopathic cataract

embryopathy
retinoic acid e.
embryotoxon
anterior e.
posterior e.
emergency light reflex
emergent
e. light
e. ray
e. ray of light
Emerson's one-piece segment bifocal
Emery lens
EMG
electromyogram
eminence
malar e.
emittance
radiant e.
emmetrope
emmetropia
emmetropic
emmetropization
Empac-Cavitron irrigation/aspiration unit
emphysema
e. of conjunctiva
e. of orbit
orbital e.
subconjunctival e.
emplaced uveitis
empty
optically e.
e. sella
e. sella syndrome
encanthis
encapsulated bleb
encephalitis
encephalocele
basal e.
orbital e.
encephalofacial angiomatosis
encephalomyelitis
encephalo-ophthalmic dysplasia
encephalopathy
Leigh's e.
Wernicke's e.
encephalotrigeminal angiomatosis
encirclement
encircling
e. band
e. band for scleral buckle
e. buckle

encircling *(continued)*
    e. element
    e. explant
    e. of globe operation
    e. implant
    e. polyethylene tube
    e. of scleral buckle
       operation
    e. silicone buckle
    e. tube
encroach
encroaching
encroachment
endarterectomy
    carotid e.
endarteritis
    e. obliterans
end-gaze nystagmus
endocapsular
endocarditis
    infective e.
endocrine
    e. exophthalmos
    e. lid retraction
    e. neoplasia
    e. ophthalmopathy
endocrine-inactive adenoma
endocryopexy
endocryophotocoagulation
endocryoretinopexy
endodiathermy
endogenous
    e. disease
    e. dyslexia
    e. endophthalmitis
    e. uveitis
endoillumination
endoilluminator
    Grieshaber e.
endolaser
    diode e.
    e. probe tip
endoneural cells
endophlebitis of retinal vein
endophotocoagulation
    argon laser e.
endophthalmitis
    bacterial e.
    bleb-associated e.
    candidal e.
    chronic e.
    endogenous e.
    exogenous e.

    fungal e.
    granulomatous e.
    infectious e.
    metastatic e.
    e. ophthalmia nodosa
    e. phacoallergica
    phacoanaphylactic e.
    e. phacoanaphylactica
    e. phacogenetica
    sterile e.
    systemic bacterial e.
    toxocariasis e.
endophthalmodonesis
endophytic
endophytum
    glioma e.
endoplasmic reticulum
EndoProbe
endoretinal
Endo-Set by Haag-Streit
Endosol
endothelial
    e. bleb
    e. cell
    e. cell basement membrane
    c. cell count
    e. cell dystrophy
    e. cell edema
    e. cell side down
    e. cell surface of cornea
    e. dystrophy
    e. dystrophy of cornea
    vesiculosus linear e.
endothelialitis
endothelioma
    Sidler-Huguenin e.
endothelium
    e. camerae anterioris bulbi
    corneal e.
    e. oculi
endotracheal tube
end-piece
end-point
    e.-p. color
    e.-p. nystagmus
    porcelain white e.-p.
end-position nystagmus
endrisone
endrysone
energy
    electromagnetic e.
    facture e.
    radiant e.

enflurane
enfoldings
ENG
electronystagmogram
electronystagmography
Englemann's disease
engorgement
venous e.
enlargement
blind spot e.
corneal e.
orbital e.
enophthalmia
enophthalmus
senescent e.
enoxacin
Enroth's sign
enstrophe
enteritis
regional e.
Enterobacter aerogenes
enterocolitis
granulomatous e.
enteropathica
acrodermatitis e.
Entero-Vioform
Enterovirus
entochoroidea
entocornea
entophthalmia
entopic phenomenon
entoptic
entoptoscope
entoptoscopy
entoretina
entrance pupil
entrapment
pupillary e.
entropion, entropium
acquired e.
acute spastic e.
atonic e.
Celsus-Hotz e.
Cibis' e.
e. cicatriceum
cicatricial e.
congenital e.
eyelid e.
e. forceps
Hotz e.
involutional e.
involutional senile e.
marginal e.

noncicatricial e.
Poulard's e.
senescent e.
senile e.
spastic e.
e. spasticum
e. uveae
uveal e.
entropionize
entry
implant e.
enucleate
enucleation
e. of eyeball operation
Foix's e.
e. scissors
e. scoop
e. spoon
e. wire snare
enucleator
Banner snare e.
Botvin-Bradford e.
Bradford snare e.
Castroviejo snare e.
Foster snare e.
snare e.
Enuclene
enzymatic
e. cleaner
e. galactosemia
e. glaucoma
e. zonulolysis
Enzymatic Cleaner for Extended Wear
enzyme
angiotensin-converting e. (ACE)
antioxidant e.
e. cleaner
e. glaucoma
enzyme-linked immunosorbent assay (ELISA)
EOG
electro-oculogram
electro-oculography
electro-olfactogram
EOM
extraocular movements
extraocular muscle
EOMI
extraocular movements intact
EOP
equivalent oxygen performance

eosinophil
eosinophilia
  angiolymphoid hyperplasia
    with e.
eosinophilic
  e. granuloma
  e. reaction
  e. response
eosin stain
ependymoma tumor
ephedrine
ephelides
epiblepharon
epibulbar
  e. dermoid cyst
  e. Fordyce nodules
  e. limbal dermoid
    choristoma
epicanthal
  e. correction
  e. fold
  e. inversus
  e. skin fold
epicanthic
epicanthine fold
epicanthus
  e. blepharophimosis
  e. caruncle
  e. inversus
  e. palpebralis
  e. supraciliaris
  e. tarsalis
epicapsular lens star
Epicar
epicauma
epicenter
epicorneascleritis
epidemic
  e. blindness
  e. conjunctivitis
  e. keratoconjunctivitis (EKC)
  e. typhus
epidermal
  e. growth factor (EGF)
  e. inclusion cyst
  e. necrolysis
epidermidis
  Staphylococcus e.
epidermidization
epidermoid
  e. carcinoma
  e. cyst

epidermolysis
  e. bullosa
  e. bullosa acquisita
epidialysis
epidiascope
Epifrin
epikeratophakia
epikeratophakic keratoplasty
epikeratoplasty
  tectonic e.
epikeratoprosthesis
epilation
epilator
epilens
epilepsy
epileptic nystagmus
E-Pilo
E-Pilo
E-Pilo-1
E-Pilo-2
E-Pilo-3
E-Pilo-4
E-Pilo-6
epimysium
Epinal
epinephrine
  e. bitartrate
  e. borate
  dipivalyl e.
  Duranest HCl with e.
  e. HCl
  lidocaine with e.
  Lidoject-1 with e.
  Marcaine HCl with e.
  Nervocaine with e.
  pilocarpine and e.
  e. and pilocarpine
  Sensorcaine with e.
  Xylocaine with e.
epipapillaris
  membrana e.
epipapillary membrane
epiphora
  atonic e.
epiretinal membrane
episclera
episcleral
  e. angioma
  e. arterial circle
  e. artery
  e. blood vessel
  e. circulation
  e. explant

e. hemangioma
e. lamina
e. nevus
e. nodule
e. rheumatic nodule
e. scarring
e. space
e. tissue
e. vein
episclerale
spatium e.
venae e.
episcleritis
circumscribed e.
gouty e.
e. multinodularis
nodular e.
e. partialis fugax
e. periodica fugax
simple e.
syphilitic e.
episclerotitis
episode
ischemic e.
epistaxis
epitarsus
e. pterygium
epithelia
epithelial
e. barrier
e. basement layer
e. basement membrane
e. basement membrane
dystrophy
e. bedewing
e. bulla
e. cell
e. cyst
e. debridement
e. diffuse keratitis
e. downgrowth
e. dystrophy
e. dystrophy of Fuchs'
e. edema
e. erosion
e. herpetic disease
e. hypertrophy
e. implantation cyst
e. inclusion cyst
e. inclusions
e. ingrowth
e. invasion
e. keratitis

e. keratopathy
e. microcyst
e. nevus
e. punctate keratitis
e. rolled edges
e. scraping
e. slide
e. tumor
epithelialization
epitheliitis
e. focal retinal pigment
pigment e.
retinal pigment e.
epitheliocapsularis
fibrillopathia e.
epithelioid cell
epithelioma, pl. **epitheliomata**
e. adenoides cysticum
Contino's e.
intraepithelial e.
Malherbe's calcifying e.
malignant ciliary e.
epitheliopathy
acute multifocal placoid
pigment e. (AMPPE)
acute multifocal posterior
pigment e.
acute multifocal posterior
placoid pigment e.
acute posterior multifocal
placoid pigment e.
(APMPPE)
pigment e.
placoid pigment e.
posterior pigment e.
retinal pigment e.
epithelioplasty
epitheliosis desquamativa
conjunctivae
epithelium, pl. **epithelia**
e. anterius corneae
ciliary e.
corneal e.
lens e.
e. lentis
nonpigmented ciliary e.
pigment e. (PE)
e. pigmentosum iridis
placoid pigmentation of e.
e. posterius corneae
retinal pigment e. (RPE)
serous pigment e.
subcapsular e.

Epitrate
epizootic keratoconjunctivitis
epoch
Eppy/N
EPS
    exophthalmos-producing
    substance
Epstein
    E. collar stud acrylic
      implant
    E. collar stud acrylic lens
Epstein-Barr virus (EBV)
Epstein's symptom
equal
    pupils round, regular,
      and e. (PRRE)
equate
equation
    Rayleigh's e.
equator
    anatomic e.
    e. bulbi oculi
    e. of crystalline lens,
      crystalline lens e.
    eyeball e.
    geometric e.
    lens e.
    e. of lens
    e. lentis
equatorial
    e. degeneration
    e. drusen
    e. lentis
    e. meridian
    e. ring scotoma
    e. staphyloma
equilateral hemianopsia
equilibrating operation
equipment
    laser e.
equivalent
    e. distance
    migraine e.
    e. oxygen percentage value
    e. oxygen performance
      (EOP)
    e. power
    e. refracting plane
    spherical e.
eraser
    e. cautery
    Mentor wet-field e.
Erbakan's inferior fornix operation

erbium laser
Erdheim-Chester disease
erect illumination
ERG
    electroretinogram
    electroretinography
ERG-Jet disposable contact lens
ergograph
ergonovine
ergot
    e. alkaloid
    e. derivative
ergotamine tartrate
Erhardt
    E. clamp
    E. lid forceps
erisiphake
erisophake
erosion
    coast e.
    corneal e.
    epithelial e.
    punctate epithelial e.
    recurrent corneal e.
    recurrent epithelial e.
    sphincter e.
ERP
    early receptor potential
ERPM
    early receptor potential mottling
erroneous projection
error
    astigmagraphic e.
    astigmatic e.
    asymmetric refractive e.'s
    field of view e.
    inborn e.
    position e.
    refractive e.
    retinal e.
    sampling e.
    velocity e.
eruptio
    zoster sine e.
eruption
    skin e.
eruptive keratoacanthoma
erysipelas
    coastal e.
erysiphake, erisiphake, erisophake
    Barraquer e.
    Bell e.
    Castroviejo e.

corneal e.
Dimitry e.
Dimitry-Bell e.
Dimitry-Thomas e.
Draeger high vacuum e.
Esposito e.
Floyd-Grant e.
Harrington e.
Johnson e.
Johnson-Bell e.
Kara e.
L'Esperance e.
Maumenee e.
New York e.
Nugent-Green-Dimitry e.
oval cup e.
Post-Harrington e.
Sakler e.
Searcy e.
Searcy oval cup e.
Simcoe nucleus e.
Storz-Bell e.
e. technique
Viers e.
Welch rubber bulb e.
Welsh e.
Welsh Silastic e.

erythema
e. chronicum migrans
e. multiforme
e. multiforme bullosum
e. multiforme conjunctivitis
e. multiforme exudativum
e. multiforme major
e. nodosum

erythematosus
discoid lupus e.
lupus e. (LE)
systemic lupus e. (SLE)

erythrocin
erythroclastic glaucoma
erythrocyte
ghost e.
e. sedimentation rate

erythrogenic
erythrolabe
erythrometer
erythrometry
erythromycin
erythrophagocytosis
erythropia
erythropsia
escape phenomenon

Escapini's cataract operation
Eschenback Optik lens
Escherichia coli
Eserine
Isopto E.
E. Salicylate
E. Sulfate

esocataphoria
esodeviation
e. accommodation
accommodative e.
nonaccommodative e.

esophoria (E)
accommodative e.
classical congenital e.
congenital e.
nonaccommodative e.

esophoric
esotropia (ET)
A-e.
e. accommodation
accommodative e.
acquired e.
alternate day e.
alternating e.
A-pattern e.
basic e.
clock-mechanism e.
congenital e.
consecutive e.
constant e.
cyclic e.
essential infantile e.
idiopathic congenital e.
infantile e.
intermittent e.
late-onset e.
left e.
mixed e.
near e. (ET')
nonaccommodative e.
nonrefractive
  accommodative e.
periodic e.
refractive accommodative e.
right e.
sensory e.
V-e.
V-pattern e.
X-e.

esotropic amblyopia
Esposito erysiphake

essential
    e. anisocoria
    e. blepharospasm
    e. hypercholesterolemic
      xanthomatosis
    e. hypertension
    e. hypotony
    e. infantile esotropia
    e. iris atrophy
    e. phthisis
    e. phthisis bulbi
    e. progressive atrophy of
      iris
    e. telangiectasia
Esser's inlay operation
ester
    cholesterol e.
    polyoxethylene sorbitan fatty
      acid e.
    sorbitan e.
Esterman scale
esthesiometer
    Cochet-Bonnet e.
esthesioneuroblastoma
Estivin
estrogen
E syndrome
ET
    esotropia
ET'
    near esotropia
etafilcon A
ETDRS
    Early Treatment Diabetic
    Retinopathy Study
ethambutol
ethanol
ethchlorvynol
ether
    dihematoporphyrin e.
    e. guard
    e. theory of light
Ethicon
    E. micropoint suture
    E. needle
    E. Sabreloc suture
    E. suture
Ethicon-Atraloc suture
ethmoid
    e. air cell
    e. bone
    e. bulla
    e. canal

    e. exenteration
    e. fistula
    e. sinuses
ethmoidal
    e. artery
    e. incisure
    e. lacrimal fistula
    e. region
    e. sinus
ethmoidalis
    lamina orbitalis ossis e.
ethmoiditis
ethmoidolacrimalis
    sutura e.
ethmoidomaxillaris
    sutura e.
ethoxyzolamide
ethyl
    e. alcohol
    e. alcohol amblyopia
    e. cyanoacrylate
    e. cyanoacrylate glue
ethylene
    e. glycol
    e. oxide
ethylenediaminetetraacetate
    calcium e.
    sodium e.
ethylenediaminetetraacetic acid (EDTA)
ethyleneglycoltetraacetate (EGTA)
ethylmercurithiosalicylate
    sodium e.
etidocaine
etoposide
etretinate
E trisomy
EUA
    exam under anesthesia
eucatropine
euchromatopsy
euploidic
euryopia
euthyphoria
euthyroid
euthyscope
euthyscopy
evagination
    optic e.
evaluation
    preoperative e.
    visual function e.
evanescent

evaporation
evasion
    macular e.
event
    independent e.
Evergreen Lasertek
    E. L. coagulator
    E. L. laser
Eversbusch's operation
eversion
    e. of eyelid
    lid e.
    e. of punctum
everted eyelid
everter
    Berens e.
    Berens lid e.
    Berke lid e.
    lid e.
    Roveda e.
    Roveda lid e.
    Schachne-Desmarres e.
    Schachne-Desmarres lid e.
    Struble e.
    Struble lid e.
    Walker e.
    Walker lid e.
evisceration
    e. of eyeball
    e. operation
    e. spoon
evisceroneurotomy
evoked
    e. nystagmus gaze
    e. potential
evolutional cataract
evulsion
evulsio nervi optici
EW
    Edinger-Westphal
Ewald's law
EWCL
    extended-wear contact lens
Ewing capsule forceps
Ewing's
    E. operation
    E. sarcoma
ex amblyopia
examination
    cytologic e.
    dark-field e.
    e. of eye
    flashlight e.

    funduscopic e.
    neurologic e.
    neuro-ophthalmologic e.
    ophthalmic e.
    serologic e.
    slit-lamp e. (SLE)
    Woods' light e.
exam under anesthesia (EUA)
ex anopsia
exanthematous conjunctivitis
excavatio
    e. disci
    e. papillae nervi optici
excavation
    atrophic e.
    glaucomatous e.
    e. of optic disk
    physiologic e.
    retinal e.
excess
    convergence e.
    divergence e.
    e. divergence
    e. esotropia convergence
excessive
    e. accommodation
    e. cyclodialysis clefts
    e. lacrimation
exchange
    air-fluid e.
    fluid-gas e.
    gas-fluid e.
    lens e.
excimer
    e. laser
    e. laser photoreactive
      keratectomy
    e. laser photorefractive
      keratectomy
excision
    Arlt-Jaesche e.
    conjunctiva-Muller muscle e.
    e. of lacrimal gland
      operation
    e. of lacrimal sac operation
    pentagonal block e.
exciting eye
exclusion of pupil
excretory duct
excursion
excycloduction
excyclophoria
excyclotropia

excyclovergence
executive
    e. bifocal
    e. lens
    e. spectacle lens
    e. trifocal
exenteration
    ethmoid e.
    Iliff's e.
    orbital e.
    e. of orbital contents
      operation
exenteratio orbitae
exercise
    antisuppression e.
    blur and clear e.
    convergent e.'s
    pleoptic e.
exertional amblyopia
Exeter ophthalmoscope
exfoliation
    e. of capsule
    e. glaucoma
    e. of lens
    e. of lens capsule
    e. syndrome
    true e.
exfoliative keratitis
exit pupil
exocataphoria
exodeviation
    comitant e.
exogenous
    e. disease
    e. endophthalmitis
    e. ochronosis
exophoria (X)
    alternating e.
    comitant e.
    concomitant e.
    constant e.
exophoric
exophthalmic
    e. goiter
    e. ophthalmoplegia
exophthalmogenic
exophthalmometer
    Hertel e.
    Luedde e.
exophthalmometric
exophthalmometry
exophthalmos, exophthalmus
    e. due to pressure

e. due to tower skull
endocrine e.
malignant e.
ophthalmoplegic e.
postural e.
pulsatile e.
pulsating e.
recurrent e.
substance e.
thyroid e.
thyrotoxic e.
thyrotropic e.
transient early e.
exophthalmos-producing substance (EPS)
exophytic
exophytum
    glioma e.
exoplant
    scleral e.
exorbitism
exotoxin
exotropia (XT)
    A-e.
    alternating e.
    A-pattern e.
    basic e.
    comitant e.
    consecutive e.
    convergence insufficiency e.
    divergence excess e.
    divergence insufficiency e.
    flick e.
    intermittent e. (X(T))
    left e.
    periodic e.
    right e.
    secondary e.
    sensory e.
    V-e.
    V-pattern e.
    X-e.
exotropic
expander
    scleral e.
experiment
    Mariotte's e.
    Scheiner's e.
experimental diabetes
explant
    encircling e.
    episcleral e.
    Molteno episcleral e.

posterior e.
segmental e.
silicone e.
silicone sponge e.
sponge e.
exploration
sclerotomy with e.
Expo Bubble
E. B. dressing
E. B. eye cover
E. B. eye shield
E. B. shield
exposure
e. keratitis
e. keratopathy
expression
nuclear e.
expressivity
expressor
Arroyo e.
Arruga e.
Bagley-Wilmer e.
Berens e.
Heath e.
Heyner e.
hook e.
e. hook
Hosford e.
Kirby hook e.
Kirby intracapsular lens e.
lens e.
e. loop
McDonald e.
meibomian gland e.
nucleus e.
ring lens e.
Rizzuti e.
Rizzuti lens e.
Smith e.
Stahl nucleus e.
Verhoeff e.
Verhoeff lens e.
Wilmer-Bagley e.
expulsive hemorrhage
extended round needle
extended-wear contact lens (EWCL)
extension
finger-like e.'s
orbital e.
Extenzyme
externa
axis oculi e.

membrana granulosa e.
membrana limitans e.
external
e. ankyloblepharon
e. axis of eye
e. canthotomy
e. exudative retinopathy
e. geniculate body
e. hordeolum
e. hydrocephalus
e. limiting membrane
e. ophthalmopathy
e. ophthalmoplegia
e. orbital fracture
e. palsy
e. pterygoid levator synkinesis
e. route
e. squint
e. strabismus
externi
insufficiency of e.
externus
axis bulbi e.
extinction
e. phenomenon
visual e.
extirpation
extorsion
extracanthic
extracapsular
e. aphakia
e. cataract extraction (ECCE)
e. cataract extraction operation
e. extraction
e. extraction of cataract
extracellular matrix
extraciliary fiber
extraconal fat reticulum
extractable nuclear antigen
extraction
Arroyo's cataract e.
Arruga's cataract e.
cataract e.
e. of cataract
Chandler-Verhoeff lens e.
extracapsular e.
extracapsular cataract e. (ECCE)
e. of extracapsular cataract
e. flap

extraction *(continued)*
> foreign body e.
> intracapsular e.
> e. of intracapsular cataract
> intracapsular cataract e.
> (ICCE)
> intraocular cataract e.
> magnetic e.
> planned extracapsular
> cataract e.

extractor
> Krwawicz cataract e.
> Look cortex e.
> Visitec cortex e.
> Welsh cortex e.

extramacular binocular vision
extramedullary
> e. course
> e. segment

extraocular
> e. movements (EOM)
> e. movements intact
> (EOMI)
> e. muscle (EOM)
> e. muscles of Tillaux

extraorbital disease
extrapyramidal system
extrarectus
extraretinal
extrascleral
extravasated
extravasation
extravisual zone
extrinsic muscles
extruded
extrusion
> implant e.
> e. needle

exudate
> circinate e.
> conjunctival e.
> cotton-wool e.
> fatty e.
> foaming e.
> hard e.
> retinal e.
> soft e.
> waxy e.

exudation
> proteinaceous aqueous e.

exudative
> e. choroiditis
> e. eye

> e. retinal detachment
> e. retinitis
> e. retinopathy
> e. senile maculopathy
> e. vitreoretinopathy

exudativum
> erythema multiforme e.

Eye
> Soothe E.
> E. Wash

eye
> accessory organs of e.
> alkali burn to e.
> amaurotic cat's e.
> anterior segment of e.
> aphakic e.
> appendage of e.
> aqueous humor e.
> artificial e.
> axial length of e.
> e. bank
> black e.
> blear e.
> Bright's e.
> bulb of e.
> bull's e.
> cat's e.
> centrally-fixing e.
> e. chamber
> e. chart
> cinema e.
> closed surgery on e.
> e. color
> compound e.
> e. contact
> contralateral e.
> contusion of e.
> crossed e.'s
> e. cup
> cyclopean e.
> cystic e.
> dark-adapted e.
> deviating e.
> disorder of e.
> doll's e.
> doll's e. maneuver
> doll's e. reflex
> doll's e. sign
> dominant e.
> donor e.
> e. dropper
> e. drops
> dry e.

examination of e.
exciting e.
external axis of e.
exudative e.
fellow e.
fibrous coat of e.
fixating e.
fixing e.
following e.
Fox's e.
fundus of e.
Gullstrand's reduced e.
Gullstrand's schematic e.
hare's e.
heavy e.
Helmholtz's schematic e.
hop e.
hot e.
e. implant conformer
e. infarction
inflammatory target site
   of e.
e. injury
internal axis of e.
iris e.
e. irrigating solution
Klieg's e.
e. knife guard
lazy e.
left e. (LE, OS)
e. lens
light-adapted e.
Listing's reduced e.
Listing's schematic e.
e. magnet
master e., master-
   dominant e.
medial angle of e.
micro movements of e.
monochromatic e.
e. movement disorder
e. movements
muscle of e.
e. muscle surgery
Nairobi's e.
e. occluder
old e.
orbicular muscle of e.
oval e.
e. pad
e. pad dressing
parietal e.
patch e.

phakic e.
photopic e.
phthisical e.
pineal e.
e. point
posterior pole of e.
e. pressing
primary e.
e. protector
pseudophakic e.
red e.
reduced e.
e. reflex
e. removed in toto
e. restored to normotensive
   pressure
right e. (OD)
e. rotated inferiorly
e. rotation
rudimentary e.
saccadic movements of e.
sagittal axis of e.
schematic e.
e. scissors
scotopic e.
secondary e.
e. shield
shipyard e.
e. size
Snellen reform e.
e. speculum
e. spot
e. spud
squinting e.
stony-hard e.
e. surgery
suspensory ligament e.
e. suture scissors
e. sweep
sympathizing e.
tension of e.
tumor of interior of e.
vertical axis of e.
e. wall
e. wash
e. was quiet
watery e.
web e.
white of e.

eyeball
e. compression reflex
dimpling of e.
e. equator

eyeball *(continued)*
    evisceration of e.
    fibrous tunic of e.
    luxation of e.
    meridian of e.
    pigmented layer of e.
    posterior pole of e.
    e. sheath
    vascular coat of e.
eyeball-heart reflex
eyebrow
    e. fixation
    e. laceration
eye-closure reflex
Eye Con 5
Eye-Cool
Eye-Cort
eyecup
eyed
eyedness
Eye-Drops
eye/ear plane
Eye-Gene
eyeglasses
eyegrounds
eyeguard
eyehole
eyeing
eyelash
    ectopic e.
    piebald e.
eyelid
    angular junction of e.
    avulsion of e.
    baggy e.
    basal cell carcinoma of e.
    capillary hemangioma of e.
    carcinoma of e.
    e. closure reflex
    e. coloboma
    e. contour
    e. crease
    e. crusting
    e. dermatochalasis
    drooping of e.
    drooping upper e.
    ecchymosis of e.
    e. ectropion
    ectropion of e.
    e. edema
    edema of e.
    e. entropion
    eversion of e.

everted e.
e. fissures
floppy e.
flutter of e.
e. flutter
e. fold
e. forceps
free margin of e.
e. fusion
glands of e.
incision into e.
inflammation of e.
insufficiency of e.'s
e. keratosis
lateral commissure of e.
levator muscle of upper e.
lower e.
e. lymphangioma
e. margin
medial commissure of e.
melanoma of e.
e. milia
e. molluscum contagiosum
    infection
e. muscle
e. myokymia
e. neurilemoma
e. neurofibroma
e. nevus
orbital portion of e.
e. papilloma
e. plaque
plastic repair of e.
ptosis of e.
e. ptosis
reconstruction of e.
e. retraction
e. retractor
e. rhytids
sluggish movements of eyes
    and e.'s
e. speculum
squamous cell carcinoma
    of e.
e. strawberry hemangioma
e. surgery
suturing of e.
e. syringoma
tarsal portion of e.
tumor of e.
e. tumor
unilateral ptosis of e.
upper e.

e. vesiculation
xanthelasma around e.
eyelids sutured closed
Eye-Mo
Eye-Pak
    E.-P. drape
    E.-P. II cover
    E.-P. II drape
    E.-P. II sheet
eyepatch
    oval e.
eyepiece
    comparison e.
    compensating e.
    demonstration e.
    huygenian e.
    negative e.
    position e.
    positive e.
    Ramsden e.
    wide-field e.
eyepoint
eye-refractometer
Eyes
    Clear E.
    Dry E.
    Easy E.

Preflex for Sensitive E.
Sensitive E.
Soft Mate Comfort Drops
    for Sensitive E.
Soft Mate Saline for
    Sensitive E.
eyes
    both e. (OU)
    cross e.
    protruding e.
    raccoon e.
Eye-Sed solution
eyeshot
eyesight
Eye-Sine
    E.-S. solution
eyespot
eyestone
eyestrain
Eye-Stream solution
eyewash
Eye Wash solution
eyewear
eyewire
eyeworm
    African e.
Eye-Zine

F
    Fahrenheit
    Faraday
    filial generation
    fluorine
    focus
    force
    free energy
    visual field

FA
    fluorescein angiography

Faber's disease

Fab fragment

Fabry's
    F. disease
    F. syndrome

face
    bird f.
    cow f.
    frog f.
    hyaloid f.
    f. line
    f. shield
    vitreous f.

face-down position

facet, facette
    corneal f.

facetectomy

facetted
    f. avascular disciform
      opacity
    f. corneal scar

faci
    no f.

facial
    f. anomalies
    f. block
    f. cleft
    f. dysplasia
    f. hemangioma
    f. hemiatrophy
    f. movement abnormality
    f. nerve
    f. nerve avulsion
    f. neuroma
    f. pain
    f. palsy
    f. paralysis
    f. perception
    f. spasm

    f. synkinesis
    f. vein
    f. vision

facialis
    vena f.

facies, pl. facies
    f. antonina
    f. bovina
    Hutchinson's f.

facility of outflow

facio-auriculovertebral spectrum

factitious
    f. blindness
    f. conjunctivitis
    f. mydriasis

factor
    antinuclear f.
    blood f. (M)
    coagulation f.
    diffusion f.
    epidermal growth f. (EGF)
    migration inhibition f.
      (MIF)
    quality f.
    rheumatoid f.
    spreading f.
    transfer f.
    vasoproliferative f.

facture energy

facultative
    f. hyperopia
    f. suppression

faculty
    fusion f.
    f. fusion

Faden's
    F. operation
    F. procedure

Faden suture

fading time

faecalis
    Streptococcus f.

Fahrenheit (F)

failure
    kidney f.
    lacrimal pump f.
    renal f.

faint flare

falciform
    f. fold of retina

falciform *(continued)*
    f. folds
    f. retinal fold
Falls-Kertesz syndrome
false
    f. blepharoptosis
    f. image
    f. macula
    f. projection
    f. ptosis
    f. vision
false-negative result
false-positive result
familial
    f. autonomic dysautonomia
    f. autonomic dysfunction
    f. colloid degeneration
    f. drusen
    f. dysautonomia
    f. exudative
    vitreoretinopathy
    f. fibrosis
    f. foveal retinoschisis
    f. hypercholesterolemic
    xanthomatosis
    f. idiocy
    f. lecithin:cholesterol acyl
    transferase deficiency
    f. lipoprotein deficiency
    f. pseudoinflammatory
    macular degeneration
    f. pseudoinflammatory
    maculopathy
    f. retinoblastoma
familiares
    cornea plana congenita f.
family study
FAN
    finger tension
fan
    sea f.
Fanconi's syndrome
fan-like
Fanta's cataract operation
fantascope
Fanta speculum
far
    f. point
    f. point of accommodation
    (fpa)
    f. point of convergence
    f. sight
Faraday (F)

Farber's disease
farinaceous
    f. epithelial keratitis
    f. keratitis
farinata
Farnsworth-Munsell
    F.-M. color test
    F.-M. 100-hue color test
    F.-M. 100-hue color vision
    test
Farnsworth's test
far-point convergence
farsighted
farsightedness
Fasanella
    F. lacrimal cannula
    F. retractor
Fasanella-Servat
    F.-S. procedure
    F.-S. ptosis operation
Fasanella's operation
fascia, pl. **fasciae**
    bulbar f.
    f. bulbi
    Crawford's f.
    f. lata
    f. lata frontalis
    f. lata frontalis sling
    f. lata musculares bulbi
    f. lata musculares oculi
    f. lata sling
    f. lata sling for ptosis
    operation
    f. lata stripper
    muscular f.
    f. musculares bulbi
    f. musculares oculi
    orbital f.
    fasciae orbitales
    palpebral f.
fascicle
fascicular
    f. keratitis
    f. ophthalmoplegia
    f. ulcer
fasciculus
    inferior f.
    inferior longitudinal f.
    longitudinal f.
    f. maculary
    medial longitudinal f.
    (MLF)
    median longitudinal f.

fasciitis
    nodular f.
    orbital f.
fashion
    McLean's f.
    stepwise f.
    in tumbling f.
fasting
    preoperative f.
fat
    f. cells
    f. embolism of retina
    f. embolus
    f. graft
    mutton f. (MF)
    orbital f.
    f. reticulum
fatigue nystagmus
fatty
    f. change
    f. exudate
Favre's
    F. disease
    F. dystrophy
FB
    foreign body
fc
    footcandle
Fc fragment
feathery clouding
Fechner intraocular lens
Federov
    F. four-loop iris clip
    F. four-loop iris clip lens
      implant
    F. lens
    F. type I intraocular lens
    F. type I lens implant
    F. type II intraocular lens
    F. type II lens implant
feeder-frond technique
feeder vessels
Fehr's macular dystrophy
Feister Dualens lens
felderstruktur fiber
Feldman
    F. adaptometer
    F. buffer solution
    F. RK optical center
      marker
fellow eye

felt
    f. disc polisher
    f. pad
fenestrae
fenestrated
    f. chain
    f. sheen macular dystrophy
fenestration
fenretinide
fentanyl
Fenzel
    F. angled manipulating
      hook
    F. insertion hook
    F. lens-manipulating hook
    F. manipulating hook
Féréol-Graux palsy
Ferguson implant
Fergus' operation
Ferree-Rand perimeter
Ferrein's canal
ferric ferrocyanide
Ferris' chart
Ferris-Smith
    F.-S. refractor
    F.-S. retractor
Ferris-Smith-Sewall
    F.-S.-S. refractor
    F.-S.-S. retractor
ferrocholinate
ferrocyanide
    ferric f.
ferrous
    f. fumarate
    f. gluconate
    f. succinate
    f. sulfate
Ferry-Porter law
Ferry's line
fetal
    f. alcohol syndrome
    f. development
    f. fibrovascular sheath
    f. fissure
    f. hydantoin syndrome
    f. trimethadione syndrome
    f. warfarin syndrome
    f. Y sutures
fetus
    harlequin f.
fever
    canicola f.
    cat-scratch f.

fever *(continued)*
drug f.
Fort Bragg f.
hay f.
Pel-Ebstein f.
pharyngoconjunctival f.
   (PCF)
Q f.
relapsing f.
rheumatic f.
Rocky Mountain spotted f.
spotted f.
uveoparotid f.
fiber
accessory f.
auxiliary f.
Bernheimer's f.'s
Brücke's f.
f. cells
chief f.
cilioequatorial f.
cilioposterocapsular f.
circular f.
circular ciliary muscle f.
collagen f.'s
cone f.
congenital medullated optic
   nerve f.'s
contiguous f.'s
continuous f.
corticonuclear f.
Edinger's f.'s
efferent f.'s
extraciliary f.
felderstruktur f.
fibrillenstruktur f.
Gratiolet's radiating f.
f.'s of Henle
interciliary f.
f. layer of axon
f. layer of Chievitz
lens f.
longitudinal f.
main f.
medullated nerve f.
meridional ciliary muscle f.
Mueller's f.
myelinated f.
myelinated nerve f.
nerve f.
oblique f.
optic nerve f.
f.'s of orbicularis oculi

f. orbicularis oculi
orbiculoanterocapsular f.
orbiculociliary f.
orbiculoposterocapsular f.
principal f.
pupilloconstrictor f.'s
Purkinje's f.'s
radial f.
Ritter's f.
rod f.
Rosenthal's f.'s
Sappey's f.
sphincter f.
sustentacular f.
trabecular f.
vitreous f.'s
von Monakow's f.
zonular f.
Fiberlite microscope
fiberoptic
f. diagnostic lens
f. light projector
f. pick
fiberscope
fibrae
f. circulares musculi ciliaris
f. lentis
f. longitudinales musculi
   ciliaris
f. meridionales musculi
   ciliaris
f. radiales musculi ciliaris
f. zonulares
Fibra Sonics phaco aspirator
fibril
fibrillar material
fibrillation
atrial f.
fibrillenstruktur fiber
fibrillogranuloma
fibrillopathia epitheliocapsularis
fibrin
f. dusting
intravitreal f.
f.-platelet embolus
postvitrectomy f.
f. pupillary block glaucoma
f. thrombus
fibrinitis
iritis f.
fibrinogen level
fibrinoid necrosis

fibrinous
    f. cataract
    f. iritis
    f. rhinitis
fibroangioma
    nasopharyngeal f.
fibroblast
fibroblastic
    f. ingrowth
    f. meningioma
fibrocystic disease
fibrocyte
fibroid cataract
fibroma
    orbital f.
fibromatosis
    orbital f.
fibronectin
    autogenous f.
fibro-osseous tumor
fibroplasia
    cicatricial retrolental f.
    retrolental f. (RLF)
fibroproliferative membrane
fibrosa
    pseudophakia f.
fibrosarcoma
    orbital f.
fibrosclerosis
    multifocal f.
fibrosis
    f. choroideae corrugans
    cyst f.
    cystic f.
    familial f.
    f. syndrome
fibrous
    f. coat of eye
    f. dysplasia
    f. fronds
    f. histiocytoma
    f. tunic
    f. tunic of eyeball
fibrovascular
    f. fronds
    f. sheath
    f. tunic
Fick
    anteroposterior axis of F.
    axis of F.
    longitudinal axis of F.
    sagittal axis of F.
    transverse axis of F.

    vertical axis of F.
    Z axis of F.
Fick's
    F. axis
    F. halo
field
    altitudinal f.
    automated visual f.
    binasal f.
    binasal quadrant f.'s
    binocular f.
    central f.'s
    checkerboard f.
    confrontation f.'s
    cribriform f.
    f. defect
    depth of f.
    f. diaphragm setting
    fixation f.
    f. of fixation
    Forel's f.
    frontal eye f.'s
    f. of gaze
    hysteric f.
    hysterical constricted f.
    keyhole f.
    f. lens
    f. loss
    peripheral f.
    receptive f.
    spiral f.
    star-shaped f.
    surplus f.
    temporal island of visual f.
    tubular visual f.'s
    f. of view
    f. of view error
    f. of vision
    visual f. (F, VF)
Fiessinger-Leroy-Reiter syndrome
fifth cranial nerve
figure
    fortification f.'s
    Purkinje's f.
    Stifel's f.
    Zöllner's f.
figure-of-eight suture
filament
    actin f.
    corneal f.
    cytoplasmic f.
    f. keratitis
    myosin f.

filamentary
    f. keratitis
    f. keratome
    f. keratopathy
filariasis
Filatov-Marzinkowsky operation
Filatov's
    F. keratoplasty
    F. operation
fil d'Arion silicone tube
filial generation (F)
filiform dystrophy
filiformis
    verruca f.
film
    absorbable gelatin f.
    aqueous layer of tear f.
    debris-laden tear f.
    gelatin f.
    precorneal f.
    precorneal tear f.
    tear f.
filter
    cobalt blue f.
    interference f.
    Millex f.
    Millipore f.
    neutral f.
    neutral density f.
    Polaroid f.
    red f.
    red free f.
    ultraviolet f.
    UV blocking f.
    Whatman f.
    Wrattan f.
filtering
    f. bleb
    f. cicatrix
    f. operation
    f. procedure
    f. wick
filtration
    f. angle
    f. surgery
fimbriated
    f. edge
    f. margin
final threshold
Fine
    F. corneal carrying case
    F. magnetic implant
    F. micropoint cautery

    F. micropoint electrocautery
    F. suture scissors
    F. suture-tying forceps
Fine-Castroviejo
    F.-C. forceps
    F.-C. suturing forceps
fine-dissecting forceps
fine iris processes
fine-toothed forceps
fine-wire speculum
finger
    f. count
    f. counting
    f. mimicking
    f. tension (FAN)
    f. vision
finger-count
finger-counting
    down to f.-c.
finger-like extensions
fingerprint
    f. corneal dystrophy
    f. dystrophy
    f. line
fingers
    counting f. (CF)
fining
finished
    f. contact lens
    f. glass
    f. lens
finite population
Fink
    F. biprong marker
    F. cataract aspirator
    F. cul-de-sac irrigator
    F. curette
    F. hook
    F. irrigating/aspirating unit
    F. irrigator
    F. lacrimal retractor
    F. muscle hook
    F. muscle marker
    F. oblique muscle hook
    F. refractor
    F. retractor
    F. tendon tucker
Fink-Jameson muscle forceps
Fink's operation
Fink-Weinstein two-way syringe
Finnoff transilluminator
first-degree relative
first-grade fusion

Fisher
    F. eye needle
    F. lid retractor
    F. spoon
    F. spud
Fisher-Arlt iris forceps
Fisher-Smith spatula
Fisher's syndrome
fishmouthing
fishmouth tear
Fison indirect binocular ophthalmoscope
fissura
    f. orbitalis inferior
    f. orbitalis superior
fissure
    calcarine f.
    choroid f.
    f. coloboma
    corneal f.
    eyelid f.'s
    fetal f.
    inferior orbital f.
    interpalpebral f.
    lid f.
    orbital f.
    orbital superior f.
    palpebral f.
    sphenoccipital f.
    sphenoidal f.
    sphenomaxillary f.
    superior orbital f. (SOF)
    water f.'s
    f. zone
fistula, pl. fistulae, fistulas
    carotid cavernous f.
    carotid cavernous sinus f.
    cavernous sinus f.
    f. of cornea
    corneal f.
    dural cavernous sinus f.
    ethmoid f.
    ethmoidal lacrimal f.
    internal lacrimal f.
    intraocular f.
    lacrimal f., f. lacrimalis
    scleral f.
    f. test
fistulizing surgery
fitting set
    diagnostic f. s.
fitting triangle
Fitz-Hugh-Curtis syndrome

fixate
fixating eye
fixation
    anomalous f.
    axis f.
    bifocal f.
    bifoveal f.
    binocular f.
    f. binocular forceps
    brow f.
    capsular f.
    central f.
    crossed f.
    f. disparity
    eccentric f.
    eyebrow f.
    f. field
    f. forceps
    four-point f.
    Guyton-Noyes f.
    f. hook
    f. instrument
    f. light
    monocular f.
    near f.
    f. nystagmus
    f. object
    f. pick
    pigtail f.
    f. point
    f. reflex
    f. ring
    split f.
    sulcus f.
    f. suture
    f. target
fixational ocular movement
fixation/anchor
    f./a. forceps
    f./a. pick
    f./a. ring
fixed
    f. dilated pupil
    f. folds
    f. forceps
    f. mydriasis
    f. point
    f. pupil
fixing eye
fixus
    strabismus f.
    vertical strabismus f.
FK506

flaccid
    f. canaliculus syndrome
    f. ectropion
Flajani's
    F. disease
    F. operation
flame
    f. hemorrhage
    f. photometer
    f. spots
flame-shaped hemorrhage
flammeus
    nevus f.
flap
    advancement f.
    bicoronal scalp f.
    Blaskovics' f.
    bridge pedicle f.
    cheek f.
    conjunctival f.
    conjunctivo-Tenon's f.
    Cutler-Beard bridge f.
    extraction f.
    fornix-based f.
    Gunderson's conjunctival f.
    Hughes tarsoconjunctival f.
    Imre's sliding f.
    limbal-based f.
    Mustarde rotational cheek f.
    f. operation cataract
    pedicle f.
    retinal f.
    scalp f.
    scleral f.
    skin f.
    sliding f.
    tarsoconjunctival f.
    Tenzel rotational cheek f.
    Truc's f.
    Van Lint's f.
flare
    aqueous f.
    cell and f. (C&F)
    f. and cell
    faint f.
Flarex
flash
    f. blindness
    f. electroretinogram
    f. keratoconjunctivitis
    f.'s of light
    f. ophthalmia

    f. picture cards
    f. visual evoked potential
flashlight
    f. examination
    f. test
flat
    f. anterior chamber
    f. chamber
    f. contact lens
    f. cornea
    f. cup
    f. eye spud
    f. hook
    f. lens
    f. and shallow
    f. top bifocal
Flatau-Schilder disease
flat-edge lens
flavimaculatus
flecked
    f. corneal dystrophy
    f. dystrophy
    f. dystrophy of cornea
    f. retina
    f. retina disease
    f. retina of Kandori
    f. retina syndrome
Fleischer's
    F. cataract
    F. dystrophy
    F. keratoconus ring
    F. ring
    F. vortex
Fleischer-Strumpell ring
fleken glaucoma
Flex-Care
flexible loop
flexible-wear
    f.-w. contact lens
    f.-w. lens
Flexlens lens
Flexner-Wintersteiner rosette
Flexsol
flick
    f. exotropia
    f. hypertropia
    f. movements
flicker
    f. perimetry
    f. phenomenon
    f. photometer

flicker-fusion
    f.-f. frequency technique
    f.-f. stimulus
Flieringa
    curved scleral-limbal incision of F.
    F. fixation ring
    F. ring
    F. scleral ring
Flieringa-Kayser
    F.-K. copper ring
    F.-K. fixation ring
Flieringa-Legrand fixation ring
flight blindness
flint
    barium f.
    f. glass
flint-glass lens
flittering scotoma
floater
    meniscus f.
    pigment f.
    vitreous f.
floor
    depression of orbital f.
    f. fracture
    orbital f.
floppy
    f. eyelid
    f. eyelid syndrome
flora
    ocular f.
Florentine's iris
florid
floriform cataract
Florinef
Floropryl
Flouren's law
floury cornea
flow
    aqueous f.
    axoplasmic f.
    laminar f.
    oxygen f.
floxuridine
Floyd-Barraquer wire speculum
Floyd-Grant erysiphake
fluconazole
flucytosine
fludrocortisone
fluff
    f. dressing
    vitreous f.

fluffed gauze dressing
fluid
    f. cataract
    cerebrospinal f. (CSF)
    f. contact lens
    intraocular f.
    f. lens
    f. mechanics
    subarachnoid f.
    subretinal f.
    viscous f.
    viscous ochre f.
    viscous xanthochromic f.
    xanthochromic f.
fluid-gas exchange
fluidless contact lens
Fluoracaine
fluorescein
    f. angiogram
    f. angiogram test
    f. angiography (FA)
    f. dilution test
    f. dye
    f. dye disappearance
    f. dye disappearance test
    f. dye and stain solution
    f. fundus angioscopy
    f. instillation test
    intravenous f. (IVF)
    sodium f.
    f. sodium
    f. staining
    f. test
fluorescein-conjugated lectin
fluorescence retinal photography
fluorescent
    f. antibody test
    f. lamp
    f. stain
    f. treponemal antibody test
Fluorescite
Fluoresoft
Fluorets
fluorexon
fluoride
    magnesium f.
fluorine (F)
Fluor-I-Strip
Fluor-I-Strip-A.T.
fluorite
fluorobiprofen
fluorocarbon
    f. in contact lens

fluorometholone
fluorometry
    noninvasive corneal redox f.
Fluor-Op
fluorophosphate
    diisopropyl f. (DFP)
fluorophotometer
fluorophotometry
    vitreous f.
Fluoroplex
fluoropolymer
fluoroquinolone
Fluorotron
    Coherent radiation F.
fluorouracil
5-fluorouracil (5-FU)
fluprednisolone
flurazepam
flurbiprofen sodium
Fluress
flush
    choroidal f.
    ciliary f.
flute needle
flutter
    eyelid f.
    f. of eyelid
    ocular f.
flux
    f. incident
    luminous f.
    oxygen f.
    radiant f.
    radiant and luminous f.
fly test
FM-100 test
FML
    FML Forte
    FML S.O.P.
FML-S
foam-appearing cytoplasm
foam cells
foaming exudate
focal
    f. choroiditis
    f. constriction
    f. depth
    f. distance
    f. granuloma
    f. illumination
    f. image point
    f. interval
    f. length

    f. point
    f. scotoma
foci
focimeter
focofilcon A
focus, pl. foci (F)
    aplanatic f.
    conjugate f.
    conjugate foci
    detectable foci
    image-space f.
    object-space f.
    principal f.
    principal foci
    real f.
    virtual f.
focusing
Föerster
    F. enucleation snare
    F. forceps
    F. iris forceps
    F. photometer
    F. photoptometer
Föerster-Fuchs black spot
Föerster's
    F. choroiditis
    F. conjunctiva
    F. disease
    F. lacrimal sac
    F. operation
    F. sacci lacrimalis
    F. spot
    F. uveitis
fogging
    f. retinoscopy
    f. system of refraction
foil sheet
Foix's
    F. enucleation
    F. syndrome
fold
    arcuate retinal f.'s
    choroidal f.
    ciliary f.'s
    concentric f.'s
    congenital retinal f.'s
    conjunctival f.
    conjunctival semilunar f.'s
    Descemet's f.'s
    epicanthal f.
    epicanthal skin f.
    epicanthine f.
    eyelid f.

falciform f.'s
falciform retinal f.
fixed f.'s
f. forceps
Hasner's f.'s
iridial f.'s
lacrimal f.'s
Lange's f.
meridional f.
mongolian f.
nasojugal f.
nasolabial f.
palpebral f.
palpebronasal f.
retinal fixed f.
retrotarsal f.
semilunar f.
star f.'s
stiff f.'s
stiff retinal f.
folding spectacles
folic
f. acid antagonist
f. acid deficiency
folinic acid
follicle
conjunctival f.
lymphoid f.
follicular
f. conjunctivitis
f. iritis
f. plugging
f. trachoma
follicularis
keratosis f.
folliculitis
f. externa
f. interna
folliculorum
Demodex f.
folliculosis
following
f. eye
f. movement
Foltz's valve
Fontana
space of F.
Fontana's
F. canal
F. space
food poisoning
footcandle (fc)
f. meter

footplate, foot plate
foramen, pl. **foramina**
Bozzi's f.
cranial foramina
cranial f.
inferior zygomatic f.
infraorbital f.
f. infraorbitale
lacerate f.
lacerate anterior f.
lacerate middle f.
lacerate posterior f.
f. lacerum anterius
optic f.
optic foramina
f. opticum
orbitomalar f.
rotundum f.
f. of sclera
Soemmering's f.
f. sphenoidalis
f. of sphenoid bone
supraorbital f.
f. supraorbitale
zygomatic f.
zygomaticofacial f.
zygomatico-orbital f.
f. zygomatico-orbitale
zygomaticotemporal f.
force (F)
muscle f.
forced
f. choice preferential
looking
f. duction
f. generation
f. generation test
forced-duction
f.-d. test
f.-d. testing
forced-eye closure
forceps
0.12 f.
Adson f.
Alabama University
utility f.
Allen-Barkan f.
Allen-Barker f.
Allen-Braley f.
Allis f.
Alvis fixation f.
Ambrose suture f.
Amenabar capsule f.

forceps *(continued)*
    angled capsule f.
    Anis f.
    Arroyo f.
    Arruga f.
    Arruga capsule f.
    Arruga-McCool capsule f.
    Asch septal f.
    Ayer chalazion f.
    Azar lens-holding f.
    Bailey chalazion f.
    Baird chalazion f.
    Ballen-Alexander f.
    Bangerter muscle f.
    Banner f.
    Bard-Parker f.
    Barkan iris f.
    Barraquer f.
    Barraquer cilia f.
    Barraquer conjunctival f.
    Barraquer corneal f.
    Barraquer corneal utility f.
    Barraquer hemostatic
      mosquito f.
    Barraquer-von Mondach
      capsule f.
    bayonet f.
    BB shot f.
    beaked f.
    Beaupre f.
    Beaupre cilia f.
    Bechert-McPherson angled
      tying f.
    Bennett f.
    Bennett cilia f.
    Berens f.
    Berens corneal transplant f.
    Berens muscle f.
    Berens ptosis f.
    Berens suturing f.
    Berke f.
    Berkeley Bioengineering
      ptosis f.
    Berke ptosis f.
    Bettman-Noyes fixation f.
    binocular fixation f.
    bipolar f.
    Birk-Mathelone micro f.
    Birks Mark II f.
    Birks Mark II Colibri f.
    Birks Mark II groove f.
    Birks Mark II grooved f.

    Birks Mark II micro
      needle-holder f.
    Birks Mark II straight f.
    Birks Mark II suture-
      tying f.
    Birks Mark II toothed f.
    Birks-Mathelone micro f.
    Bishop-Harman f.
    Bishop-Harman foreign
      body f.
    Bishop-Harman tissue f.
    Blaydes f.
    Blaydes corneal f.
    Blaydes lens-holding f.
    blepharochalasis f.
    Bonaccolto f.
    Bonaccolto fragment f.
    Bonaccolto jeweler f.
    Bonaccolto magnet tip f.
    Bonaccolto utility f.
    bone-biting f.
    Bonn f.
    Bonn iris f.
    Bonn suturing f.
    Boruchoff f.
    Botvin f.
    Botvin iris f.
    Bracken f.
    Bracken fixation f.
    Bracken iris f.
    Bronson-Magnion f.
    Bruining f.
    Calibri f.
    Callahan fixation f.
    capsule f.
    capsule fragment f.
    capsulorrhexis f.
    Cardona corneal
      prosthesis f.
    Cardona threading f.
    Castroviejo f.
    Castroviejo-Arruga f.
    Castroviejo capsule f.
    Castroviejo clip-applying f.
    Castroviejo-Colibri f.
    Castroviejo corneal-
      holding f.
    Castroviejo corneoscleral f.
    Castroviejo fixation f.
    Castroviejo lid f.
    Castroviejo scleral fold f.
    Castroviejo suture f.
    Castroviejo suturing f.

Castroviejo tying f.
Castroviejo wide grip handle f.
Catalano f.
Catalano corneoscleral f.
Catalano tying f.
chalazion f.
Chandler f.
Chandler iris f.
Choyce lens-inserting f.
Cilco lens f.
cilia f.
Clark capsule fragment f.
Clark-Verhoeff capsule f.
Clayman lens-holding f.
Clayman lens implant f.
Clayman lens-inserting f.
clip-applying f.
Cohan corneal f.
Cohen corneal f.
Coleman-Taylor IOL f.
Colibri f.
Colibri micro f.
conjunctiva f.
cornea-holding f.
corneal fixation f.
corneal prosthesis f.
corneal splinter f.
corneoscleral f.
Cozen-McPherson tying f.
Crawford f.
cross-action capsule f
Culler fixation f.
curved tying f.
Dallas lens-inserting f.
Danberg f.
Danberg iris f.
Dan chalazion f.
Dan-Gradle cilia f.
Davis f.
delicate serrated straight dressing f.
Desmarres f.
Desmarres chalazion f.
disk f.
Dixon-Thorpe vitreous foreign body f.
Dodick lens-holding f.
double-pronged f.
Douglas cilia f.
Draeger f.
dressing f.
Drews cilia f.

Drews-Sato tying f.
Eber needle-holder f.
Ehrhardt lid f.
Elschnig f.
Elschnig capsule f.
Elschnig fixation f.
Elschnig-O'Brien f.
Elschnig-O'Connor f.
Elschnig-O'Connor fixation f.
entropion f.
Erhardt lid f.
Ewing capsule f.
eyelid f.
Fine-Castroviejo f.
Fine-Castroviejo suturing f.
fine-dissecting f.
Fine suture-tying f.
fine-toothed f.
Fink-Jameson muscle f.
Fisher-Arlt iris f.
fixation f.
fixation/anchor f.
fixation binocular f.
fixed f.
Föerster f.
Föerster iris f.
fold f.
foreign body f.
Francis f.
Francis chalazion f.
Francis spud chalazion f.
Fuchs f.
Fuchs capsule f.
Fuchs extracapsular f.
Fuchs iris f.
Furniss cornea-holding f.
Gaskin fragment f.
Gelfilm f.
Gifford fixation f.
Gifford iris f.
Gill-Arruga capsular f.
Gill-Hess f.
Gill-Hess iris f.
Gill iris f.
Gills-Welsh capsule f.
Girard corneoscleral f.
Gradle f.
Gradle cilia f.
Graefe f.
Graefe dressing f.
Graefe eye dressing f.
Graefe fixation f.

forceps *(continued)*
Graefe iris f.
Graefe tissue f.
Grayson corneal f.
Grayton corneal f.
Grazer blepharoplasty f.
Green f.
Green capsule f.
Green chalazion f.
Green fixation f.
Grieshaber diamond
  coated f.
Grieshaber iris f.
f. guard
Guist fixation f.
Gunderson muscle f.
Guyton-Clark fragment f.
Guyton-Noyes fixation f.
Halberg contact lens f.
Halsted curved mosquito f.
Halsted curved mosquito
  hemostatic f.
Halsted mosquito
  hemostatic f.
Harman f.
Harman fixation f.
Harms corneal f.
Harms-Tubingen tying f.
Harms tying f.
Hartmann f.
Hartmann hemostatic f.
Hartmann mosquito
  hemostatic f.
Hasner lid f.
Heath f.
Heath chalazion f.
hemostatic f.
Hertel stone f.
Hess f.
Hess-Barraquer f.
Hessburg lens f.
Hessburg lens-inserting f.
Hess-Horwitz f.
Heyner f.
Hirschman lens f.
Hirschman lens-inserting f.
Holth f.
Hoskins f.
Hoskins beaked Colibri f.
Hoskins-Dallas intraocular
  lens-inserting f.
Hoskins fine straight f.
Hoskins fixation f.

Hoskins-Luntz f.
Hoskins micro straight f.
Hoskins miniaturized micro
  straight f.
Hoskins-Skeleton fine f.
Hoskins-Skeleton micro
  grooved broad-tipped f.
Hoskins straight micro
  iris f.
Hoskins suture f.
host tissue f.
House miniature f.
Hubbard f.
Hubbard corneoscleral f.
Hunt chalazion f.
Hyde f.
Hyde corneal f.
Hyde double curved f.
Ilg capsule f.
Ilg curved micro tying f.
Ilg insertion f.
intraocular f.
Iowa State fixation f.
iris f.
I-tech intraocular foreign
  body f.
I-tech splinter f.
I-tech tying f.
Jacob capsule fragment f.
Jaffe suturing f.
Jameson f.
Jameson muscle f.
Jansen-Middleton
  septotomy f.
Jensen intraocular lens f.
Jensen lens f.
Jensen lens-inserting f.
Jervey capsule fragment f.
Jervey iris f.
jeweler f.
Jones f.
Judd f.
Kalt f.
Katena f.
Katzin-Barraquer f.
Keeler extended round
  tip f.
Keeler intraocular foreign
  body grasping f.
Kelman-McPherson f.
Kelman-McPherson
  corneal f.
Kelman-McPherson tying f.

Kerrison f.
Kevorkian-Younge f.
King-Prince muscle f.
Kirby f.
Kirby capsule f.
Kirby corneoscleral f.
Kirby iris f.
Kirby tissue f.
Knapp f.
Koby cataract f.
Kraff intraocular utility f.
Kraff lens-inserting f.
Kraff suturing f.
Kraff tying f.
Kraff-Utrata
  capsulorrhexis f.
Kraff-Utrata intraocular
  utility f.
Kraft f.
Kratz lens-inserting f.
Kremer two-point fixation f.
Kronfeld f.
Kronfeld suturing f.
Krukenberg pigment
  spindle f.
Kuhnt f.
Kuhnt fixation f.
Kulvin-Kalt f.
Lambert f
Lambert chalazion f.
large-angled f.
Leakey chalazion f.
Leigh capsule f.
lens-holding f.
lens-threading f.
Lester fixation f.
lid f.
Lieberman-Polack double
  corneal f.
Lindstrom lens-insertion f.
Linn-Graefe iris f.
Lister f.
Littauer cilia f.
Llobera fixation f.
Lordan chalazion f.
Lucae dressing f.
Machemer diamond dust-
  coated foreign body f.
Machemer's diamond dust-
  coated foreign body f.
Malis f.
Manhattan f.

Manhattan Eye & Ear
  suturing f.
marginal chalazion f.
Maumenee f.
Maumenee capsule f.
Maumenee-Colibri corneal f.
Maumenee corneal f.
Maumenee Suregrip f.
Max Fine f.
McCullough f.
McCullough suturing f.
McGregor conjunctival f.
McGuire f.
McGuire marginal
  chalazion f.
McLean f.
McLean capsule f.
McLean muscle recession f.
McPherson f.
McPherson angled f.
McPherson bent f.
McPherson corneal f.
McPherson irrigating f.
McPherson micro iris f.
McPherson micro suture f.
McPherson tying f.
McPherson tying iris f.
McQueen vitreous f.
Mentor-Maumenee
  Suregrip f.
Metico f.
micro Colibri f.
miniature f.
Moehle f.
Moehle corneal f.
Moore lens f.
Moore lens-inserting f.
mosquito hemostatic f.
muscle f.
Neubauer f.
Nevyas lens f.
New Orleans Eye & Ear
  fixation f.
New York Eye & Ear
  Hospital fixation f.
Noble f.
Noyes f.
Nugent f.
Nugent fixation f.
Nugent rectus f.
Nugent superior rectus f.
O'Brien f.
O'Brien-Elschnig fixation f.

forceps *(continued)*
    O'Brien fixation f.
    Ochsner f.
    Ochsner cartilage f.
    Ochsner tissue f.
    Ochsner tissue/cartilage f.
    O'Connor-Elschnig
     fixation f.
    O'Connor iris f.
    O'Connor lid f.
    O'Connor sponge f.
    O'Gawa suture-fixation f.
    Ogura cartilage f.
    Ogura tissue f.
    Ogura tissue/cartilage f.
    Osher foreign body f.
    Paton anterior chamber lens
     implant f.
    Paton capsule f.
    Paton corneal transplant f.
    Paton suturing f.
    Paton tying/stitch
     removal f.
    Paufique suturing f.
    Pavlo-Colibri corneal f.
    Penn-Anderson fixation f.
    Penn-Anderson scleral
     fixation f.
    Perritt f.
    Perritt double-fixation f.
    Peyman-Green vitreous f.
    Phillips fixation f.
    Pierse f.
    Pierse corneal f.
    Pierse corneal Colibri-
     type f.
    Pierse fixation f.
    Pierse-Hoskins f.
    Pierse-type Colibri f.
    Pley f.
    Pley extracapsular f.
    Pollock f.
    Primbs suturing f.
    Prince f.
    Prince muscle f.
    ptosis f.
    Puntenny f.
    pupil spreader/retractor f.
    Quevedo fixation f.
    Quevedo suturing f.
    Quire mechanical finger f.
    Reese f.
    Reese muscle f.

    Reisinger lens-extracting f.
    Rhein fine foldable lens-
     insertion f.
    ring f.
    Ritch-Krupin-Denver eye
     valve insertion f.
    Rizzuti fixation f.
    Rizzuti-Furness cornea-
     holding f.
    Rizzuti rectus f.
    Rizzuti scleral fixation f.
    Rolf f.
    roller f.
    Russian f.
    Rycroft tying f.
    Sachs tissue f.
    Sanders-Castroviejo
     suturing f.
    Sandt f.
    Sauer f.
    Sauer suture f.
    Sauer suturing f.
    Schaaf f.
    Schaaf foreign body f.
    Schaefer fixation f.
    Scheie-Graefe fixation f.
    Schepens f.
    Schweigger f.
    Schweigger capsule f.
    Schweigger extracapsular f.
    scleral twist-grip f.
    Scott lens-insertion f.
    Sewall f.
    Sheets lens-inserting f.
    Sheets-McPherson tying f.
    Shepard f.
    Shepard intraocular lens f.
    Shepard intraocular utility f.
    Shepard lens-inserting f.
    Shepard-Reinstein f.
    Shepard tying f.
    Shields f.
    silicone rod and sleeve f.
    silicone sponge f.
    Simcoe lens implant f.
    Simcoe lens-inserting f.
    Simcoe nucleus f.
    Simcoe posterior chamber
     lens f.
    Sinskey micro tying f.
    Sinskey-Wilson foreign
     body f.
    Skeleton fine f.

sleeve spreading f.
Smart f.
Smart-Leiske cross-action
  intraocular lens f.
Smith-Leiske cross-action
  intraocular lens f.
Snellen entropion f.
Snyder corneal spring f.
Sparta micro f.
Spencer chalazion f.
Spero f.
splaytooth f.
Starr fixation f.
Stern-Castroviejo f.
Stern-Castroviejo locking f.
Stern-Castroviejo suturing f.
Stevens f.
Stevens iris f.
stitch-removal f.
Storz-Bonn suturing f.
Storz capsule f.
Storz cilia f.
Storz corneal f.
Storz-Utrata f.
strabismus f.
Strow corneal f.
superior rectus f.
suturing f.
Takahashi f.
Takahashi iris retractor f.
Tennant-Colibri corneal f.
Tennant lens f.
Tennant lens-inserting f.
Tennant titanium
  suturing f.
Tennant-Troutman superior
  rectus f.
Tenner titanium suturing f.
Tenzel f.
Terson capsule f.
Terson extracapsular f.
Thomas f.
Thomas fixation f.
Thornton fixation f.
Thorpe f.
Thorpe-Castroviejo
  corneal f.
Thorpe-Castroviejo
  fixation f.
Thorpe-Castroviejo vitreous
  foreign body f.
Thorpe conjunctival f.
Thorpe corneal f.

Thorpe foreign body f.
Thrasher lens implant f.
three-toothed f.
titanium suturing f.
Troutman f.
Troutman-Barraquer corneal
  fixation f.
Troutman-Barraquer corneal
  utility f.
Troutman-Castroviejo
  corneal fixation f.
Troutman-Llobera fixation f.
Troutman rectus f.
Troutman tying f.
tying f.
tying/stitch removal f.
Utrata f.
Utrata-Kershner
  capsulorrhexis cystome f.
Verhoeff f.
Verhoeff capsule f.
Vickerall round ringed f.
Vickers f.
vitreous f.
vitreous foreign body f.
von Graefe f.
von Graefe fixation f.
von Graefe iris f.
von Graefe tissue f.
von Mondak f.
von Mondak capsule
  fragment clot f.
Wadsworth lid f.
Wainstock suturing f.
Waldeau f.
Waldeau fixation f.
Watzke f.
Weaver chalazion f.
Welsh pupil-spreader f.
Whitney superior rectus f.
Wies chalazion f.
Wilde f.
Wilkerson f.
Wilkerson intraocular lens-
  insertion f.
Wills f.
Wills Hospital utility f.
Wills utility eye f.
Wolfe f.
Worth f.
Worth strabismus f.
Wullstein-House cup f.

forceps *(continued)*
    Ziegler f.
    Ziegler cilia f.
Fordyce's nodule
forebrain dysplasia
foreign
    f. body (FB)
    f. body bur
    f. body cell
    f. body extraction
    f. body forceps
    f. body locator
    f. body needle
    f. body sclerotomy
    f. body spud
Forel's field
Forker retractor
form
    f. sense
    f. vision
formaldehyde
    buffered f.
formation
    balloon cell f.
    midbrain reticular f.
    paramedian pontine
      reticular f. (PPRF)
    pontine paramedian
      reticular f.
    sac f.
    star f.
forme fruste
FormFlex
    F. lens
    F. lens loupe
formula
    Hoffer-Colenbrander f.
    lens maker's f.
    SRK f.
fornix, pl. **fornices**
    f. approach
    inferior f.
    inferior conjunctival f.
    lacrimal f.
    f. reformation
    f. sacci lacrimalis
    superior f.
    superior conjunctival f.
fornix-based flap
Forsius-Eriksson syndrome
forskolin
Forssman's carotid syndrome
Fort Bragg fever

Forte
    AK-Sulf F.
    FML F.
    Inflamase F.
    Lipo-Tears F.
    Liquifilm F.
    Naphcon F.
    Ocu-Pred F.
    Pred F.
    Predair F.
    Prednefrin F.
    Sulfair F.
fortification
    f. figures
    f. spectrum
fortified topical preparation
fortuitum
    Mycobacterium f.
forward traction test
foscarnet sodium
Foscavir
fossa, pl. **fossae**
    f. glandulae lacrimalis
    hyaloid f.
    f. hydoidea
    lacrimal f.
    lacrimal gland f.
    lacrimal sac f.
    lenticular f.
    optical f.
    patellar f.
    f. sacci lacrimalis
    trochlear f.
    f. trochlearis
    f. tumor
fossette
Foster
    F. enucleation snare
    F. Kennedy's syndrome
    F. snare enucleator
    F. suture
Fould's entropion operation
four base-out prism testing
four-dot test
four-loop
    f.-l. iris fixated implant
    f.-l. lens
four-loop
    f.-l. iris clip implant
four-mirror
    f.-m. goniolens
    f.-m. goniolens lens
four-point fixation

fourth
    f. cranial nerve
    f. nerve palsy
fovea, pl. **foveae**
    central f.
    f. centralis
    trochlear f.
    f. trochlearis
foveal
    f. avascular zone
    f. cyst
    f. dystopia
    f. flicker fusion frequency
    f. image
    f. reflex
    f. vision
foveate
foveation
foveola, pl. **foveolae**
    f. ocularis
    retinal f.
foveolar reflex
foveomacular
    f. retinitis
    f. retinopathy
    f. vitelliform dystrophy
Foville's syndrome
Foville-Wilson syndrome
Fox
    F. aluminum shield
    F. conformer
    F. eye shield
    F. implant
    F. irrigating/aspirating unit
    F. shield
    F. speculum
    F. sphere implant
Fox's
    F. eye
    F. operation
FP
    fundus photos
fpa
    far point of accommodation
fraction
    Snellen f.
fracture
    apex f.
    blow-out f.
    blow-out f. of orbit
    combined f.
    comminuted orbital f.
    depressed f.

    external orbital f.
    floor f.
    midfacial f.
    naso-orbital f.
    f. of orbit
    orbital f.
    orbital blow-out f.
    orbital floor f.
    orbital rim f.
    orbital wall f.
    roof f.
    zygomatic f.
fragilitas ossium
fragmatome
    CooperVision f.
    Gill-Hess f.
    Girard f.
Fragmatome flute syringe
fragment
    Cooper blade f.
    Fab f.
    Fc f.
    Hoskins razor blade f.
fragmentation/aspiration handpiece
fragmentor
    Lieberman f.
frame
    celluloid f.
    cellulose acetate f.
    cellulose nitrate f.
    Lucite f.
    molded f.
    MTL trial f.
    nylon f.
    optical f.
    Optyl f.
    Perspex f.
    plastic f.
    Plexiglas f.
    polymethyl methacrylate f.
    rimless f.
    f. scotoma
    spectacle f.
    Stryker f.
    trial f.
    xylonite f.
    zyl f.
    zylonite f.
framework
    scleral f.
    uveal f.
framing
Franceschetti-Klein syndrome

Franceschetti's
F. coreoplasty operation
F. corepraxy operation
F. deviation operation
F. disease
F. dystrophy
F. keratoplasty operation
F. mandibulofacial
 dysostosis
F. operation
F. pupil deviation operation
F. syndrome
Franchesseti
oculodigital sign of F.
Francis
F. chalazion forceps
F. forceps
F. spud
F. spud chalazion forceps
Francis' disease
Francisela tularensis
François
central cloudy dystrophy
 of F.
dermochondral corneal
 dystrophy of F.
dyscephalic syndrome of F.
F. dystrophy
F. syndrome
Frankfort horizontal plane
Franklin
F. bifocal
F. glasses
F. spectacles
Franklin-style bifocal lenses
Fraser's syndrome
Fraunfelder's "no touch" technique
Fraunhofer's
F. diffraction
F. line
freckle
Hutchinson's f.'s
iris f.'s
free
f. energy (F)
f. margin of eyelid
f. running mode
f. skin autograft
f. tenotomy
Freeman
F. punctum plug
F. solution
Freeman-Sheldon syndrome

Freer
F. chisel
F. elevator
F. periosteal elevator
freeze
Keeler-Amoils f.
freeze-thaw cryotherapy
Frelex lens
French
F. catheter
F. hook spatula
F. lacrimal dilator
F. lacrimal probe
F. lacrimal spatula
F. needle holder
F. pattern spatula
**Frenkel's anterior ocular traumatic
syndrome**
Frenzel lens
frequency
critical corresponding f.
 (CCF)
critical flicker fusion f.
foveal flicker fusion f.
fusion f.
Fresnel
F. lens
F. membrane
F. optics
F. press-on prism
F. prism
Fresnel's principle
Frey
F. implant
F. tunneled implant
Frey's syndrome
Fricke's operation
Fridenberg's stigometric card test
Friedenwald
F. funduscope
F. ophthalmoscope
Friedenwald-Guyton operation
Friedenwald's
F. operation
F. syndrome
Friede's operation
Friedman
F. clip
F. hand-held Hruby lens
F. tantalum clip
Friedman-Hruby lens
Friedmann visual field analyzer

Friedreich's
  F. ataxia
  F. syndrome
Frigitronics
  Cilco F.
  F. cryosurgery apparatus
  F. cryosurgical unit
  F. freeze-thaw cryopexy
    probe
  F. nitrous oxide cryosurgery
    apparatus
  F. vitrector
frill
  plaited f.
Frin
  Isopto F.
fringe
  interference f.
  Moiré's f.
Fritz vitreous transplant needle
frog cortex remover
frog face
fronds
  fibrous f.
  fibrovascular f.
  sea f.
  vascular f.
frons
  f. cranii
  f. of cranium
front
  f. build-up implant
  f. surface toric contact lens
  f. vertex
frontal
  f. axis
  f. bone
  f. craniotomy
  f. diploic vein
  f. eye fields
  f. incisure
  f. nerve
  f. sinus
  f. sinusitis
  f. triangle
  f. tuber
frontalis
  facies orbitalis ossis f.
  fascia lata f.
  incisura f.
  incisura ethmoidalis ossis f.
  margo supraorbitalis ossis f.
  f. muscle

  f. muscle sling
  pars orbitalis ossis f.
  f. sling technique
  sulcus orbitales lobi f.
  vena diploica f.
frontispiece
frontolacrimalis
  sutura f.
frontolacrimal suture
frontosphenoid suture
Frost
  F. scissors
  F. suture
Frost-Lang operation
frozen globe
fruste
  forme f.
  keratoconus f.
FTA-absorption test
5-FU
  5-fluorouracil
Fuchs
  F. capsule forceps
  F. extracapsular forceps
  F. forceps
  F. iris forceps
  F. lancet type keratome
  F. retinal detachment
    syringe
  F. two-way syringe
Fuchs'
  F. adenoma
  F. aphakic keratopathy
  F. atrophy
  F. black spot
  F. canthorrhaphy operation
  F. coloboma
  F. combined corneal
    dystrophy
  combined dystrophy of F.
  F. crypt
  F. cyclitis
  F. dimple
  F. dystrophy
  F. endothelial corneal
    dystrophy
  F. endothelial dystrophy
  F. endothelial-epithelial
    dystrophy
  F. epithelial corneal
    dystrophy
  F. epithelial dystrophy
  epithelial dystrophy of F.

Fuchs' *(continued)*
    F. epithelial-endothelial
      dystrophy
    F. heterochromia
    F. heterochromic cyclitis
    F. heterochromic
      iridocyclitis
    F. inferior coloboma
    F. iris bombe transfixation
      operation
    F. keratitis
    lamella of F.
    F. operation
    F. spot
    F. spot coloboma
    F. spur
    F. syndrome
    F. uveitis
Fuchs-Kraupa syndrome
fucosidosis
fugax
    amaurosis partialis f.
    episcleritis partialis f.
    saburral amaurosis f.
Fukala's operation
Ful-Glo
Ful-Glo-Strips
full-dimpled Lucite implant
Fuller silicone sponge
full-thickness
    f.-t. autograft
    corneal f.-t.
    f.-t. corneal graft
    f.-t. graft
full versions and ductions
fulminant
    f. glaucoma
    f. myasthenia gravis
    f. ocular toxoplasmosis
Ful-Vue
    F.-V. bifocal
    F.-V. ophthalmoscope
    F.-V. spot retinoscope
    F.-V. streak retinoscope
fumarate
    ferrous f.
fumigatus
    Aspergillus f.
function
    bandpass f.
    cone f.
    Easterman's visual f.
    modulation transfer f.

    motor f.
    rod f.
    spread f.
    transfer f.
    visual f.
functional
    f. amblyopia
    f. blindness
    f. defect
    f. visual loss
fundal reflex
fundectomy
fundus, pl. **fundi**
    albinotic f.
    f. albipunctalis
    albipunctate f.
    f. albipunctatus
    blond fundi
    f. camera
    coloboma of f.
    f. contact lens
    f. diabeticus
    f. of eye
    f. flavimaculatus
    f. focalizing lens
    Kowa f.
    f. laser lens
    leopard f.
    f. microscopy
    mottling of f.
    normal f.
    f. oculi
    pepper and salt f.
    f. photos (FP)
    f. polycythemicus
    prismatic f.
    f. reflex
    salt and pepper f.
    tessellated f.
    f. tigré
    tigroid f.
    tomato-ketchup f.
    f. xerophthalmicus
Funduscein
Funduscein-10
Funduscein-25
funduscope
    Friedenwald f.
funduscopic examination
funduscopy
fundusectomy
fungal
    f. blepharitis

f. corneal ulcer
f. endophthalmitis
f. infection
f. keratitis
f. uveitis
fungating
fungi
Fungizone
fungoides
mycosis f.
fungus, pl. **fungi**
funnel
muscular f.
vascular f.
funnel-shaped retinal detachment
Furadantin
furnacemen's cataract
Furniss cornea-holding forceps
furosemide
furrow
corneal marginal f.
f. degeneration
f. dystrophy
f. keratitis
marginal f.
palpebral f.
scleral f.
superior palpebral f.
Fusarium
F. solani
fuscu
lamina f.
membrana f.
fuscin
fused
f. bifocal
f. bifocal lens
f. multifocal lens
fusiform
f. aneurysm
f. cataract

fusion
amplitude of f.
f. area
binocular f.
f. breakpoint
central f.
color f.
eyelid f.
faculty f.
f. faculty
first-grade f.
flicker-f.
f. frequency
f. grade
motor f.
peripheral f.
f. reflex
second-grade f.
sensory f.
third-grade f.
f. tube
f. with accommodation
f. with amplitude
Worth's concept of f.
fusional
f. convergence
f. convergence amplitude
f. divergence
f. divergence amplitude
f. movement
f. reserve
f. vergence
fusional area
Panum's f. a.
fusion-free
f.-f. position

GABA
γ-aminobutyric acid
Gaffee speculum
Gaillard-Arlt suture
galactocerebroside
galactokinase
galactose cataract
galactosemia
g. cataract
enzymatic g.
β-galactosidase
galactosyl ceramide lipidosis
Galassi's pupillary phenomenon
Galen's vein
galeropia
galeropsia
Galezowski lacrimal dilator
Galilean
G. magnification changer
G. telescope
Galin
G. bleb cup
G. intraocular implant lens
G. lens
Gallic cryoenucleator
gallium
g. citrate contrast
g. citrate contrast material
g. scan
g. scanning
Galt aspirating cannula
galvanic nystagmus
Gamboscope
game
E g.
gamma
g. angle
g. crystallin
ganciclovir sodium
ganglion, pl. ganglia
basal g.
g. cell
g. cell layer
cervical g.
ciliary g.
gasserian g.
g. layer of optic nerve
g. layer of retina
lenticular g.

long root of ciliary g.
motor root of ciliary g.
oculomotor root of
ciliary g.
ophthalmic g.
optic g.
orbital g.
retinal g.
Schacher's g.
sensory root of ciliary g.
short root of ciliary g.
g. stratum of optic nerve
superior cervical g.
ganglioneuroma
ganglionic
g. layer of optic nerve
g. layer of retina
g. stratum of optic nerve
g. stratum of retina
ganglionitis
ganglioside
gangliosidosis
G_{M1} g.
G_{M2} g.
generalized g.
juvenile GM_1 g.
juvenile GM_2 g.
gangliosus ciliaris
gangraenescens
granuloma g.
gangrenosa
vaccinia g.
gangrenosum
ecthyma g.
gangrenous rhinitis
Gans
G. cannula
G. cyclodialysis cannula
Gantrisin
Ganzfeld
G. electroretinograph
G. stimulation
Garamycin
Garcia-Ibanez camera
Garcia-Novito
G.-N. eye implant
G.-N. implant
Gardner's syndrome
gargoylism

garter
Goffman eye g.
Gas
gas
g. bubble
g. discharge lamp
hexafluoride g.
inspired g. (I)
intraocular g.
laughing g.
mustard g.
octofluoropropane g.
perfluoropropane g.
sulfur g.
g. tamponade
tear g.
gas-fluid exchange
Gaskin fragment forceps
gas-permeable
g.-p. contact lens
g.-p. lens
g.-p.-permeable daily cleaner
Gass
G. cannula
G. cataract aspirating
cannula
G. corneoscleral punch
G. dye applicator
G. irrigating/aspirating unit
G. muscle hook
G. retinal detachment hook
G. scleral marker
G. scleral punch
G. sclerotomy punch
G. vitreous aspirating
cannula
gasserian ganglion
Gaucher's disease
gauge
blade g.
coin g.
depth g.
Marco radius g.
radius g.
Reichert radius g.
Shepard incision depth g.
Stahl lens g.
V-groove g.
Gaule's
G. pit
G. spot
Gault's reflex
gaussian optical system

Gaussian's distribution
Gayet's operation
gaze
apraxia of g.
cardinal direction of g.
cardinal position of g.
g. center
conjugate g.
diagnostic positions of g.
disconjugate g.
distant g.
downward g.
dysconjugate g.
eccentric g.
evoked nystagmus g.
g. evoked tinnitus
field of g.
horizontal g.
left g.
midline position of g.
g. movement
near g.
near fixation position of g.
g. nystagmus
g. palsy
parallelism of g.
paralysis of g.
g. paretic nystagmus
ping-pong g.
primary position of g.
right g.
spasticity of conjugate g.
upward g.
vertical g.
gaze-evoked nystagmus
gaze-holding
G-banding
GCA
giant cell arteritis
Geiger
G. cautery
G. electrocautery
Gel
G. Clean
Gonio G.
gel
acoustical conductive g.
Aquasonic 100 g.
silica g.
vitreous g.
gelatin
g. disk
g. film

gelatinous
g. material
g. scleritis
gelatinous-appearing limbal hypertrophy
Gel-Clean
Gelfilm
G. cap
G. forceps
G. implant
G. plate
G. retinal implant
Schepens G.
Gelfoam
gene
dominant g.
g. locus
nonpenetrant g.
penetrant g.
syntenic g.'s
general
g. anesthesia
g. anesthetic
g. cataract
generalized
g. gangliosidosis
g. vaccinia
generating spectacle lens
generation
filial g. (F)
forced g.
Genesis lens
genetic
g. counseling
g. disease
g. screening
geneticist
genetics
biochemical g.
clinical g.
molecular g.
Geneva lens measure
geniculate
g. body
g. hemianopsia
g. nucleus
geniculocalcarine
g. radiation
g. tract
genome
Genoptic S.O.P.
genotype
Gentacidin

Gentafair
Gentak
gentamicin, gentamycin
gentian violet marking pen
Gentrasul
geographic
g. choroidopathy
g. helicoid peripapillary choroidopathy
g. herpes simplex corneal ulcer
g. keratitis
g. lesions
g. peripapillary choroiditis
geometric
g. axis
g. center
g. equator
g. optics
g. perspective
Geopen
Georgariou's cyclodialysis operation
German
G. Hefner candle
G. measles
germicide
germinoblast
gerontopia
gerontoxon lentis
Gerstmann's syndrome
gestational
g. diabetes
g. diabetes mellitus
Geuder
G. implanter
G. keratoplasty needle
G_{M2} gangliosidosis
G_{M1} gangliosidosis
Ghormley double cannula
ghost
Bidwell's g.
g. cell glaucoma
g. cells
dendritic g.'s
g. erythrocyte
g. image
g. ophthalmoscope
g. vessel
Gianelli's sign
giant
g. axonal neuropathy
bipolar g.
g. cell

177

giant *(continued)*
- g. cell arteritis (GCA)
- g. cyst of retina
- g. drusen
- g. epithelial cell
- g. papillae
- g. papillary conjunctivitis (GPC)
- g. papillary hypertrophy (GPH)
- g. retinal break
- g. tear

Giardet corneal transplant scissors
Gibralter headrest
Gibson
- G. irrigating/aspirating unit

Giemsa stain
Gierke's disease
Gifford
- G. applicator
- G. corneal curette
- G. curette
- G. fixation forceps
- G. iris forceps
- G. needle holder

Gifford-Galassi reflex
Gifford's
- G. delimiting keratotomy operation
- G. operation
- G. reflex
- G. sign

gigantism
- pituitary g.

Gilchrist's disease
Gill
- G. blade
- G. corneal knife
- G. counterpressor
- G. incision spreader
- G. intraocular implant lens
- G. iris forceps
- G. knife
- G. scissors

Gill-Arruga capsular forceps
Gill-Fine corneal knife
Gill-Hess
- G.-H. blade
- G.-H. forceps
- G.-H. fragmatome
- G.-H. iris forceps
- G.-H. knife
- G.-H. scissors

Gillies'
- G. operation
- G. scar correction operation

Gills
- G. double irrigating-aspirating cannula
- G. double Luer-Lok cannula
- G. irrigating-aspirating cannula

Gills-Welsh
- G.-W. aspirating cannula
- G.-W. capsule forceps
- G.-W. capsule polisher
- G.-W. curette
- G.-W. double-barreled irrigating-aspirating cannula
- G.-W. guillotine port
- G.-W. irrigating-aspirating cannula
- G.-W. knife
- G.-W. olive-tip cannula
- G.-W. scissors
- G.-W. spatula
- G.-W. Vannas angled micro scissors

Gills-Welsh-Vannas scissors
Gilmore
- G. intraocular implant lens
- G. lens

Girard
- G. anterior chamber needle
- G. cataract aspirating needle
- G. corneoscleral forceps
- G. corneoscleral scissors
- G. fragmatome
- G. irrigating cannula
- G. irrigating tip
- G. phacofragmatome needle
- G. phakofragmatome
- G. scleral-expander ring
- G. Ultrasonic unit

Girard's
- G. keratoprosthesis operation
- G. procedure

Girard-Swan knife-needle
Giraud-Teulon law
girdle
- limbal g.
- limbus g.
- Vogt's limbal g.
- Vogt's white limbal g.

girth hitch
Gish micro YAG laser
Givner lid retractor
glabella
glabellar
glabellum
Gladstone-Putterman
    G.-P. entropion clamp
    G.-P. transmarginal rotation
      entropion clamp
gland
    acinar lacrimal g.
    apocrine g.
    Baumgarten's g.
    Bruch's g.
    Ciaccio's g.
    ciliary g.
    conjunctival g.
    drainage of lacrimal g.
    harderian g.
    Harder's g.
    Henle's g.
    inferior lacrimal g.
    Krabbe's disease g.
    Krause's g.
    Krause's lacrimal g.
    lacrimal g.
    Manz's g.
    meibomian g.
    Moll's g.
    Mueller's g.
    nasolacrimal g.
    palpebral g.
    pineal g.
    pituitary g.
    Rosenmüller's g.
    salivary g.
    sebaceous g's of
      conjunctiva g.
    superior lacrimal g.
    sweat g.
    tarsal g.
    tarsoconjunctival g.
    trachoma g.
    g. trachoma
    Waldeyer's g.
    g. of Wolfring
    Wolfring's g.
    Wolfring's lacrimal g.
    Zeis g.'s
    g. of Zeis
    zeisian g.
glanders

glands of eyelid
glandula
    g. lacrimalis
    g. lacrimalis inferior
    g. lacrimalis superior
glandulae
    g. ciliares conjunctivales
    g. conjunctivales
    g. lacrimales accessoriae
    g. mucosae conjunctivae
    g. sebaceae conjunctivales
    g. tarsales
glandular fossa of frontal bone
glare
    blinding g.
    dazzling g.
    direct g.
    peripheral g.
    specular g.
    g. test
    veiling g.
glarometer
glass
    g. bifocal
    Chavasse g.
    Crookes g.
    crown g.
    finished g.
    flint g.
    High-Lite g.
    g. lens
    optical g.
    semifinished g.
    g. sphere implant
glassblower's cataract
Glasscock scissors
glasses
    bifocal g.
    cataract g.
    contact g.
    crutch g.
    Difei g.
    Franklin g.
    Grafco magnifying g.
    Hallauer g.
    hemianopic g.
    hyperbolic g.
    magnifying g.
    Masselon g.
    presbyopia g.
    reading g.
    safety g.

glasses *(continued)*
    striated g.
    trifocal g.
glassine strands
glass-rod
    g.-r. negative phenomenon
    g.-r. positive phenomenon
glassworker's cataract
glassy
    g. membrane
    g. sheets
glaucoma
    absolute g.
    g. absolutum
    acute g.
    acute angle-closure g.
      (AACG)
    acute chronic g.
    acute congestive g.
    air-block g.
    alpha-chymotrypsin g.
    alpha-chymotrypsin-
      induced g.
    angle-closure g. (ACG)
    angle-recession g.
    aphakic g.
    apoplectic g.
    auricular g.
    capsular g.
    chamber-deepening g.
    chronic g.
    chronic angle-closure g.
    chronic narrow-angle g.
    chronic open-angle g.
      (COAG)
    chronic simple g.
    α-chymotrypsin-induced g.
    ciliary block g.
    closed-angle g.
    combined g.
    combined-mechanism g.
    compensated g.
    congenital g.
    congestive g.
    g. consummatum
    Contino's g.
    contusion g.
    contusion angle g.
    corticosteroid-induced g.
    cyclocongestive g.
    90-day g.
    Donders' g.
    drug-induced g.

    enzymatic g.
    enzyme g.
    erythroclastic g.
    exfoliation g.
    fibrin pupillary block g.
    g. field defect
    fleken g.
    g. fulminans
    fulminant g.
    ghost cell g.
    hemolytic g.
    hemorrhagic g.
    herpes zoster g.
    hypersecretion g.
    g. imminens
    infantile g.
    inflammatory g.
    intermittent angle-closure g.
    juvenile g.
    latent angle-closure g.
    lens exfoliation g.
    lens-induced g.
    lenticular g.
    low-pressure g.
    low-tension g.
    malignant g.
    melanomalytic g.
    monocular g.
    mydriatic test for g.
    mydriatic test for angle-
      closure g.
    narrow-angle g. (NAG)
    neovascular g. (NVG)
    neovascular angle-closure g.
    noncongestive g.
    obstructive g.
    ocular hypertension g.
    ocular hypertensive g.
    open-angle g. (OAG)
    g. pencil
    phacogenic g.
    phacolytic g.
    phacomorphic g.
    phakogenic g.
    phakolytic g.
    phakomorphic g.
    pigmentary g.
    pigmentary dispersion g.
    primary g.
    primary angle-closure g.
    primary infantile g.
    primary open-angle g.
      (POAG)

prodromal g.
pseudoexfoliative capsular g.
pseudoglaucoma g.
pupil block g.
pupillary block g.
recessed-angle g.
recession-angle g.
retrobulbar hemorrhage g.
scleral shell g.
secondary g.
simple g., g. simplex
simplex g.
steroid g.
steroid-induced g.
g. surgery
trabeculitis g.
traumatic g.
uveitic g.
vitreous block g.
wide-angle g.
glaucomatocyclitic crisis
glaucomatous
g. atrophy
g. cataract
g. cul-de-sac
g. cup
g. cupping
g. excavation
g. habit
g. halo
g. nerve-fiber bundle
scotoma
g. optic nerve damage
(GOND)
g. pannus
g. ring
Glaucon
glaucosis
Glaucotest
glaukomflecken of Vogt
glia
glial
g. cell
g. proliferation
g. ring
glide
Hessburg intraocular lens g.
intraocular lens g.
lens g.
Sheets g.
Sheets lens g.
glioblastoma multiforme

gliocyte
retinal g.
glioma
astrocytic g.
chiasmal g.
g. endophytum
g. exophytum
hypothalamic g.
intracranial g.
optic g.
g. of optic chiasm
optic nerve g.
orbital g.
peripheral g.
g. of retina
retinal g.
g. sarcomatosum
telangiectatic g.
gliomatosis
gliomatous
glioneuroma
gliosarcoma
retinal g.
gliosis
neonatal g.
premacular g.
retinal g.
traumatic g.
gliotic
g. membrane
g. strip
glissade
glissadic
global
globe
contact burns of g.
contusion of g.
disorganized g.
frozen g.
luxation of g.
ruptured g.
globoid cell leukodystrophy
globosa
cornea g.
globule, pl. globuli, globules
morgagnian g.
Morgagni's g.
ora g.
globulin
glomerulonephritis
glory
morning g.

glower
Nernst g.
glucocorticoid
systemic g.
topical g.
gluconate
ferrous g.
Glucose-40
glucose
g. 6-phosphate
dehydrogenase
β-glucuronidase
glue
butyl cyanoacrylate g.
ethyl cyanoacrylate g.
histoacryl g.
methyl cyanoacrylate g.
g. patch
g. patch leak
glued-on hard contact lens
glutaraldehyde
glutathione
glycerin
glycerine
glyceringlycerol
glycerol
anhydrase g.
glyceryl monostearate
glycogen
g. granule
g. storage disease
glycogenesis
hepatorenal g.
glycohemoglobin
glycol
ethylene g.
polyethylene g. (PEG)
propylene g.
glycolipid
g. lipidosis
g. metabolism
glycosaminoglycan
glycoside
cardiac g.
digitalis g.
glycosphingolipid lipidosis
Glyrol
goblet cell
Goffman eye garter
goggle
night-vision g.
pinhole g.
plethysmographic g.

goiter
exophthalmic g.
gold
g. dust retinopathy
g. salts
g. sodium thiomalate
g. sphere implant
gold-198 (^{198}Au)
Goldberg's syndrome
Goldenhar's syndrome
Goldmann
G. applanation tonometer
G. contact lens
G. contact lens prism
G. diagnostic contact lens
G. fundus contact lens
G. goniolens
G. implant
G. lens
G. macular contact lens
G. multi-mirrored lens
G. prism
G. serrated knife
G. three-mirror implant
G. three-mirror lens
G. three-mirror prism
G. tonometer
Goldmann-Favre
G.-F. disease
G.-F. dystrophy
G.-F. syndrome
Goldmann-Larson
G.-L. foreign body
G.-L. foreign body
operation
Goldmann's
G. coherent radiation
G. kinetic perimetry
G. kinetic technique
G. perimeter
G. perimetry
G. static technique
Goldmann-Weeker dark
adaptometer
Gold-Mules implant
Goldstein
G. anterior chamber syringe
G. cannula
G. golf club spud
G. lacrimal sac retractor
G. lacrimal syringe
G. refractor

G. retractor
G. syringe
golf-club
g.-c. eye spud
g.-c. spud
Golgi
G. apparatus
G. II neuron
G. I neuron
G. neurons
Golgi's complex
Goltz-Gorlin syndrome
Goltz syndrome
Gomez-Marquez
G.-M. lacrimal operation
Gonak Gonioscopic
GOND
glaucomatous optic nerve
damage
gondii
Toxoplasma g.
gonia
gonial
gonin
G. cautery
G. marker
Gonin-Amsler marker
Gonin's
G. cautery operation
G. operation
goniodysgenesis
goniofocalizing lens
Gonio Gel
goniogram
Becker g.
goniolaser
Thorpe four-mirror g.
goniolens
Allen-Thorpe g.
Barkan g.
four-mirror g.
Goldmann g.
Koeppe g.
g. lens
single-mirror g.
Thorpe-Castroviejo g.
Thorpe four-mirror g.
Zeiss g.
goniometer
Bailliart g.
goniophotocoagulation
goniophotography
gonioplasty

gonioprism
Posner g.
Posner diagnostic g.
Posner surgical g.
Swan-Jacob g.
goniopuncture knife
gonioscope
Jacob-Swann g.
Lovac g.
Sussman four-mirror g.
Thorpe surgical g.
Troncoso g.
Zeiss g.
Gonioscopic
Gonak G.
gonioscopic
g. implant
g. lens
g. prism
gonioscopy
indentation g.
Goniosol
goniospasis
goniosynechia
goniosynechiae
goniotomy
g. knife
g. knife cannula
g. needle holder
g. operation
gonoblennorrhea
gonococcal
g. bacillus
g. conjunctivitis
g. disease
gonococcus
gonorrhea
gonorrheal
g. conjunctivitis
g. ophthalmia
gonorrhoeae
Neisseria g.
Good retractor
Goppert's sign
gossamer scarring
gouge
lacrimal sac g.
spud g.
g. spud
Todd g.
West g.
Gould intraocular implant lens

183

gout
    g. conjunctivitis
gouty
    g. diabetes
    g. episcleritis
    g. episcleritis disease
    g. iritis
Gower's sign
GP
GPC
    giant papillary conjunctivitis
GPH
    giant papillary hypertrophy
graceful swirling rods
grade
    fusion g.
Gradenigo's syndrome
gradient method
grading
    Broders' g.
Gradle
    G. cilia forceps
    G. corneal trephine
    G. electrode
    G. forceps
    G. operation
    G. refractor
    G. retractor
Gradle's keratoplasty operation
graduated tenotomy
Graefe
    G. cataract knife
    G. cystitome
    G. cystitome knife
    G. dressing forceps
    G. eye dressing forceps
    G. fixation forceps
    G. forceps
    G. hook
    G. iris forceps
    G. knife
    G. needle
    G. strabismus hook
    G. tissue forceps
Graefe's
    G. disease
    G. operation
    G. sign
    G. syndrome
Graether
    G. button-hook
    G. collar-button

    G. collar-button micro iris retractor
    G. collar-button retractor
    G. mushroom hook
    G. refractor
    G. retractor
Grafco
    G. eye shield
    G. magnifying glasses
graft
    Amsler's corneal g.
    annular corneal g.
    autogenous dermis fat g.
    bone g.
    g. carrier spoon
    conjunctival g.
    conjunctival patch g.
    corneal g.
    crescent g.
    crescent corneal g.
    dermis-fat g.
    dermis patch g.
    donor g.
    fat g.
    full-thickness g.
    full-thickness corneal g.
    g. infection
    lamellar g.
    lamellar corneal g.
    Marquez-Gomez conjunctival g.
    mucous membrane g.
    mushroom g.
    mushroom corneal g.
    Mustarde's g.
    patch g.
    pattern-cut corneal g.
    penetrating g.
    penetrating corneal g.
    penetrating full-thickness corneal g.
    g. preservation solution
    scleral patch g.
    skin g.
    Tudor-Thomas g.
    Wolfe's g.
graft-host interface
grafting
    surgical patch g.
graft-versus-host disease
gramicidin
    neomycin, polymixin B, and g.

gram-negative
- g.-n. bacteria
- g.-n. media
- g.-n. rods

gram-positive
- g.-p. bacteria
- g.-p. cocci

Gram's stain

granular
- g. cell myoblastoma
- g. conjunctivitis
- g. corneal dystrophy
- g. dystrophy
- g. lid
- g. ophthalmia
- g. trachoma

granularity

granule
- Birbeck g.'s
- cone g.
- dense core g.'s
- glycogen g.
- Langerhans' g.'s
- pigment g.'s
- rod g.
- scintillating g.'s

granulocytic
- g. leukemia
- g. sarcoma

granuloma
- caseating orbital g.
- cholesterol g.
- chorioretinal g.
- choroidal g.
- conjunctival g.
- eosinophilic g.
- focal g.
- g. gangraenescens
- g. inguinale
- g. iridis
- lethal midline g.
- midline g.
- orbital g.
- palisading orbital g.
- pyogenic g.
- reparative giant cell g.
- sclerosing orbital g.
- g. venereum

granulomatosis
- allergic g.
- lymphoid g.
- lymphomatoid g.
- Wegener's g.

granulomatous
- g. endophthalmitis
- g. enterocolitis
- g. uveitis

granulosa
- *Echinococcus g.*

graph
- shadow g.

graphics

graphite

grating
- g. acuity
- Arden g.'s
- Cambridge low-contrast g.'s

Gratiolet's radiating fiber

Graves'
- G. disease
- G. ophthalmopathy
- G. orbitography

gravidarum
- retinitis g.

gravidic
- g. retinitis
- g. retinopathy

gravid retinitis

gravis
- fulminant myasthenia g.
- myasthenia g.

gray
- g. atrophy
- g. cataract
- g. line
- g. plaque

graying
- g. of macula
- macular g.

grayline incision

gray-scale ultrasonogram

Grayson corneal forceps

Grayson-Wilbrandt
- G.-W. anterior corneal dystrophy
- G.-W. dystrophy

Grayson-Wilbrandt corneal dystrophy

Grayton corneal forceps

gray-white corneal scar

Grazer blepharoplasty forceps

grease

greater
- g. ring
- g. ring of iris
- g. wing of the sphenoid

Greaves' operation
Green
- G. calipers
- G. capsule forceps
- G. cataract knife
- G. chalazion forceps
- G. corneal dissector
- G. corneal knife
- G. corneal marker
- G. curette
- G. dissector
- G. double spatula
- G. eye shield
- G. fixation forceps
- G. forceps
- G. hook
- G. iris replacer
- G. knife
- G. lens spatula
- G. muscle hook
- G. muscle tucker
- G. needle holder
- G. refractor
- G. replacer
- G. replacer spatula
- G. shield
- G. spatula
- G. strabismus hook
- G. strabismus tucker
- G. trephine

green
- argon g.
- g. blindness
- g. cataract
- indocyanine g.
- monochromatic g.
- g. vision

Green-Kenyon corneal marker
Green's cataract
Greig's syndrome
Grey-Hess screen
grid
- Amsler's g.
- Bernell's g.

Gridley intraocular lens
Grieshaber
- G. blade
- G. corneal trephine
- G. diamond coated forceps
- G. endoilluminator
- G. iris forceps
- G. keratome
- G. knife
- G. micro-bipolar coagulator
- G. needle
- G. needle holder
- G. ophthalmic needle
- G. power injector system
- G. ruby knife
- G. trephine
- G. ultrasharp knife
- G. vertical cutting scissors
- G. vitreous scissors

Grieshaber's ultrasharp microsurgery
Grieshaber-type corneal trephine
Griffith's sign
Grimsdale's operation
grinding
- bicentric g.
- slab-off g.

grip
- scleral g.

griseofulvin
Grocco's sign
Groenholm
- G. refractor
- G. retractor

Groenouw's
- G. corneal dystrophy
- G. dystrophy
- G. type I dystrophy
- G. type II dystrophy
- G. type II maculopathy

Grolman photographic system
Grönblad-Strandberg syndrome
groove
- Blessig's g.
- corneal lamellar g.
- corneoscleral g.
- infraorbital g.
- lacrimal g.
- lamellar g.
- limbal g.
- nasolacrimal g.
- optic g.
- g. suture
- Verga's lacrimal g.

grooved
- g. director
- g. incision
- g. silicone implant
- g. silicone sponge

Gross
- G. retractor
- G. stereopsis

Grossmann's operation
round-glass appearance
round glass sheet
roup
case g.
control g.
rowth
g. hormone
g. hormone deficiency
scaffold for new vessel g.
rowth-onset diabetes
ruber's syndrome
runert's spur
runing magnet
S-9
GS-9 blade
GS-9 needle
SA-9 blade
t
gutta (drop)
tt
guttae (drops)
uanethidine
uard
cataract knife g.
ether g.
eye knife g.
forceps g.
Hansen keratome g.
keratome g.
knife g.
scalpel g.
uardian
G. scalpel with depth
resistor
G. scalpel with myoguard
depth resistor
uarnieri's inclusion body
udden
commissure of G.
udden's commissure
ueder keratoplasty needle
uibor
G. duct tube
G. shield
G. Silastic tube
G. tube
uibor's chart
uide
Clayman g.
uillain-Barré syndrome

guillotine
g. cutting tip
g. vitrectomy instruments
guillotine-type cutter
Guist
G. enucleation hemostat
G. enucleation scissors
G. fixation forceps
G. hemostat
G. implant
G. scissors
G. speculum
G. sphere implant
Guist-Bloch speculum
Gullstrand
G. lens
G. loupe
G. ophthalmoscope
G. slit lamp
Gullstrand's
G. law
G. reduced eye
G. schematic eye
gumma, pl. gummas, gummata
gun
BB g.
gun-barrel field defect
Gunderson muscle forceps
Gunderson's conjunctival flap
Gunn
Marcus G. (MG)
Gunn's
G. dot
G. jaw-winking phenomenon
G. pupil
G. pupillary reflex
G. sign
G. syndrome
gustatolacrimal reflex
gustatory sweating
Guthrie
G. fixation hook
G. hook
gutta, pl. guttae
g. amaurosis
g. serena
gutta (drop) (gt)
guttae (drops) (gtt)
Guttat.
guttatim (drop by drop)
guttata
absent g.
g. of cornea

187

guttata *(continued)*
    cornea g.
    corneal g.
    g. senilis choroiditis
guttate choroidopathy
guttatim (drop by drop) (Guttat.)
gutter dystrophy of cornea
guttering
    corneal g.
    limbal g.
    limbus g.
Gutzeit's dacryostomy operation
guy suture
Guyton
    G. corneal transplant
      trephine
    G. electrode
Guyton-Clark fragment forceps
Guyton-Friedenwald suture
Guyton-Lundsgaard
    G.-L. cataract knife
    G.-L. keratome
    G.-L. knife
    G.-L. scalpel
    G.-L. sclerotome

Guyton-Maumenee speculum
Guyton-Minkowski Potential Acuit Meter
Guyton-Noyes
    G.-N. fixation
    G.-N. fixation forceps
Guyton-Park
    G.-P. eye speculum
    G.-P. lid speculum
    G.-P. speculum
Guyton's
    G. operation
    G. ptosis operation
gymnastics
    ocular g.
gyrata
    atrophia g.
gyrate
    g. atrophy
    g. atrophy of choroid and
      retina
gyrosa
gyrus
    angular g.

H
- Hauch
- henry
- Holzknecht unit
- hydrogen
- hyperopia
- hyperopic
- hyperphoria

HA
- hyaluronic acid

Haab
- H. knife needle
- H. magnet
- H. needle
- H. scleral resection knife

Haab's
- H. reflex
- II. striae

Haag-Streit
- Endo-Set by H.-S.
- H.-S. fluorescein dye
- H.-S. slit lamp

habit
- glaucomatous h.

habitus
- acromegalic h.

Haemophilus
- *H. aegypticus*
- *H influenzae*

haemorrhagica
- retinitis h.

Haenel's symptom
Haenig irrigating scissors
Hagberg-Santavuori syndrome
Hague cataract lamp
Haidinger brush
Haik implant
hair
- h. bulb incubation test
- h. follicle tumor

hairy-cell leukemia
halation
Halberg
- H. contact lens forceps
- H. indirect ophthalmoscope
- H. trial clip
- H. trial clip occluder

Halberstaedter-Prowazek inclusion body
half-glass spectacles

half-thickness
- dissected h.-t.

half vision
Hallauer
- H. glasses
- H. spectacles

Hall dermatome
Haller
- circle of H.

halleri
- circulus arteriosus h.

Hallermann-Streiff-Francois syndrome
Hallermann-Streiff syndrome
Haller's
- H. layer
- H. membrane

Hallervorden-Spatz syndrome
Hallgren's syndrome
Hallpike maneuver
hallucination
- hypnagogic h.
- hypnopompic h.
- irritative h.
- release h.
- visual h.

halo
- h. demonstrator
- Fick's h.
- glaucomatous h.
- parafoveal h.
- pigmentary h.
- h. saturninus
- senescent h.
- senile h.
- h. sheathing
- h. symptom
- h. vision
- visual h.

halogen ophthalmoscope
halogram
halometer
halometry
haloperidol
halos
halothane
Halpin's operation
Halsey needle holder
Halsted
- H. curved mosquito forceps

189

Halsted *(continued)*
    H. curved mosquito
      hemostatic forceps
    H. hemostat
    H. mosquito hemostatic
      forceps
    H. strabismus scissors
Haltia-Santavuori type of Batten's
    syndrome
hamartoblastoma
hamartoma
    astrocytic h.
    melanocytic h.
    orbit h.
    orbital h.
    uveal tract h.
    vascular h.
hamartomatosis
hammock pupil
hamular procedure
hamulus
    h. lacrimalis
    trochlear h.
hand
    h. motion (HM)
    h. movement (HM)
hand-held
    h.-h. eye magnet
    h.-h. fundus camera
    h.-h. Hruby lens
    h.-h. magnet
    h.-h. rotary prism
handle
    Beaver h.
    Elliot trephine h.
hand motion at 3 feet (HM/3ft)
hand-motion visual acuity test
hand-movement visual acuity test
handpiece
    Avit h.
    B-mode h.
    Cavitron I/A h.
    fragmentation/aspiration h.
    Kelman irrigating h.
    phacoemulsification h.
Hand-Schüller-Christian disease
Hanna trephine
Hannover's canal
Hansel's stain
Hansen
    H. keratome
    H. keratome guard
Hansen's disease

haploid
haplopia
haploscope
    mirror h.
haploscopic vision
hapten
haptic
    h. contact
    h. loop
    violet h.
Harada-Ito procedure
Harada's
    H. disease
    H. syndrome
hard
    h. cataract
    h. contact lens (HCL)
    h. drusen
    h. exudate
hardened spectacle lens
hardening of lens
harderian gland
Harder's gland
Hardesty
    H. tendon hook
    H. tenotomy hook
hard-finger tension
hardware
Hardy
    H. Lensometer
    H. punch
Hardy-Rand-Littler
    H.-R.-L. plate
    H.-R.-L. screening plate
Hardy-Rand-Ritter (HRR)
    H.-R.-R. test
hare's eye
harlequin fetus
Harman
    H. eye dressing
    H. fixation forceps
    H. forceps
Harman's operation
harmonious
    h. abnormal retinal
      correspondence
    h. correspondence
    h. retinal correspondence
Harms
    H. corneal forceps
    H. trabeculotome
    H. trabeculotomy probe
    H. tying forceps

Harms-Dannheim trabeculotomy operation
Harms-Tubingen tying forceps
Harrington
    H. erysiphake
    H. retractor
    H. tonometer
Harrington-Flocks
    H.-F. multiple pattern
    H.-F. test
Harrison
    H. retractor
    H. scissors
Harrison-Stein nomogram
Hartinger Coincidence refractionometer
Hartmann
    H. forceps
    H. hemostatic forceps
    H. mosquito hemostatic forceps
Hart pediatric three-mirror lens
Hartstein
    H. irrigating/aspirating unit
    H. irrigating iris retractor
    H. irrigator
    H. refractor
    H. retractor
Hashimoto's thyroiditis
Hasner
    H. lid forceps
    valve of H.
Hasner's
    H. folds
    H. operation
    H. valve
Hassall-Henle
    H.-H. bodies
    H.-H. wart
Hassall's body
HATTS
    hemagglutination treponemal test for syphilis
    HATTS test
Hauch (H)
hay
    h. fever
    h. fever conjunctivitis
Hay-Wells syndrome
haze
    aerial h.
    stromal h.
    vitreous h.

H band
HBr
    tropicamide and hydroxyamphetamine H.
HCL
    hard contact lens
HCl
    hydrochloride
    antazoline phosphate and naphazoline HCl
    apraclonidine HCl
    dapiprazole HCl
    dipivefrin HCl
    Duranest HCl
    Marcaine HCl
    pheniramine maleate and naphazoline HCl
    pilocarpine HCl
    proparacaine HCl
head
    Medusa h.
    h. mirror
    optic nerve h.
    h. posture
    h. shaking
    h. titubation
    h. tremors
    h. turning
headache
    brain tumor h.
    cluster h.
    cough h.
    migraine h.
    muscle contraction h.
    postherpetic h.
    posttraumatic h.
    sinus h.
head-nodding
headrest
    Gibralter h.
head-tilt test
head-turning reflex
Healon solution
hearing loss
heat-generated cataract
Heath
    H. chalazion curette
    H. chalazion forceps
    H. curette
    H. dilator
    H. expressor
    H. forceps
heat-ray cataract

heavy
> h. eye
> h. ion irradiation
> h. ion radiation

Hebra
> H. blade
> H. curette
> H. hook

hedger cataract
Heerfordt's
> H. disease
> H. syndrome

hefilcon A
Heidenhaim's syndrome
height
> contact lens h.
> orbital h.
> sagittal h.

Heine's
> H. cyclodialysis
> H. operation

Heisrath's operation
helcoma
helicoid choroidopathy
heliotrope
helium-ion aiming laser
helium-neon aiming laser
helium neon beam
Helmholtz
> H. keratometer
> H. ophthalmoscope
> H. theory of
>   accommodation
> H. theory of color vision

Helmholtz's
> H. line
> H. schematic eye

helminthic disease
helper/inducer
> h./i. T cell
> T-cell h./i.

HEMA
> hydroxyethylmethacrylate

hemagglutination
> h. test
> h. treponemal test
> h. treponemal test for
>   syphilis (HATTS)

hemangioblastoma
hemangioendothelioma
> orbital h.

hemangioma
> capillary h.

cavernous h.
choroidal h.
conjunctival h.
episcleral h.
eyelid strawberry h.
facial h.
orbital h.
racemose h.
strawberry h.
uveal tract h.
venous h.

hemangiomatosis
hemangiopericytoma
> meningeal h.
> orbital h.

hematic cyst
hematin
> acid h.

hematocrit
hematogenous pigmentation
hematologic testing
hematoma
> orbital h.
> subdural h.

hematopoietic metastasis
hematopsia
hematoxylin stain
hemeralopia
hemeranopia
hemiamblyopia
hemianopia (*var. of* hemianopsia)
hemianopic
> h. glasses
> h. scotoma
> h. spectacles

hemianopsia, hemianopia
> absolute h.
> altitudinal h.
> bilateral h.
> bilateral homonymous h.
> binasal h.
> binocular h.
> bitemporal h.
> bitemporal fugax h.
> complete h.
> congenital h.
> congruous h.
> crossed h.
> double homonymous h.
> equilateral h.
> geniculate h.
> heteronymous h.
> homonymous h.

horizontal h.
incomplete h.
incongruous h.
lateral h.
lower h.
nasal h.
pseudo-h.
quadrant h.
quadrantic h.
relative h.
temporal h.
true h.
unilateral h., uniocular h.
upper h.
vertical h.
hemianoptic
hemianosmia
hemiatrophy
facial h.
hemichromatopsia
hemicrania
hemicraniosis
hemidecussate
hemifacial
h. atrophy
h. blepharospasm
h. microsomia
h. spasm
hemifield slide phenomenon
hemiopalgia
hemiopia
hemiopic
h. hypoplasia
h. pupillary reaction
hemiparesis
hemiplegia
alternating oculomotor h.
hemiscotosis
hemisphere
cerebellar h.
h. eye implant
h. implant
h. projection perimetry
silicone h.
hemispherical
hemizygous
hemochromatosis
hemocytic mesenchyme
hemodialysis
hemoglobin
h. A
h. C

h. electrophoresis
h. S
hemoglobinopathy
sickle h.
sickle cell h.
hemolytic
alpha h.
beta h.
h. glaucoma
h. jaundice
β-hemolytic streptococcus
hemophilia
hemophthalmia, hemophthalmus
hemophthalmos
hemorrhage
arachnoid h.
blot h.
blot-and-dot h.'s
cerebellar h.
choroidal h.
conjunctival h.
disk drusen h.
dot h.
dot-and blot h.
eight-ball h.
expulsive h.
flame h.
flame-shaped h.
intraocular h.
nasal h.
ochre h.
preretinal h.
punctate h.
retinal h.
retinopathy h.
retrobulbar h.
round h.
salmon-patch h.
splinter h.
subarachnoid h.
subconjunctival h.
subhyaloid h.
subjunctival h.
subretinal h.
suprachoroidal h.
vitreal h.
vitreous h. (VH)
vitreous break-through h.
white-centered h.
yellow-ochre h.
hemorrhagic
h. conjunctivitis
h. disorder

hemorrhagic *(continued)*
    h. glaucoma
    h. iritis
    h. retinopathy
    h. sarcoma
hemostasis
hemostat
    Corboy h.
    Guist h.
    Guist enucleation h.
    Halsted h.
    Kelly h.
hemostatic forceps
Hemovac
Henderson-Patterson inclusion body
HeNe beam
Henle
    fibers of H.
Henle's
    H. body
    H. fiber layer
    H. gland
    H. layer
    H. membrane
    H. warts
Henoch-Scönlein purpura
henry (H)
Hensen's body
heparan sulfate
hepatitis
    h. B
    h. B surface antigen
hepatolenticular degeneration
hepatoma
hepatorenal glycogenesis
heptachromic
herapathite
Herbert's
    H. operation
    H. peripheral pit
    H. pit
hereditaria
    atrophia bulborum h.
    degeneratio
    hyaloideoretinas h.
hereditary
    h. anterior membrane
    dystrophy
    h. benign intraepithelial
    dyskeratosis
    h. benign intraepithelial
    dyskeratosis syndrome

    h. benign intraepithelial
    syndrome
    h. cerebellar ataxia
    h. degeneration
    h. endothelial dystrophy
    h. epithelial corneal
    dystrophy
    h. epithelial dystrophy
    h. hemorrhagic macular
    dystrophy
    h. hemorrhagic telangiectasia
    h. macular dystrophy
    h. mucoepithelial dysplasia
    h. progressive arthro-
    ophthalmopathy
    h. renal-retinal dysplasia
    h. spherocytosis
    h. telangiectasia
    h. vitelliform dystrophy
heredity maculopathy
heredodegeneration
    macular h.
heredodegenerative
    h. atrophy
    h. neurologic syndrome
heredofamilial optic atrophy
heredogenerative neurologic
syndrome
heredomacular degeneration
Hering-Bielschowsky after-image
test
Hering-Hellebrand deviation
Hering's
    H. after-image mechanism
    H. law
    H. law of equal innervation
    H. law of equivalent
    innervation
    H. test
    H. theory of color vision
Hermann grid illusion
Hermansky-Pudlak syndrome
hernia
    h. of iris
    orbital h.
    vitreous h.
herniation
    vitreous h.
heroin
herpes
    h. corneae
    h. epithelial tropic
    ulceration

h. follicular
keratoconjunctivitis
h. iridis
h. iridocyclitis
h. keratitis
neonatal h.
ocular h.
h. ophthalmicus
h. panuveitis
h. simplex
h. simplex blepharitis
h. simplex cellulitis
h. simplex conjunctivitis
h. simplex corneal ulcer
h. simplex iridocyclitis
h. simplex keratitis
h. simplex
keratoconjunctivitis
h. simplex keratouveitis
h. simplex retinitis
h. simplex scleritis
h. simplex uveitis
h. simplex virus (HSV)
h. uveitis
h. zoster
h. zoster conjunctivitis
h. zoster glaucoma
h. zoster iridocyclitis
h. zoster keratitis
h. zoster keratoconjunctivitis
h. zoster ophthalmicus
herpesvirus
herpetic
h. keratitis
h. keratoconjunctivitis
h. metakeratitis
h. stromal keratitis
h. ulcer
herpetiformis
dermatitis h.
herpetoid lesion
Herplex Liquifilm
Herrick lacrimal plug
Herring's law of motor
correspondence
Hertel
H. exophthalmometer
H. stone forceps
Hertwig-Magendie
H.-M. phenomenon
H.-M. syndrome

Hertzog
H. lens spatula
H. pliable probe
Hess
H. diplopia screen
H. forceps
H. screen
H. screen test
H. spoon
Hess'
H. eyelid operation
H. operation
H. ptosis operation
Hess-Barraquer forceps
Hessburg
H. corneal shield
H. eye shield
H. intraocular lens glide
H. lacrimal needle
H. lens
H. lens forceps
H. lens-inserting forceps
H. subpalpebral lavage
system
Hessburg-Barron
H.-B. suction trephine
H.-B. trephine
H.-B. vacuum trephine
Hess-Horwitz forceps
Hess-Lee screen
hetacillin
heterochromia
atrophic h.
binocular h.
h. cataract
congenital h.
h. cyclitis
Fuchs' h.
h. iridis, h. of iris
monocular h.
simple h.
sympathetic h.
h. uveitis
heterochromic
h. cataract
h. cyclitis
h. Fuchs' cyclitis
h. iridocyclitis
h. uveitis
heterogeneity
heterogeneous donor material

heterogenous
    h. donor material
    h. keratoplasty
heterograft
heterokeratoplasty
heterometropia
heteronymous
    h. diplopia
    h. hemianopsia
    h. image
    h. parallax
heterophoralgia
heterophoria
heterophoric position
heterophthalmia, heterophthalmos,
  heterophthalmus
heteropsia
heteroptics
heteroscope
heteroscopy
heterotropia, heterotropy
    circadian h.
    comitant h.
    concomitant h.
    h. maculae
    noncomitant h.
    paralytic h.
heterotropic deviation
heterozygote
heterozygous
hexachloride
    benzene h.
hexachromic
Hexadrol
hexafluoride
    h. gas
    sulfur h.
hexahydrate
    trisodium
      phosphonoformate h.
hexametaphosphate
    sodium h.
hexamethonium chloride
hexosaminidase
hex procedure
hexylcaine
Heyer-Schulte microscope
Heyner
    H. cannula
    H. curette
    H. dilator
    H. double cannula
    H. double needle

    H. expressor
    H. forceps
    H. needle
Hg
    mercury
HGH laser
HGM
    HGM argon green laser
    HGM intravitreal laser
Hgroton
HHH
    hyperornithinemia,
      hyperammonemia, and
      homocitrullinuria
    HHH syndrome
Hidex glass lens
Hiff's
    H. operation
    H. ptosis
high
    h. convex
    h. hyperopia
    h. intensity illuminator
    h. myopia
High-Lite glass
high-tension suturing technique
Hildreth
    H. cautery
    H. electrocautery
Hillis
    H. refractor
    H. retractor
Hill retractor
Hill's
    H. operation
    H. procedure
Hilton
    H. self-retaining infusion
      cannula
    H. sutureless infusion
      cannula
Hippel-Lindau syndrome
Hippel's
    H. disease
    H. operation
hippus
    respiratory h.
Hirschberg
    H. magnet
    H. reflex
Hirschberg's
    H. method
    H. test

Hirschman
    H. hook
    H. lens forceps
    H. lens-inserting forceps
    H. micro iris hook
    H. spatula
    H. speculum
histamine
histidine
histiocyte
histiocytic
    h. disorder
    h. lymphoma
histiocytoma
    fibrous h.
histiocytosis
histiocytosis X
Histoacryl
histoacryl
    h. glue
    h. glue patch
histocompatibility
histogram
histopathology
Histoplasma
    H. capsulatum
    II. duboisii
histoplasmic choroiditis
histoplasmin skin test
histoplasmosis
    h. maculopathy
    ocular h.
    presumed ocular h.
    h. syndrome
history
    case h.
    neuro-ophthalmologic case h.
histo spots
hitch
    girth h.
HIV
    human immunodeficiency virus
hivialis ophthalmia
HIV-specific antibodies
Hl
    latent hyperopia
HLA
    human leukocyte antigen
    HLA typing
HLA-A29
    H.-A. antigen
HLA-B5 antigen
HLA-B7 antigen

HLA-B15 antigen
HLA-B27 antigen
HM
    hand motion
    hand movement
Hm
    manifest hyperopia
HM/3ft
    hand motion at 3 feet
HMS Liquifilm
hockey-end temple
hockey stick
Hodgkin's disease
Hoffer
    H. forward-cutting knife
    cannula
    H. optical center marker
Hoffer-Colenbrander formula
Hoffer-Laseridge intraocular lens
Hogan's operation
Hoglund's sign
holder
    Alabama-Green needle h.
    Arruga needle h.
    baby Barraquer needle h.
    Barraquer curved h.
    Barraquer needle h.
    Belin double-ended
    needle h.
    Birks Mark II Instruments
    micro cross-action h.
    Birks Mark II micro cross-
    action h.
    Birks Mark II micro lock-
    type needle h.
    Birks Mark II needle h.
    Bodkin thread h.
    Boyce needle h.
    Boynton needle h.
    Castroviejo-Barraquer
    needle h.
    Castroviejo blade h.
    Castroviejo-Kalt needle h.
    Castroviejo needle h.
    Clerf needle h.
    Cohan needle h.
    Corboy needle h.
    Crile needle h.
    Dean knife h.
    Derf needle h.
    Ellis needle h.
    French needle h.
    Gifford needle h.

holder *(continued)*
  goniotomy needle h.
  Green needle h.
  Grieshaber needle h.
  Halsey needle h.
  Ilg micro needle h.
  Ilg needle h.
  I-tech cannula h.
  I-tech needle h.
  Jaffe needle h.
  Kalt needle h.
  Keeler Catford micro jaws
    needle h.
  McIntyre fish-hook
    needle h.
  McPherson needle h.
  needle h.
  Neumann razor blade
    fragment h.
  Paton needle h.
  Schaefer sponge h.
  Stangel modified Barraquer
    microsurgical needle h.
  Stephenson needle h.
  Stevens needle h.
  Tilderquist needle h.
  Troutman needle h.
  Vickers needle h.
holding clip
hole
  cystoid macular h.
  iatrogenic retinal h.
  idiopathic macular cyst
    and h.
  impending macular h.
  macular h.
  retinal h.
  senescent macular h.
hole of retina
holes
  macular h.
Holladay posterior capsule polisher
Hollenhorst's plaque
hollowing
  acoustical h.
  h. and shadowing
hollow-sphere implant
Holmes-Adie
  H.-A. pupil
  H.-A. syndrome
Holmgren method
Holmgren's
  H. color test

H. skein
H. wool skein test
Holofax
hologram
Holth
  H. forceps
  H. punch
  H. scleral punch
Holthouse-Batten superficial
  choroiditis
Holth's
  H. iridencleisis
  H. operation
  H. sclerectomy
Holt-Oram syndrome
Holzknecht unit (H)
Homatrocel
Homatropine
  Isopto H.
homatropine
  h. dilatation
  h. hydrobromide
  h. refraction
Homén's syndrome
homeostasis
Homer-Wright rosette
homocitrullinuria
  hyperornithinemia,
    hyperammonemia, and h.
    (HHH)
homocystinuria
homogeneous donor material
homogenous
  h. donor material
  h. keratoplasty
homograft
homokeratoplasty
homolateral
homologous
homonymous
  h. crescent
  h. diplopia
  h. field defect
  h. hemianopic scotoma
  h. hemianopsia
  h. hemiopic hypoplasia
  h. image
  h. parallax
  h. quadrantanopsia
homoplastic keratomileusis
homotropic antibody
homozygous

Honan
   H. balloon
   H. cuff
   H. manometer
honey bee lens
honeycomb
   h. dystrophy
   h. macula
hook
   Amenabar discission h.
   anchor h.
   angled discission h.
   Azar lens-manipulating h.
   Berens h.
   Berens scleral h.
   Birks Mark II h.
   boat h.
   Bonn micro iris h.
   Catalano muscle h.
   corneal h.
   Culler muscle h.
   discission h.
   Drews-Sato suture pickup h.
   h. expressor
   expressor h.
   Fenzel angled
     manipulating h.
   Fenzel insertion h.
   Fenzel lens-manipulating h.
   Fenzel manipulating h.
   Fink h.
   Fink muscle h.
   Fink oblique muscle h.
   fixation h.
   flat h.
   Gass muscle h.
   Gass retinal detachment h.
   Graefe h.
   Graefe strabismus h.
   Graether button-h.
   Graether mushroom h.
   Green h.
   Green muscle h.
   Green strabismus h.
   Guthrie h.
   Guthrie fixation h.
   Hardesty tendon h.
   Hardesty tenotomy h.
   Hebra h.
   Hirschman h.
   Hirschman micro iris h.
   Hunkeler ball-point h.
   iris h.

   Jaeger h.
   Jaffe lens-manipulating h.
   Jaffe micro iris h.
   Jameson h.
   Jameson muscle h.
   Katena boat h.
   Kennerdell muscle h.
   Kennerdell nerve h.
   Kirby h.
   Kirby muscle h.
   Knapp h.
   Knapp iris h.
   Kratz K push-pull iris h.
   Kuglen h.
   Kuglen manipulating h.
   Manson double-ended
     strabismus h.
   Maumenee iris h.
   McIntyre irrigating h.
   McReynolds h.
   McReynolds lid
     retracting h.
   muscle h.
   Nugent h.
   oblique muscle h.
   Ochsner h.
   O'Connor flat h.
   O'Connor sharp h.
   O'Connor tenotomy h.
   ophthalmic h.
   Osher h.
   Praeger iris h.
   retinal detachment h.
   Russian four-pronged
     fixation h.
   scleral h.
   Scobee muscle h.
   Scobee oblique muscle h.
   sharp h.
   Sheets micro iris h.
   Shepard iris h.
   Shepard micro iris h.
   Shepard reversed iris h.
   Sinskey h.
   Sinskey lens h.
   Sinskey lens-manipulating h.
   Sinskey micro iris h.
   Sinskey micro lens h.
   skin h.
   Smith expressor h.
   Smith lid h.
   h. spatula
   spatula h.

hook *(continued)*
   squint h.
   Stevens h.
   Stevens tenotomy h.
   St. Martin-Franceschetti
    cataract h.
   strabismus h.
   suture pickup h.
   Tennant h.
   Tennant anchor lens-
    insertion h.
   Tennant lens-
    manipulating h.
   tenotomy h.
   Tomas iris h.
   Tomas suture h.
   twist fixation h.
   Tyrell iris h.
   Tyrell tympanic
    membrane h.
   Visitec angled lens h.
   Visitec micro h.
   Visitec micro double iris h.
   Visitec micro iris h.
   Visitec straight lens h.
   von Graefe h.
   von Graefe muscle h.
   von Graefe strabismus h.
   Wiener h.
   Wiener corneal h.
   Wiener scleral h.
   Y h.
hook-shaped cataract
hook-type implant
Hoopes corneal marker
hop eye
Hopkins Rod Lens Telescope
Hopmann's polyp
Horay's operation
hordeolum
   external h.
   h. externum
   internal h.
   h. internum
   h. meibomianum
horizontal
   h. band pallor
   h. cells
   h. deviation
   h. diplopia
   h. gaze
   h. gaze center
   h. hemianopsia

   h. mattress suture
   h. meridian
   h. nystagmus
   h. plane
   h. prism bars
   h. raphe
hormone
   adrenocorticotropic h.
   (ACTH)
   growth h.
   thyroid-releasing h. (TRH)
   thyrotropin-releasing h.
   (TRH)
horn
   cutaneous h.
   lateral h.
   medial h.
Horner-Bernard syndrome
Horner's
   H. law
   H. muscle
   H. ptosis
   H. pupil
   H. syndrome
Horner-Trantas
   H.-T. dots
   H.-T. spot
horopter
   Vieth-Mueller h.
horopteric
horror fusionis
horseshoe tear
Horton's syndrome
Horvath's operation
Hosford
   H. expressor
   H. lacrimal dilator
   H. spud
Hoskins
   H. beaked Colibri forceps
   H. fine straight forceps
   H. fixation forceps
   H. forceps
   H. micro straight forceps
   H. miniaturized micro
    straight forceps
   H. razor blade fragment
   H. razor fragment blade
   H. straight micro iris
    forceps
   H. suture forceps
Hoskins-Castroviejo corneal
  scissors

Hoskins-Dallas intraocular lens-inserting forceps
Hoskins-Luntz forceps
Hoskins-Skeleton
    H.-S. fine forceps
    H.-S. micro grooved broad-tipped forceps
Hoskins-Westcott tenotomy scissors
host tissue forceps
hot eye
HOTV test
Hotz
    H. entropion
    H. entropion operation
Hotz-Anagnostakis operation
Hough drape
House
    H. knife
    H. lacrimal dilator
    H. miniature forceps
    H. myringotomy knife
House-Bellucci alligator scissors
House-Dieter nipper
Houser
    H. cul-de-sac irrigator T-tube
    H. cul-de-sac irrigator tube
House-Urban-Pentax camera
Hovius'
    H. canal
    H. circle
    H. membrane
    H. plexus
Howard abrader
Hoya
    H. HDR objective refractometer
    H. MRM objective refractometer
HRR
    Hardy-Rand-Ritter
Hruby
    H. contact lens
    H. implant
    H. lens
HS
    Pilopine HS
hSOD
    human superoxide dismutase
HSV
    herpes simplex virus
HT
    hypertropia

Ht
    total hyperopia
Hubbard
    H. corneoscleral forceps
    H. forceps
Hudson's line
Hudson-Stähli
    H.-S. line
    H.-S. line of corneal pigmentation
hue
    salmon patch h.
Hueck's ligament
Huey scissors
Hughes
    H. implant
    H. tarsoconjunctival flap
Hughes'
    H. modification of Burch technique
    H. operation
human
    h. immunodeficiency virus (HIV)
    h. leukocyte antigen (HLA)
    h. superoxide dismutase (hSOD)
Hummelsheim's
    H. operation
    H. procedure
humor, gen. humoris
    aqueous h.
    h. aquosus
    h. cristallinus
    crystalline h.
    ocular h.
    plasmoid h.
    plasmoid aqueous h.
    vitreous h.
humoral immunity
Humorsol
Humphrey
    H. automatic refractor
    H. field analyzer
    H. Instruments vision analyzer
    H. Instruments Vision Analyzer Overrefraction System
    H. lens analyzer
    H. retina imager
    H. ultrasonic pachometer
    H. visual field analyzer

Humphrey's perimeter
Hunkeler
    H. ball-point hook
    H. lens
Hunt
    H. chalazion forceps
    H. chalazion scissors
Hunter-Hurler syndrome
Hunter's
    H. disease
    H. syndrome
Huntington's disease
Hunt-Transley operation
Hurler's
    H. disease
    H. syndrome
Hurler-Scheie
    H.-S. compound
    H.-S. syndrome
Huschke's valve
Hutchinson's
    H. disease
    H. facies
    H. freckles
    H. patch
    H. pupil
    H. sign
    H. syndrome
    H. triad
Hutchinson-Tays central guttate
  choroiditis
huygenian eyepiece
hyaline
    h. artery
    h. bodies
    h. cast
    h. degeneration
    h. mass
    h. material
    h. membrane
    h. plaque
hyalinization
hyalinosis cutis et mucosae
hyalitis
    h. anterior membrane
    h. artery
    asteroid h.
    h. punctata
    punctate h.
    h. suppurativa
    suppurative h.
Hyall
hyalocyte

hyaloid
    h. artery
    h. asteroid
    h. body
    h. canal
    h. corpuscle
    h. face
    h. fossa
    h. membrane
    h. posterior membrane
    h. system
hyaloidal fibrovascular proliferation
hyaloidea
    membrana h.
    stella lentis h.
hyaloideocapsular ligament
hyaloideoretinal degeneration
hyaloideus
    canalis h.
hyaloiditis
hyaloidotomy
hyalomucoid
hyalonyxis
hyalosis
    asteroid h.
    punctate h.
hyaluronate
    chondroitin sulfate and
      sodium h.
    sodium h.
    h. sodium
    h. sodium with chondroitin
hyaluronic acid (HA)
hyaluronidase
hydatid disease
hydatoid
Hyde
    H. astigmatism ruler
    H. corneal forceps
    H. double curved forceps
    H. forceps
    H. irrigating/aspirating unit
    H. irrigator/aspirator unit
Hydeltrasol
hydoidea
    fossa h.
Hydracon
    H. contact lens
    H. lens
hydralazine
Hydrasoft contact lens
hydrate
    chloral h.

hydration
hydraulic retinal reattachment
hydroa vacciniforme
hydroblepharon
hydrobromide
    homatropine h.
    hydroxyamphetamine h.
Hydrocare preserved saline
hydrocephalus
    external h.
    internal h.
    obstructive h.
hydrochloric acid
hydrochloride (HCl)
    benoxinate h.
    betaxolol h.
    cocaine h.
    cyclopentolate h.
    diphenhydramine h.
    hydromorphone h.
    levobunolol h.
    lidocaine h.
    meperidine h.
    oxymorphone h.
    phenacaine h.
    phencyclidine h.
    phenmetrazine h.
    phenoxybenzamine h.
    phenylephrine h.
    phenylpropanolamine h.
    piperocaine h.
    procaine h.
    proparacaine h.
    protriptyline h.
    quinacrine h.
    tetracaine h.
    thioridazine h.
    trifluoperazine h.
    trifluperidol h.
hydrochlorothiazide
hydrocortisone
    h. acetate
    bacitracin, neomycin,
      polymixin B, and h.
    neomycin, polymyxin B,
      and h.
    h. suspension
Hydrocortone
Hydrocurve lens
hydrocystoma
    apocrine h.
hydrodelamination
hydrodelineation

hydrodiascope
hydrodissection
HydroDIURIL
hydrogel
    h. contact lens
    h. lens
hydrogen (H)
    h. peroxide
hydrolysis
    h. of solution
hydrometric chamber
hydromorphone hydrochloride
Hydron
    American H.
    H. lens
Hydronol
hydrophila
    Aeromonas h.
hydrophilic contact lens
hydrophobic contact lens
hydrophthalmia, hydrophthalmos,
    hydrophthalmus
    anterior h.
    posterior h.
    total h.
hydropic degeneration
hydrops
    acute h.
    h. of iris
    meningeal h.
hydroquinone
Hydrosight lens
hydroxide
    calcium h.
    potassium h. (KOH)
    sodium h.
hydroxyamphetamine
    h. HBR
    h. HBr and topicamide
    h. hydrobromide
hydroxychloroquine sulfate
hydroxyethl cellulose
hydroxyethylmethacrylate (HEMA)
hydroxypropyl methylcellulose
hydroxyzine pamoate
Hy-Flow
hyfrecator
hygroblepharic
Hymenolepsis nana
Hyoscine
    Isopto H.
hyoscine
    scopolamine h.

hyoscyamine
Hyoscyamus niger
hyperactivity
hyperacuity
hyperacusia
hyperacusis
hyperammonemia
hyperbaric oxygen
hyperbetalipoproteinemia
hyperbilirubinemia
hyperbolic glasses
hypercalcemia
hypercalcemic
hypercapnia
hypercholesterolemic xanthomatosis
hyperchylomicronemia
hypercupremia
hyperdeviation
    dissociated h.
hyperelastica
    cutis h.
hyperemia
    ciliary h.
    conjunctival h.
hyperemic
hyperesophoria
hyperesthesia
    optic h.
    h. optica
hypereuryopia
hyperexophoria
hyperfluorescence
    choroidal h.
hyperglycemia
hyperhidrosis
hyperkeratosis
hyperkeratotic disorder
hyperkinesia
hyperkinesis
hyperlipidemia
hyperlipoproteinemia
hypermaturation
hypermature cataract
hypermetrope
hypermetropia
    index h.
hypermetropic astigmatism
hyperope
hyperophthalmopathic syndrome
hyperopia, hypermetropia (H)
    absolute h.
    axial h.
    curvature h.

facultative h.
high h.
index h.
h. index
latent h. (Hl)
manifest h. (Hm)
refractive h.
relative h.
total h. (Ht)
hyperopic (H)
    h. astigmatism
hyperornithinemia
hyperornithinemia,
  hyperammonemia, and
  homocitrullinuria (HHH)
hyperosmotic agent
hyperostosis
    infantile cortical h.
hyperparathyroidism
hyperphoria (H)
    circumduction h.
    left h.
    right h.
hyperpituitarism
hyperplasia
    iris epithelial h.
    lymphoid h.
    pseudoepitheliomatous h.
    pseudosarcomatous
      endothelial h.
    retinal epithelial pigment h.
hyperplastic vitreous
hyperprebetalipoproteinemia
hyperpresbyopia
hyperprolactinemia
Hypersal
hypersecretion
    h. glaucoma
hypersensitivity
    antibody-dependent
      cytotoxic h.
    cell-mediated h.
    delayed h.
    delayed-type h.
    immediate type h.
    h. reaction
hypertelorism
    canthal h.
    ocular h.
    orbital h.
hypertension
    adrenal h.
    arterial h.

essential h.
idiopathic h.
malignant h.
ocular h. (OHT)
hypertensive
  h. iridocyclitis
  h. neuroretinopathy
  h. oculopathy
  h. retinitis
  h. retinopathy
hyperthermia
  malignant h.
hyperthyroidism
  ophthalmic h.
hyperthyroid stare
hypertonia oculi
hypertonic
  h. agent
  h. osmotherapy
  h. solution
hypertrophic
  h. interstitial neuropathy
  left h.
  h. rhinitis
hypertrophy
  epithelial h.
  gelatinous-appearing
   limbal h.
  giant papillary h. (GPH)
  retinal pigment epithelial h.
  RP h.
hypertropia (HT)
  alternating h.
  constant h.
  dissociated h.
  dissociated double h.
   (DDH)
  double h.
  double dissociated h.
  flick h.
  left h. (LHT)
  right h.
hyperviscosity
  h. syndrome
hypervitaminosis
  vitamin A h.
  vitamin D h.
hypha, pl. **hyphae**
hyphal
hyphema
  black-ball h.
  eight-ball h.
  layered h.

microscopic h.
postsurgical h.
spontaneous h.
total h.
traumatic h.
uveitis glaucoma h. (UGH)
hyphemia
hypnagogic hallucination
hypnopompic hallucination
hypocalcemia
hypocalcemic cataract
hypochlorite
  calcium h.
  sodium h.
hypochromic
Hypoclear
hypocyclosis
hypoesophoria
hypoexophoria
hypofluorescence
hypogammaglobulinemia
  X-linked h.
hypoglycemia
  neonatal h.
hypoglycemic cataract
hypokalemia
hypolipoproteinemia
hypolysinemia
hypometric saccade
hypoparathyroidism
hypoperfusion
  aortic h.
hypophoria
hypophosphatasia
  congenital h.
hypophyseal, hypophysial
  h. artery
hypophysectomy
hypophysis
hypopituitarism
hypoplasia
  bow-tie h.
  hemiopic h.
  homonymous hemiopic h.
  macular h.
  optic nerve h.
  thymic h.
hypoplastic disk
hypopyon
  h. keratitis
  keratoiritis h.
  recurrent h.
  h. ulcer

hyposcleral
Hypotears
Hypotears PF
hypotelorism
    ocular h.
    orbital h.
hypotensive
    h. agent
    h. retinopathy
hypothalami
    pars optica h.
hypothalamic glioma
hypothalamic-pituitary-thyroid axis
hypothalamus
hypothesis
    Lyon h.
    h. testing
hypothyroidism
hypotonia, hypotony
    h. oculi
hypotonic solution
hypotonus

hypotony
    essential h.
    ocular h.
hypotropia
    alternating h.
    constant h.
hypovitaminosis
hypoxia
    orbital h.
hypoxic eyeball syndrome
hypsiconchous
hysteria
hysteric
    h. amaurosis
    h. amblyopia
    h. field
hysterical
    h. amblyopia
    h. blindness
    h. constricted field
    h. nystagmus
hysteropia

I
    inspired gas
    iodine
    luminous intensity
I&A
    irrigating-aspirating
    irrigation-aspiration
    irrigation and aspiration
        Simcoe I&A system
I/A
    irrigating/aspirating
    irrigation/aspiration
        I/A machine
Ialo photocoagulator
ianthinopsia
iatrogenic
        i. break
        i. retinal break
        i. retinal hole
        i. retinal tear
ibuprofen
ICCE
    intracapsular cataract extraction
ICD
    intercanthal distance
ICE
    iridocorneal endothelial syndrome
        ICE syndrome
ice ball
Iceland spar
I-cell disease
I-Chlor
ichthyosis
        congenital i.
        i. cornea
ICR rat model
icteric
icterus
        scleral i.
IDDM
    insulin-dependent diabetes
        mellitus
identical point
identification
        nasal mucosal i.
IDI corneoscope
idiocy
        amaurotic i.
        amaurotic familial i.
        familial i.

idiopathic
        i. arteritis of Takayasu
        i. congenital esotropia
        i. hypertension
        i. lipid keratopathy
        i. macular cyst and hole
        i. preretinal membrane
        i. vitreitis
        i. vitritis
idioretinal light
idiosyncrasy
        drug i.
idoxuridine (IDU)
I-Drops
IDU
    idoxuridine
IFA
    indirect fluorescent antibody
I-Gent
ignipuncture
I-Homatrine
IK
    interstitial keratitis
I-knife
    Alcon I-k
ileitis
Ilg
        I. capsule forceps
        I. curved micro tying
          forceps
        I. insertion forceps
        I. lens loop
        I. micro needle holder
        I. needle
        I. needle holder
        I. probe
        I. push/pull
Iliff
        I. lacrimal probe
        I. lacrimal trephine
        I. probe
        I. trephine
Iliff-Haus operation
Iliff-House sclerectomy
Iliff-Park speculum
Iliff's
        I. approach
        I. exenteration
        I. operation

Iliff-Wright
    I.-W. fascia needle
    I.-W. needle
I-Liqui Tears
illacrimation
illaqueation
illiterate eye chart
illuminance
illuminated suction needle
illuminating
illumination
    axial i.
    background i.
    central i.
    coaxial i.
    contact i.
    critical i.
    dark-field i.
    dark-ground i.
    direct i.
    erect i.
    focal i.
    Köhler i.
    lateral i.
    narrow-slit i.
    oblique i.
    slit i.
    vertical i.
Illuminator
    Luxo Surgical I.
illuminator
    high intensity i.
illumining
illusion
    Hermann grid i.
    Kuhnt's i.
    i. of movement
    oculogravic i.
    oculogyral i.
    optical i.
    passive i.
Ilotycin
I-Lube
image
    accidental i.
    astigmatic i.
    catatropic i.
    i. degradation
    direct i.
    i. displacement
    false i.
    foveal i.

    ghost i.
    heteronymous i.
    homonymous i.
    incidental i.
    inversion of i.
    inverted i.
    i. jump
    i. of mires
    mirror i.
    negative i.
    ocular i.
    optical i.
    i. point
    Purkinje's i.
    Purkinje-Sanson i.
    Purkinje-Sanson mirror i.
    real i.
    retinal i.
    Sanson's i.
    spectacular i.
    specular i.
    stigmatic i.
    true i.
    unequal retinal i.
    virtual i.
    visual i.
imager
    Humphrey retina i.
image-space
    i.-s. focus
imaging
    cine-magnetic resonance i.
    magnetic resonance i. (MRI)
    posterior visual pathway i.
    i. technology
imbalance
    binocular i.
Imbert-Fick principle
imbrication
    retinal i.
imipramine
immature
    i. cataract
    i. neuroglia
immediate type hypersensitivity
immersion
    i. lens
    i. method
imminens
    glaucoma i.
immitis
    Coccidioides i.

immobilization
    Treponema pallidum i.
    (TPI)
immune
    i. complex
    i. complex disease
    i. mechanism
    i. reaction
    i. response
    i. system
immunity
    adaptive i.
    cell-mediated i. (CMI)
    humoral i.
immunization
immunodeficiency
    severe combined i. (SCID)
immunodeficiency syndrome
immunodiagnosis
immunodiagnostic method
immunofluorescence
    anticomplement i.
immunofluorescent
    i. assay
    i. staining
immunoglobulin
immunoglobulin E
immunohistochemical technique
immunohistochemistry
immunologic
    i. abnormality
    i. memory
    i. reaction
immunological conjunctivitis
immunology
    ocular i.
immunomodulation
immunopathology
immunopotentiation
immunosuppression
immunosuppressive
    i. agent
    i. drug
immunotherapy
    desensitization i.
impact resistance
impairment
    adduction i.
    cortical visual i.
impatency
    congenital i.
impending macular hole

imperfecta
    osteogenesis i.
impetigo
    i. contagiosa
impinge
impinged
impingement
impinging
Implant
implant
    acorn-shaped i.
    acorn-shaped eye i.
    acrylic i.
    Allen-Braley i.
    Allen orbital i.
    Alpar i.
    Arroyo i.
    Arruga i.
    Arruga-Moura-Brazil i.
    Barkan infant i.
    Barraquer i.
    Berens i.
    Berens conical i.
    Berens pyramidal i.
    Berens-Rosa i.
    Berens-Rosa scleral i.
    Binkhorst i.
    Binkhorst collar stud lens i.
    Binkhorst four loop iris-
      fixated i.
    Binkhorst two-loop
      intraocular lens i.
    Biomatrix ocular i.
    Boberg-Ans i.
    Boberg-Ans lens i.
    Bonaccolto monoplex
      orbital i.
    Bonaccolto orbital i.
    Boyd i.
    Boyd orbital i.
    Brawner i.
    Brawner orbital i.
    Brown-Dohlman Silastic
      corneal i.
    build-up i.
    Bunker i.
    Cardona focalizing fundus i.
    Cardona focalizing fundus
      lens i.
    Cardona goniofocalizing i.
    Castroviejo i.
    Castroviejo acrylic i.
    Choyce i.

implant *(continued)*
    Choyce Mark VIII i.
    Cogan-Boberg-Ans i.
    Cogan-Boberg-Ans lens i.
    conical i.
    conus shell type eye i.
    conventional shell i.
    Cooper i.
    Copeland i.
    corneal i.
    cosmetic contact shell i.
    Cryo-Barrages vitreous i.
    curl backshell i.
    Cutler i.
    Dannheim i.
    Dannheim eye i.
    45-degree bent reform i.
    Dermostat i.
    Doherty i.
    Doherty sphere i.
    encircling i.
    i. entry
    Epstein collar stud acrylic i.
    i. extrusion
    Federov four-loop iris clip
      lens i.
    Federov type I lens i.
    Federov type II lens i.
    Ferguson i.
    Fine magnetic i.
    four-loop iris clip i.
    four-loop iris fixated i.
    Fox i.
    Fox sphere i.
    Frey i.
    Frey tunneled i.
    front build-up i.
    full-dimpled Lucite i.
    Garcia-Novito i.
    Garcia-Novito eye i.
    Gelfilm i.
    Gelfilm retinal i.
    glass sphere i.
    Goldmann i.
    Goldmann three-mirror i.
    Gold-Mules i.
    gold sphere i.
    gonioscopic i.
    grooved silicone i.
    Guist i.
    Guist sphere i.
    Haik i.
    hemisphere i.

    hemisphere eye i.
    hollow-sphere i.
    hook-type i.
    Hruby i.
    Hughes i.
    Intracanalicular Collagen i.
    intraocular i.
    intraocular lens i.
    Iowa i.
    Iowa orbital i.
    Ivalon sponge i.
    Jordan i.
    keratolens i.
    King i.
    King orbital i.
    Koeppe i.
    Koeppe gonioscopic i.
    Krupin-Denver long-value i.
    Kryptok i.
    Landegger i.
    Landegger orbital i.
    Lemoine i.
    Lemoine orbital i.
    lens i.
    i. lens
    Levitt i.
    Lincoff i.
    Lincoff scleral sponge i.
    Lovac fundus contact
      lens i.
    Lovac six-mirror i.
    Lovac six-mirror gonioscopic
      lens i.
    Lucite i.
    Lucite sphere i.
    Lyda-Ivalon-Lucite i.
    i. magnet
    magnetic i.
    McCannel i.
    McGhan i.
    Medical Optics PC11NB
      intraocular lens i.
    Medical Workshop
      intraocular lens i.
    Medicornea Kratz
      intraocular lens i.
    Melauskas acrylic i.
    Melauskas orbital i.
    meridional i.
    methyl methacrylate i.
    i. migration
    Molteno i.
    motility i.

Mueller i.
Muhlberger orbital i.
Mules i.
Nocito i.
Nocito eye i.
O'Malley i.
O'Malley self-adhering
   lens i.
optic i.
orbital i.
orbital floor i.
peanut i.
Pierce I/A tripod i.
i. placement
plastic sphere i.
Platina intraocular lens i.
Plexiglas i.
polyethylene i.
posterior chamber lens i.
   (PCLI)
posterior tube shunt i.
Precision Cosmet intraocular
   lens i.
primary lens i.
pseudophake i.
Radin-Rosenthal i.
Radin-Rosenthal eye i.
Rayner-Choyce i.
retinal Gelfilm i.
reverse-shape i.
Ridley i.
Ridley anterior chamber
   lens i.
Ridley Mark II i.
Ridley Mark II lens i.
Rodin i.
Rodin orbital i.
Rosa-Berens i.
Rosa-Berens orbital i.
Ruedemann i.
Ruedemann eye i.
Ruiz plano fundus i.
Ruiz plano fundus lens i.
Schepens hollow
   hemisphere i.
scleral i.
secondary lens i.
segmental i.
semishell i.
Severin i.
Shearing posterior chamber
   intraocular lens i.
shelf-type i.

shell i.
Sichi i.
Sichi orbital i.
Silastic i.
Silastic scleral buckler i.
silicone i.
silicone mesh i.
i. sleeve
sleeve i.
sling for i.
Smith orbital floor i.
Snellen i.
Snellen conventional
   reform i.
solid silicone with Supramid
   mesh i.
sphere i.
spherical i.
i. sponge
sponge i.
Stone i.
Stone-Jordan i.
Strampelli i.
Strampelli lens i.
subperiosteal i.
Supramid i.
Supramid-Allen i.
Supramid lens i.
surface i.
tantalum mesh i.
Teflon i.
temporary intracanalicular
   collagen i.
Tennant i.
Tensilon i.
i. tire
tire i.
Troncoso gonioscopic i.
Troncoso gonioscopic lens i.
Troutman i.
tunneled i.
Ultex i.
Ultex lens i.
Uribe i.
Uribe orbital i.
VA magnetic i.
VA magnetic orbital i.
Varigray i.
Varilux i.
Varilux lens i.
Vitallium i.
Volk conoid i.
Volk conoid lens i.

implant *(continued)*
  Walter Reed i.
  Wheeler i.
  Wheeler eye sphere i.
  wire mesh i.
implantation
  in-the-bag i.
  intraocular lens i.
  i. lens
implanter
  Geuder i.
implantoptic
Implens intraocular lens
impletion
impression
  basilar i.
  i. cytology
  i. tonometer
imprint
improvement
  no i. (NI)
  pinhole no i. (PHNI)
Imre's
  I. keratoplasty
  I. lateral canthoplasty
  I. lateral canthoplasty
    operation
  I. operation
  I. sliding flap
  I. treatment
inadequacy
  blink i.
I-Naphline
inattention
  visual i.
inborn
  i. error
  i. error of metabolism
incandescent lamp
incarceration
  iris i.
incidence
  i. rate
incident
  i. angle
  flux i.
  i. light
  i. point
  ray i.
  i. ray of light
incidental
  i. color
  i. image

incipient cataract
incision
  Agnew-Verhoeff i.
  chord i.
  conjunctival i.
  corneal i.
  corneoscleral i.
  corridor i.
  cutdown i.
  grayline i.
  grooved i.
  i. into eyelid
  limbal i.
  posterior i.
  relaxing i.
  i. spreader
  Swan i.
  T-i.
  i. terminus
  trap i.
  trapezoidal i.
  von Noorden's i.
incisura, pl. **incisurae**
  i. ethmoidalis ossis frontalis
  i. frontalis
  i. lacrimalis
  i. maxillae
  i. supraorbitalis
incisure
  ethmoidal i.
  frontal i.
  lacrimal i.
  supraorbital i.
inclinometer
inclusion
  i. blennorrhea
  i. body
  i. conjunctivitis
  i. cyst
  i. disease
  epithelial i.'s
  lipid-like i.'s
  mascara particle i.'s
incomitance
incomitant
  i. strabismus
  i. vertical deviation
  i. vertical strabismus
incomplete
  i. achromatopsia
  i. hemianopsia
incongruent nystagmus

incongruous
  i. field defect
  i. hemianopsia
incontinentia pigmenti
increment
  i. threshold spectral
    sensitivity
incrementally
incrustation
  zinc i.'s
incycloduction
incyclophoria
incyclotropia
incyclovergence
indentation
  i. gonioscopy
  i. operation
  prominent i.
  i. tonometer
  i. tonometry
independent event
index, gen **indicis**, pl. **indices**,
  indexes
  i. amblyopia
  i. ametropia
  i. case
  i. hypermetropia
  hyperopia i.
  i. hyperopia
  myopia i.
  i. myopia
  i. of refraction (n)
  i. of refraction
indicator
  Berens-Tolman ocular
    hypertension i.
  i. yellow
indirect
  binocular i.
  i. fluorescent antibody (IFA)
  i. fluorescent antibody test
  i. ophthalmoscope
  i. ophthalmoscopy
  i. pupillary reaction
  i. vision
Indocin ophthalmic solution
indocyanine green
indomethacin
  i. toxicity keratopathy
induced anisophoria
induction
industrial spectacles
inelastic

I-Neocort
inert material for intraocular lens
infant
  i. Karickhoff laser lens
  premature i.
  i. three-mirror laser lens
infantile
  i. cataract
  i. cortical hyperostosis
  i. esotropia
  i. glaucoma
  i. optic atrophy
  i. purulent conjunctivitis
  i. Refsum disease
infantilism
  Lorain's i.
infarct
infarction
  cerebral i.
  eye i.
  myocardial i.
  retinochoroidal i.
infection
  anaerobic ocular i.
  bacterial i.
  chlamydial i.
  dental i.
  eyelid molluscum
    contagiosum i.
  fungal i.
  graft i.
  mycotic i.
  trematode i.
  vaccinia i.
infectiosus
  conjunctivitis necroticans i.
infectious
  i. conjunctivitis
  i. dacryoadenitis
  i. disease
  i. eczematoid dermatitis
  i. endophthalmitis
  i. mononucleosis
  i. ophthalmoplegia
  i. polyneuritis
infective endocarditis
Infectrol
inferior
  i. altitudinal defect
  i. arcade
  i. arcuate bundle
  arcus palpebralis i.
  arteriola macularis i.

inferior *(continued)*
    arteriola nasalis retinae i.
    arteriola temporalis
      retinae i.
    i. canaliculus
    i. conjunctival fornix
    i. conus
    i. fasciculus
    fissura orbitalis i.
    i. fornix
    i. fornix reformation
    glandula lacrimalis i.
    i. lacrimal gland
    i. longitudinal fasciculus
    i. macular arteriole
    i. meatus nasi
    i. muscle
    musculus tarsalis i.
    i. nasal artery
    i. nasal vein
    i. oblique (IO)
    i. oblique extraocular
      muscles
    i. oblique muscle
    i. oblique overaction
    i. ophthalmic vein
    i. orbital fissure
    i. orbital rim
    i. palpebra
    i. palpebral vein
    i. pole
    i. punctum
    i. rectus (IR)
    i. rectus extraocular muscles
    i. rectus muscle
    i. tarsal muscle
    i. tarsus
    i. tarsus palpebra
    i. temporal arcade
    i. temporal artery
    i. temporal vein
    vena ophthalmica i.
    venula macularis i.
    venula nasalis retinae i.
    venula temporalis retinae i.
    i. zone of retina
    i. zygomatic foramen
inferiores
    venae palpebrales i.
inferioris
    pars orbitalis gyri
      frontalis i.

inferiorly
    eye rotated i.
inferonasal artery
inferonasally
inferotemporal
    i. arcade
    i. artery
inferotemporally
infiltrate
    corneal i.
    corneal punctate i.
    crystalline i.
    leukemic i.
    plasmacytoid i.
    subepithelial punctate
      corneal i.
    white stromal i.
infiltrates in cornea
infiltration
    choroidal i.
    leukemic i.
    lymphoid i.
    mononuclear cell i.
infinite distance
infinity
Inflamase
    I. Forte
    I. Mild
inflammation
    i. of eyelid
    ocular i.
inflammatory
    i. bowel disease
    i. cells
    i. changes of retina
    i. ectropion
    i. glaucoma
    i. mediator
    i. optic neuropathy
    i. retinopathy
    i. target site
    i. target site of eye
inflection, inflexion
inflow
    aqueous i.
influenza
influenzae
    Haemophilus i.
infraciliary
infraduct
infraduction
infraepitrochlear nerve
infranasal

infranasally
infranuclear
    i. disorder
    i. pathway
infraorbital
    i. anesthesia
    i. artery
    i. canal
    i. foramen
    i. groove
    i. margin
    i. margin of maxilla
    i. nerve
    i. region
    i. sulcus of maxilla
    i. suture
infraorbitale
    foramen i.
infraorbitalis
    nervus i.
    sutura i.
infrapalpebralis
    sulcus i.
infrapalpebral sulcus
infrared
    i. cataract
    i. radiation
    i. slit lamp
infratentorial arteriovenous
  malformation
infratrochlear nerve
infravergence
infraversion
infundibular cyst
infusion
    i. cannula
    i. suction cutter vitreous
      cutter
ingrowth
    epithelial i.
    fibroblastic i.
inguinale
    granuloma i.
INH
  isoniazid
inhalational agent
inhalation anesthetic
inheritance
    autosomal recessive i.
    dominant i.
    polygenic i.
    recessive i.
    X-linked i.

inhibition
    lateral i.
inhibitional
    i. palsy
    i. palsy of contralateral
      antagonist
inhibitor
    anticholinesterase i.
    carbonic anhydrase i.
    collagenase i.
    sympathetic i.
injection
    ciliary i.
    circumcorneal i.
    conjunctival i.
    intravitreal i.
    i. molding
    peribulbar i.
    periocular i.
    retrobulbar i.
    subconjunctival i.
    Van Lint's i.
injector
    automatic twin syringe i.
    Dyonics syringe i.
injury
    chemical i.
    concussion i.
    contrecoup i.
    coup i.
    eye i.
    levator i.
    microwave radiation i.
    ocular i.
    penetrating i.
    radiation i.
inlay
    corneal i.'s
inner
    i. canthus
    i. limiting membrane
    i. nuclear layer
    i. plexiform layer
    i. punctate choroidopathy
    i. retina
    i. segment
innervate
innervation
    Hering's law of equal i.
    Hering's law of
      equivalent i.
    reciprocal i.

innervation *(continued)*
Sherrington's law of
reciprocal i.
innocens
diabetes i.
InnoMed Corporation
Innovar
INNOVA System 920
INO
internuclear ophthalmoplegia
inositus
diabetes i.
input
nerve i.
i. nerve
input/output (I/O)
inserter
Lens-Eze i.
insertion
tendinous i.
tensor i.
insipidus
diabetes i.
inspired gas (I)
instillation
instilled
Institute
American National
Standards I. (ANSI)
Dartmouth Eye I.
instrument
Daisy irrigation-aspiration i.
fixation i.
optical centering i.
vitrectomy i.
instrument/apparatus
Squid i./a.
instrumentation
Instruments
AO Reichert I.
instruments
American Hydron i.
Argyll-Robertson i.
Ascon i.
Ayerst i.
Birks Mark II i.
Carl Zeiss i.
guillotine vitrectomy i.
IOLAB titanium i.
Karl Ilg i.
Kerato-Kontours i.
Rizzuti-Bonaccolto i.
Rizzuti-Fleischer i.

Rizzuti-Kayser-Fleischer i.
Rizzuti-Lowe i.
Rizzuti-Maxwell i.
Rizzuti-Soemmering i.
Sutherland Rotatable
Microsurgery i.
Thomas Kapsule i.
Thomas Kapsule i.
insufficiency
carotid artery i.
convergence i.
cortical visual i.
divergence i.
i. of externi
i. of eyelids
muscular i.
insular scotoma
insulin
i. pump CPI90-100
insulin-deficient diabetes
insulin-dependent
i.-d. diabetes mellitus
(IDDM)
Insulin pump CP190-100
intact
extraocular movements i.
(EOMI)
intake
caloric i.
integrity
break in retinal i.
intensity
luminous i. (I)
radiant i.
interaction
contour i.
drug i.
spatial i.
intercalary staphyloma
intercanthal distance (ICD)
intercanthic
intercellular space
interciliary fiber
intercilium
interface
graft-host i.
i. opacity
parallel i.
i. phenomena
interfasciale
spatium i.
interfascial space

interference
    i. filter
    i. fringe
    i. visual acuity test
interferometer
    electron i.
interferometry
    electron i.
    laser i.
interferon
interior eye tumor
interlamellar space
interleukin
intermediate
    i. posterior curve (IPC)
    i. uveitis
intermedics
    I. intraocular tonometer
    I. lens
    I. Phaco I/A Unit
    Pharmacia I.
intermedius nerve
intermittent
    i. angle-closure glaucoma
    i. esotropia
    i. exotropia (X(T))
    i. strabismus
    i. tropia
intermuscular
    i. membrane
    i. septum
interna
    axis oculi i.
    membrana granulosa i.
    membrana limitans i.
internal
    i. axis of eye
    i. blockage
    i. capsule syndrome
    i. carotid artery
    i. hordeolum
    i. hydrocephalus
    i. lacrimal fistula
    i. limiting membrane
    i. ophthalmopathy
    i. ophthalmoplegia
    i. ostium
    i. palsy
    i. squint
    i. strabismus
internuclear
    i. ophthalmoplegia (INO)
    i. paralysis

internus
    axis bulbi i.
interpalpebral
    i. fissure
    i. zone
interpolation
interpretation
interpupillary
    i. distance (IPD)
interrogans
    Leptospira i.
interrupted nylon suture
Intersol
Interspace YAG laser lens
interstitial
    i. keratitis (IK)
    i. neovascularization
    i. pneumonitis
interthalamic commissure
intervaginale
    spatium i.
intervaginal space of optic nerve
interval
    focal i.
    i. of Sturm
    Sturm's i.
intestinal disorder
in-the-bag
    i.-t.-b. implantation
    i.-t.-b. lens
intima
intimal
intorsion
intortor
intoxication with alcohol
intoxification amaurosis
intra-axonal
intracameral suture
Intracanalicular Collagen implant
intracanicular
intracapsular
    i. cataract extraction (ICCE)
    i. cataract extraction
      operation
    i. extraction
    i. extraction of cataract
intracavernous
intracellular
intracorneal
intracranial
    i. glioma
    i. pressure
intracytoplasmic inclusion body

intradermal nevus
intraepithelial
  i. cyst
  i. dyskeratosis
  i. epithelioma
  i. neoplasia
  i. plexus
intralesional
intramarginal sulcus
intramedullary segment
intranuclear
intraocular
  i. administration
  i. air
  i. cataract extraction
  i. cysticercus
  i. distance
  i. fistula
  i. fluid
  i. forceps
  i. foreign body
  i. gas
  i. gas bubble
  i. hemorrhage
  i. implant
  i. lens (IOL)
  i. lens dialer
  i. lens dislocation
  i. lens glide
  i. lens implant
  i. lens implantation
  i. lymphoma
  i. melanoma
  i. muscle (IOM)
  i. neuritis
  i. optic neuritis
  i. pressure (IOP)
  i. silicone oil tamponade
  i. tension
intraoperative adjustment
IntraOptics lensometer
intraorbital
  i. anesthesia
  i. foreign body
  i. margin of orbit
  i. nerve dysfunction
intrapapillary drusen
intraretinal microvascular
  abnormality (IRMA)
intrascleral
  i. nerve loop
  i. plexus
intrasellar tumor

intrasheath tenotomy
intrastromal laser
intratemporal segment
intrathecal
intravenous
  i. agent
  i. fluorescein (IVF)
  i. thyrotropin-releasing
    hormone test
intravitreal
  i. fibrin
  i. injection
intravitreous
intrinsic
  i. light
  i. muscle
  i. ocular muscle
introducer
  Carter sphere i.
  silicone i.
  sphere i.
  Weaver trocar i.
intubation
  Silastic i.
  silicone i.
intumescent cataract
invaginated
invagination
invasion
  epithelial i.
invasive adenoma
inverse
  i. astigmatism
  i. ocular bobbing
inversion
  i. of image
inversus
  blepharophimosis i.
  epicanthal i.
  situs i.
inverted
  i. image
  i. posture
investigation
  neurophthalmological i.
invisible bifocal
involution
involutional
  i. ectropion
  i. entropion
  i. ptosis
  i. senile ectropion

i. senile entropion
i. senile ptosis
inward rectifier
IO
inferior oblique
I/O
input/output
Iocare
I. balanced salt solution
I. titanium needle
Iodide
Phospholine I.
iodide
echothiophate i.
metubine i.
potassium i.
iodine (I)
radioactive i.
iodochlorhydroxyquin
iodopsin
iodoquinol
IOL
intraocular lens
Kearney side-notch IOL
IOLAB
I. 108 B lens
I. I&A photocoagulator
I. intraocular lens
I. irrigating/aspirating
photocoagulator
I. irrigating/aspirating unit
I. irrigating needle
I. needle
I. taper-cut needle
I. taper-point needle
I. titanium instruments
I. titanium needle
IOM
intraocular muscle
ION
ischemic optic neuropathy
ion
irradiation i.
laser i.
i. laser
ionic surfactant
ionizing radiation
iontophoresis
IOP
intraocular pressure
Ioptex
I. intraocular lens

I. laser intraocular lens
I. TabOptic lens
iothalamate meglumine/sodium
Iowa
I. implant
I. orbital implant
I. State fixation forceps
I/P
iris and pupil
I-Paracaine
I-Parescein
IPC
intermediate posterior curve
IPD
interpupillary distance
ipecac
I-Pentolate
I-Phrine
I-Picamide
I-Pilocarpine
I-Pilopine
I-Pred
I-Prednicet
ipsilateral
i. antagonist
i. centrocecal scotoma
IR
inferior rectus
Irene lens
I-Rescein
iridal
iridalgia
iridauxesis
iridectasis
iridectome
iridectomesodialysis
iridectomize
iridectomy
argon laser i.
basal i.
Bethke's i.
buttonhole i.
Castroviejo's i.
central i.
Chandler's i.
complete i.
Elschnig's i.
Elschnig's central i.
laser i.
i. operation
optic i.
optical i.
patent i.

219

iridectomy *(continued)*
    peripheral i. (PI)
    preliminary i.
    preparatory i.
    pupil-to-root i.
    i. scissors
    sector i.
    stenopeic i.
    superior sector i.
    therapeutic i.
iridectopia
iridectropium
iridemia
iridencleisis
    Holth's i.
    i. operation
iridentropium
irideremia
irides
iridescent vision
iridesis
iridiagnosis
iridial, iridian, iridic
    i. angle
    i. folds
iridica
    stella lentis i.
iridis
    angulus i.
    ectopia i.
    epithelium pigmentosum i.
    facies anterior i.
    facies posterior i.
    granuloma i.
    herpes i.
    ligamentum pectinatum i.
    margo ciliaris i.
    margo pupillaris i.
    melanosis i.
    plicae i.
    rubeosis i.
    i. rubeosis
    sinus circularis i.
    spatia anguli i.
    sphincter i.
    xanthelasmatosis i.
    xanthomatosis i.
iridization
iridoavulsion
iridocapsular
    i. intraocular lens
    i. lens
iridocapsulitis

iridocapsulotomy
    i. scissors
iridocele
iridochoroiditis
iridocoloboma
iridoconstrictor
iridocorneal
    i. angle
    i. dysgenesis
    i. endothelial syndrome
    i. endothelial syndrome (ICE)
    i. mesodermal dysgenesis
iridocornealis
    angular i.
    angulus i.
    ligamentum anguli i.
    ligamentum pectinatum
     anguli i.
    spatia anguli i.
iridocorneosclerectomy
iridocyclectomy
iridocyclitis
    Fuchs' heterochromic i.
    herpes i.
    herpes simplex i.
    herpes zoster i.
    heterochromic i.
    hypertensive i.
    i. masquerade syndrome
    posttraumatic i.
    i. septica
    varicella i.
iridocyclochoroidectomy
    Peyman's i.
iridocyclochoroiditis
iridocycloretraction
iridocystectomy
iridodesis
iridodiagnosis
iridodialysis operation
iridodiastasis
iridodilator
iridodonesis
iridoendothelial syndrome
iridogoniocyclectomy
iridogoniodysgenesis
iridokeratitis
iridokinesis, iridokinesia
iridokinetic
iridoleptynsis
iridology
iridolysis
iridomalacia

iridomesodialysis
iridomotor
iridoncosis
iridoncus
iridoparalysis
iridopathy
iridoperiphakitis
iridoplasty
iridoplegia
    i. accommodation
    complete i.
    i. reflex
    sympathetic i.
iridoptosis
iridopupillary
iridorhexis
iridoschisis
iridoschisma
iridosclerotomy
iridosteresis
iridotasis operation
iridotomy
    Abraham i.
    Castroviejo's i.
    Castroviejo's radial i.
    laser i.
    i. lens
    i. operation
    radial i.
    i. scissors
iridovitreosynechiae
Irigate
I-Rinse
iris, pl. irides
    angle of i.
    arterial circle of greater i.
    arterial circle of lesser i.
    i. atrophy
    i. bombé
    i. capture
    ciliary margin of i.
    circle of greater i.
    circle of lesser i.
    coloboma of i.
    i. coloboma
    congenital cleft of i.
    i. contraction reflex
    cosmetic i.
    i. crypt
    i. cyst
    i. dehiscence
    detached i.
    i. diameter

i. diastasis
i. dilator
i. ectasia
embryonal epithelial cyst
    of i.
i. epithelial hyperplasia
i. eye
Florentine's i.
i. forceps
i. freckles
i. frill
greater ring of i.
hernia of i.
i. hook
i. hook cannula
hydrops of i.
i. incarceration
i. knife needle
leiomyoma of i.
lesser ring of i.
major arterial circle of i.
melanoma of i.
i. neurofibroma
i. nodule
notch of i.
i. pearl
pectinate ligament of i.
pigmented epithelium of i.
pigmented layer of i.
i. pits
plateau i.
i. process
prolapse of i.
i. prolapse
i. and pupil (I/P)
pupillae muscle of i.
pupillary margin of i.
i. repositor
i. retraction syndrome of
    Campbell
ring of i.
i. ring
i. roll
i. root
i. scissors
shredded i.
i. spatula
i. sphincter
i. stroma
stroma of i.
i. support
i. suture
i. sweep

iris *(continued)*
    i. synechia
    transfixion of i.
    tremulous i.
    i. tuck
    umbrella i.
iris-fixated lens
iris-nevus syndrome
Iri-Sol
irisopsia
iris-supported lens
iritic
iritides
iritis
    i. blennorrhagique à
      rechutes
    i. blenorrhagique à rechutes
    i. catamenialis
    diabetic i.
    Doyne's i.
    Doyne's guttate i.
    i. fibrinitis
    fibrinous i.
    follicular i.
    i. glaucomatosa
    gouty i.
    hemorrhagic i.
    i. nodosa
    nodular i.
    i. obturans
    i. papulosa
    plastic i.
    purulent i.
    quiet i.
    i. recidivans staphylococcal
      allergica
    i. recidivans staphylococco-
      allergica
    i. roseata
    serous i.
    spongy i.
    sympathetic i.
    syphilitic i.
    tuberculous i.
    uratic i.
iritoectomy
iritomy
IRMA
    intraretinal microvascular
      abnormality
iron
    i. deposit
    i. deposition

    i. Fleischer ring
    i. line
iron-ferry line
iron-Hudson-Stähli line
iron-leaking bleb
iron-stocker line
irotomy
irradiance
irradiation
    cataract i.
    i. cataract
    heavy ion i.
    i. ion
irregular
    i. astigmatism
    i. nystagmus
    i. pupil
irregularity
    surface i.
irreversible amblyopia
irrigating
    i. anterior chamber vectis
    i. cannula
    i. cystitome
    i. solution
    i. vectis
irrigating/aspirating,
  irrigation/aspiration (I/A)
    i. cannula
    i. unit
    i. vectis
irrigation-aspiration, irrigating-
  aspirating (I&A)
    i.-a. system
    i.-a. unit
irrigation and aspiration (I&A)
irrigator
    anterior chamber i.
    Birch-Harman i.
    Bishop-Harman i.
    Bishop-Harman anterior
      chamber i.
    cul-de-sac i.
    Fink i.
    Fink cul-de-sac i.
    Hartstein i.
    Randolph i.
    Sylva anterior chamber i.
irritative
    i. hallucination
    i. miosis
Irvine
    I. irrigating/aspirating unit

I. probe-pointed scissors
I. scissors
Irvine-Gass syndrome
Irvine's operation
ischemia
    carotid i.
    choroidal i.
    i. retinae
    retinal i.
    transient i.
    transient vertebrobasilar i.
ischemic
    i. atherosclerosis
    i. chiasmal syndrome
    i. choroidal atrophy
    i. disk
    i. episode
    i. ocular syndrome
    i. oculomotor palsy
    i. optic atrophy
    i. optic neuropathy (ION)
    i. papillitis
    i. papillopathy
    i. retinae
    i. retinopathy
I-Scrub
iseikonia
iseikonic lens
isethionate
    propamidine i.
Ishihara
    I. I-Temp cautery
    I. IV slit lamp
    I. plate
    I. pseudoisochromatic plate
Ishihara's
    I. color test
    I. test
    I. test for color blindness
island
    isolated i.
    Traquair's i.
Ismotic
isobar
isobutyl 2-cyanoacrylate
Isocaine
isocarboxazid
isochromatic plate
isochromosome
isocoria
isoflurophate
isoiconia
isoiconic

iso-iconic lens
I-Sol
isolated island
isomerase
    retinal i.
    retinene i.
isometropia
isoniazid (INH)
    i. therapeutic test
isophoria
isopia
isopropanol
isopropyl alcohol Isopto Alkaline
isoproterenol
isopter
    nasal i.
    sloping i.'s
Isopto
    I. Alkaline
    I. Atropine
    I. Carbachol
    I. Carpine
    I. Cetamide
    I. Cetapred
    I. Eserine
    I. Frin
    I. Homatropine
    I. Hyoscine
    I. P-ES
    I. Prednisolone
    I. Sterofrin
    I. Tears
isoscope
isosorbide
isotonic solution
isotope scan
isotretinoin
I-Sulfacet
I-Sulfalone
Isuprel
I-tech
    I.-t. cannula
    I.-t. cannula holder
    I.-t. cannula tray
    I.-t. Castroviejo bladebreaker
    I.-t. intraocular foreign body
      forceps
    I.-t. needle holder
    I.-t. splinter forceps
    I.-t. tying forceps
I-Temp cautery
Ito procedure
itraconazole

I-Trol
I-Tropine
Ivalon sponge implant
ivermectin
IVEX system
IVF
    intravenous fluorescein

IV slit lamp
Iwanoff's
    I. cysts
    I. retinal edema
I-Wash
I-White
Ixodes dammini

J
joule
jack-in-the-box phenomenon
Jackson
J. cross cylinder
J. lacrimal intubation set
Jacob capsule fragment forceps
Jacob's
J. membrane
J. ulcer
Jacobson's retinitis
Jacob-Swann
J.-S. gonioscope
J.-S. gonioscopic prism
Jacoby
border tissue of J.
Jacod's syndrome
Jacquart's angle
Jadassohn-type anetoderma
Jaeger
J. grading system
J. hook
J. keratome
J. lid plate
J. retractor
J. system
Jaeger's
J. test
J. test types
J. visual test
Jaesche-Arlt operation
Jaesche's operation
Jaffe
J. Cilco lens
J. intraocular spatula
J. lens-manipulating hook
J. lens spatula
J. lid retractor
J. lid retractor set
J. lid speculum
J. micro iris hook
J. needle holder
J. spatula
J. suturing forceps
Jaffe-Bechert nucleus rotator
Jaffe-Givner lid retractor
Jahnke's syndrome
Jaime's
J. lacrimal operation
J. operation

Jamaican optic neuropathy
Jameson
J. calipers
J. forceps
J. hook
J. muscle forceps
J. muscle hook
Jameson's operation
Janelli clip
Jansen-Middleton septotomy forceps
Jansky-Bielschowsky
J.-B. disease
J.-B. syndrome
Jardon eye shield
Jarisch-Herxheimer reaction
jaundice
congenital hemolytic j.
hemolytic j.
neonatal j.
jaundiced
Javal ophthalmometer
Javal-Schiotz ophthalmometer
jaw
j. claudication
Keeler Catford needle
holder with micro j.'s
j. muscle pain
j. winking
jaw-winking
j.-w. phenomenon
j.-w. syndrome
JCAHPO
Joint Commission on Allied
Health Personnel in
Ophthalmology
Jedmed A-scan
Jedmed/DGH A-scan
Jellinek's sign
Jendrassik's sign
Jenning's test
Jensen
J. capsule scratcher
J. intraocular lens forceps
J. lens forceps
J. lens-inserting forceps
J. polisher/scratcher
Jensen's
J. choroiditis
J. choroiditis juxtapapillaris

Jensen's *(continued)*
    J. disease
    J. jerk nystagmus
    J. juxtapapillaris choroiditis
    J. operation
    J. procedure
    J. retinitis
    J. transposition procedure
Jensen-Thomas irrigating-aspirating cannula
jequirity ophthalmia
jerk
    macro square-wave j.'s
    j. nystagmus
    square-wave j.'s
Jervey
    J. capsule fragment forceps
    J. iris forceps
Jeune syndrome
jeweler
    j. forceps
    j. tweezers
J loop
J-loop
    J.-l. PC lens
    J.-l. posterior chamber
    intraocular lens
Joal lens
Jodassohn
    nevus sebaceus of J.
Joffroy's sign
John Green calipers
Johnson
    J. double cannula
    J. erysiphake
    J. evisceration knife
Johnson-Bell erysiphake
Johnson's
    J. operation
    J. syndrome
Johnson-Tooke corneal knife
joint
    sacroiliac j.
Joint Commission on Allied Health Personnel in Ophthalmology (JCAHPO)
Joint Review Committee for Ophthalmic Medical Personnel (JRCOMP)
Jones
    J. dilator
    J. forceps
    J. keratome

    J. punctum dilator
    J. Pyrex tube
    J. tear duct tube
    J. towel clamp
    J. tube
Jones'
    J. dye test
    J. operation
    J. repair
    J. test
    J. tube procedure
Jordan implant
Joseph
    J. device
    J. elevator
joule (J)
JRCOMP
    Joint Review Committee for
    Ophthalmic Medical Personnel
J-shaped
    J.-s. irrigating/aspirating
    cannula
    J.-s. sella
Judd forceps
Judson-Smith manipulator
jump
    image j.
junction
    basal j.
    corneoscleral j.
    mucocutaneous j.
    parieto-occipital-temporal j.
    sclerocorneal j.
    scotoma j.
    j. scotoma
junctional
    j. bay
    j. nevus
    j. scotoma
    j. scotoma of Traquair
    j. zone
Jung-Schaffer intraocular lens
Just Tears
juvenile
    j. arcus
    j. cataract
    j. corneal epithelial
    dystrophy
    j. developmental cataract
    j. diabetes
    j. epithelial dystrophy
    j. glaucoma
    j. GM$_2$ gangliosidosis

j. GM$_1$ gangliosidosis
j. iris xanthogranuloma
j. melanoma
j. nevoxanthoendothelioma
j. optic atrophy
j. pilocytic astrocytoma
j. reflex
j. retinoschisis
j. rheumatoid arthritis
j. xanthogranuloma (JXG)
juvenilis
angiopathia retinae j.

juxtafoveal
juxtapapillaris
Jensen's choroiditis j.
juxtapapillary
j. leakage
j. nerve fiber layer
juxtaposition
juxtapupillary choroiditis
JXG
juvenile xanthogranuloma

K

K
kelvin
phylloquinone
potassium
Kainair
Kaiser speculum
kallikrein
Kalt
K. corneal needle
K. forceps
K. needle holder
K. spoon
Kamerling Capsular 90 lens
kanamycin
Kandori
flecked retina of K.
Kaposi
xeroderma of K.
Kaposi's sarcoma
kappa angle
Kara
K. cataract-aspirating
cannula
K. cataract needle
K. erysiphake
Karakashian-Barraquer scissors
Karickhoff
K. double cannula
K. laser lens
Karl Ilg instruments
karyotype
Kasabach-Merritt syndrome
Katena
K. boat hook
K. double-edged sapphire
blade
K. forceps
K. iris spatula
K. Products
K. trephine
katophoria
katotropia
Katzin
K. scissors
K. trephine
Katzin-Barraquer forceps
Katzin's operation
Kaufman
K. medium
K. type II retractor

K. type II vitrector
K. vitrector
K. vitreophage
Kaufman's media
Kawasaki's disease
Kayser-Fleischer
K.-F. cornea ring
K.-F. ring
KCS
keratoconjunctivitis sicca
Kearney
K. side-notch IOL
K. side-notch lens
Kearns-Sayre syndrome
Keeler
K. Catford micro jaws
needle holder
K. Catford needle holder
with micro jaws
K. cryoextractor
K. cryophake
K. cryophake unit
K. cryosurgical unit
K. extended round tip
forceps
K. intraocular foreign body
grasping forceps
K. intravitreal scissors
K. lancet tip
K. loupe
K. micro round tip
K. microscissors
K. micro spear tip
K. micro tip
K. ophthalmoscope
K. panoramic lens
K. panoramic loupe
K. prism
K. Pulsair tonometer
K. puncture tip
K. razor tip
K. retinoscope
K. retractable blade
K. ruby knife
K. specular microscope
K. tonometer
K. triple facet tip
K. ultrasonic cataract
removal lancet

Keeler-Amoils
    K.-A. curved cataract probe
    K.-A. freeze
    K.-A. glaucoma probe
    K.-A. long-shank probe
    K.-A. long-shank retinal
      probe
    K.-A. Machemer retinal
      probe
    K.-A. micro curved cataract
      probe
    K.-A. Ophthalmic
    Cryosystem
    K.-A. ophthalmic curved
      cataract probe
    K.-A. ophthalmic long-shank
      probe
    K.-A. ophthalmic Machemer
      retinal probe
    K.-A. ophthalmic micro
      curved cataract probe
    K.-A. ophthalmic retinal
      probe
    K.-A. ophthalmic straight
      cataract probe
    K.-A. ophthalmic vitreous
      probe
    K.-A. retinal probe
    K.-A. straight cataract probe
    K.-A. vitreous probe
Keeler-Fison tissue retractor
Keeler-Keislar lacrimal cannula
Keeler-Meyer diamond knife
Keeler-Pierse
    K.-P. eye speculum
    K.-P. speculum
Keeler-Rodger iris retractor
Keeler's pantoscope
Keflin
Kefzol
Keith-Wagener
    K.-W. changes (KW)
    K.-W. classification
    K.-W. retinopathy
Keith-Wagener-Barker classification
Keizer-Lancaster
    K.-L. eye speculum
    K.-L. lid retractor
    K.-L. speculum
Kelly-Descemet membrane punch
Kelly hemostat
Kelman
    K. air cystitome

    K. aspirator
    K. cannula
    K. cryoextractor
    K. cryophake
    K. cryosurgical unit
    K. cyclodialysis cannula
    K. cystitome
    K. flexible tripod lens
    K. iris retractor
    K. irrigating/aspirating unit
    K. irrigating handpiece
    K. knife
    K. lens
    K. Multiflex II lens
    K. Omnifit II intraocular
      lens
    K. Omnifit lens
    K. PC 27LB CapSul lens
    K. phacoemulsification unit
    K. Quadriflex anterior
      chamber intraocular lens
Kelman-Cavitron
    K.-C. I/A unit
    K.-C. irrigating/aspirating
      unit
Kelman-McPherson
    K.-M. corneal forceps
    K.-M. forceps
    K.-M. tying forceps
Kelman's operation
keloid
kelvin (K)
Kenacort
Kenalog
Kennedy's syndrome
Kennerdell
    K. muscle hook
    K. nerve hook
KeraCorneoScope
Kerascan
keratalgia
keratan sulfate
keratectasia
keratectomy
    Castroviejo's k.
    excimer laser
      photoreactive k.
    excimer laser
      photorefractive k.
    k. operation
    photorefractive k. (PRK)
    phototherapeutic k. (PTK)

k. scissors
superficial k.
keratic precipitate (KP)
keratination
keratinization
keratinous
keratitic precipitate
keratitis
    Acanthamoeba k.
    acne rosacea k.
    actinic k.
    aerosol k.
    alphabetical k.
    annular k.
    arborescens k.
    artificial silk k.
    avascular k.
    bacterial k.
    band k.
    k. band
    k. bandelette
    band-shaped k.
    bank k.
    k. bullosa
    candidal k.
    catarrhal ulcerative k.
    chronic superficial k.
    Cogan's interstitial k.
    corneal k.
    deep k.
    deep punctate k.
    deep pustular k.
    dendriform k., dendritic k.
    dendritic herpes zoster k.
    desiccation k.
    diffuse deep k.
    Dimmer's k.
    Dimmer's nummular k.
    disciform k.
    disciform herpes simplex k.
    k. disciformis
    epithelial k.
    epithelial diffuse k.
    epithelial punctate k.
    exfoliative k.
    exposure k.
    farinaceous k.
    farinaceous epithelial k.
    fascicular k.
    filament k.
    filamentary k.
    k. filamentosa
    Fuchs' k.

fungal k.
furrow k.
geographic k.
herpes k.
herpes simplex k.
herpes zoster k.
herpetic k.
herpetic stromal k.
hypopyon k.
interstitial k. (IK)
lagophthalmic k.
lattice k.
k. lesion
letter-shaped k.
k. linearis migrans
luetic interstitial k.
Lyme disease k.
lymphogranuloma
  venereum k.
marginal k.
metaherpetic k.
microbial k.
k. molluscum contagiosum
mumps k.
mycotic k.
necrogranulomatous k.
neuroparalytic k.
neurotrophic k.
nonulcerative interstitial k.
nummular k.
k. nummularis
oyster shuckers' k.
paddy k.
parenchymatous k.
k. periodica fugax
k. petrificans
phlyctenular k.
polymorphic superficial k.
k. post vaccinulosa
k. profunda
pseudodendritic k.
k. punctata leprosa
k. punctata profunda
k. punctata subepithelialis
punctate k., k. punctata
purulent k.
k. pustuliformis profunda
pyknotic k.
radiation k.
k. ramificata superficialis
reaper's k.
reticular k.
ribbon-like k.

keratitis *(continued)*
  rosacea k.
  k. rosacea
  Schmidt's k.
  sclerosing k.
  scrofulous k.
  secondary k.
  serpiginous k.
  k. sicca
  striate k.
  stromal k.
  subepithelial k.
  superficial k.
  superficial linear k.
  superficial punctate k.
   (SPK)
  suppurative k.
  syphilitic k.
  Thygeson's k.
  Thygeson's superficial
   punctate k.
  trachomatous k.
  trophic k.
  tuberculous k.
  ulcerative k.
  k. urica
  k. vaccinia
  vaccinial k.
  varicella k.
  vascular k.
  vasculonebulous k.
  vesicular k.
  xerotic k.
  zonular k.
keratoacanthoma
  eruptive k.
keratocele
keratocentesis operation
keratoconjunctivitis
  adenoviral k.
  allergic k.
  atopic k.
  atopic eczema k.
  epidemic k. (EKC)
  epizootic k.
  flash k.
  herpes follicular k.
  herpes simplex k.
  herpes zoster k.
  herpetic k.
  limbic k.
  limbic vernal k.
  phlyctenular k.

  shipyard k.
  k. sicca (KCS)
  staphylococcal k.
  staphylococcal allergic k.
  superior limbic k. (SLK)
  Theodore's k.
  ultraviolet k.
  vernal k.
  viral k.
  welder's k.
keratoconus
  anterior k.
  k. dystrophy
  k. fruste
  posterior k.
  Sato's k.
keratocyte
keratoderma
  k. blennorrhagica
keratodermatocele
keratoectasia
keratoepithelioplasty
keratoglobus
keratohelcosis
keratohemia
keratoid
keratoiridocyclitis
keratoiridoscope
keratoiritis hypopyon
Kerato-Kontours instruments
keratokyphosis
keratolens implant
keratoleptynsis
keratoleukoma
Keratolux fixation device
keratolysis
keratoma
  solar k.
keratomalacia
keratomas
keratomata
keratome
  Agnew k.
  Bard-Parker k.
  Beaver k.
  Berens k.
  Berens partial k.
  Castroviejo k.
  Castroviejo angled k.
  Czermak k.
  filamentary k.
  Fuchs lancet type k.
  Grieshaber k.

k. guard
Guyton-Lundsgaard k.
Hansen k.
Jaeger k.
Jones k.
Kirby k.
Lancaster k.
Martinez k.
McReynolds k.
Rowland k.
Storz k.
Wiener k.
keratometer
Bausch & Lomb k.
Helmholtz k.
k. mires
Storz k.
Terry k.
keratometric
keratometry
surgical k.
keratomileusis
homoplastic k.
myopic k.
k. operation
keratomy
prospective evaluation of
radial k. (PERK)
keratomycosis
keratonosus
keratonyxis
keratopathy
aphakic bullous k.
band k
band-shaped k.
Bietti's k.
bullous k.
calcific band k.
chloroquine k.
climatic k.
climatic droplet k.
crystalline k.
dendritic k.
epithelial k.
exposure k.
filamentary k.
Fuchs' aphakic k.
idiopathic lipid k.
indomethacin toxicity k.
Labrador k.
lamellar k.
linear k.
lipid k.

neuroparalytic k.
neurotrophic k.
pearl diver's k.
phenothiazine k.
plaque k.
punctate k.
punctate epithelial k. (PEK)
striate k.
superficial k.
superficial punctate k.
Thygeson's superficial
punctate k.
trigeminal neuropathic k.
urate k.
urate band k.
uveitic band k.
vesicular k.
vortex k.
keratophakia
keratophakic keratoplasty
keratoplasty
allopathic k.
Arroyo's k.
Arruga's k.
autogenous k.
Elschnig's k.
epikeratophakic k.
Filatov's k.
heterogenous k.
homogenous k.
Imre's k.
keratophakic k.
lamellar k. (LKP)
lamellar refractive k.
layered k.
Morax's k.
nonpenetrating k.
k. operation
optic k.
optical k.
partial k.
Paufique's k.
penetrating k. (PK, PKP)
perforating k.
photorefractive k. (PRK)
punctate epithelial k.
refractive k.
k. scissors
Sourdille's k.
superficial lamellar k.
tectonic k.
thermal k. (TKP)
total k.

keratoprosthesis
keratorefractive
keratorhexis, keratorrhexis
keratorus
keratoscleritis
keratoscope
  Klein k.
  wire-loop k.
keratoscopy
keratosis
  actinic k.
  eyelid k.
  k. follicularis
  k. follicularis spinulosa
    decalvans
  k. palmoplantaris
  seborrheic k.
  senescent k.
  senile k.
  solar k.
keratostomy
keratotome
keratotomy
  arcuate transverse k.
  astigmatic k.
  delimiting k.
  laser k.
  k. operation
  radial k. (RK)
  refractive k.
  Ruiz trapezoidal k.
  trapezoidal k.
keratotorus
keratouveitis
  herpes simplex k.
  stromal k.
kerectasis
kerectomy
keroid
Kerrison
  K. forceps
  K. rongeur
Kestenbaum's
  K. capillary count
  K. procedure
  K. rule
  K. sign
ketamine
ketanserin
ketoconazole
ketorolac
ketosis-prone diabetes
ketosis-resistant diabetes

Kevorkian-Younge forceps
keyhole
  k. bridge
  k. field
  k. pupil
  k. vision
Key's operation
Keystone
  K. test
  K. View steopsis test
Khodadoust line
Khosia cautery
kibisitome
kidney failure
Kiloh-Nevin syndrome
Kimmelstiel-Wilson
  K.-W. disease
  K.-W. syndrome
Kimura
  K. platinum spatula
  K. spatula
Kimura's disease
Kimwipes
kindergarten eye chart
kinescope
kinetic
  k. echography
  k. perimeter
  k. perimetry
  k. strabismus
King
  K. corneal trephine
  K. implant
  K. orbital implant
King-Prince
  K.-P. knife
  K.-P. muscle forceps
King's operation
kinin
Kirby
  K. angulated iris spatula
  K. capsule forceps
  K. cataract knife
  K. corneoscleral forceps
  K. cylindrical zonal
    separator
  K. dislocator
  K. flat zonal separator
  K. forceps
  K. hook
  K. hook expressor
  K. intracapsular lens
    expressor

K. intracapsular lens loupe
K. intracapsular lens spoon
K. intraocular lens loupe
K. intraocular lens scoop
K. iris forceps
K. iris spatula
K. keratome
K. knife
K. lens
K. lens dislocator
K. lens loupe
K. lid retractor
K. loupe
K. muscle hook
K. refractor
K. retractor
K. scissors
K. tissue forceps
Kirby-Bauer disk sensitivity test
Kirby's operation
Kirisawa's uveitis
Kirschner wire
Kirsch's test
Kishi lens
kissing choroidals
Kit
    Massachusetts Vision K.
    (MVK)
Kjer's
K. dominant atrophy
K. dominant optic atrophy
K. optic atrophy
Klebsiella
    K. pneumoniae
Kleen
    Velva K.
Klein
K. curved cannula
K. keratoscope
K. punch
Klein-Tolentino ring
Klieg's eye
Klinefelter's syndrome
Klippel-Feil
K.-F. anomaly
K.-F. syndrome
Klippel-Trenaunay-Weber syndrome
Kloti
K. cutter
K. vitreous cutter
Klumpke's paralysis
Knapp
    K. blade

K. cataract knife
K. eye speculum
K. forceps
K. hook
K. iris hook
K. iris probe
K. iris repositor
K. iris scissors
K. iris spatula
K. knife
K. knife-needle
K. lacrimal sac retractor
K. lens spoon
K. needle
K. probe
K. refractor
K. retractor
K. scissors
K. scoop
K. spatula
K. speculum
Knapp-Culler speculum
Knapp-Imre operation
Knapp's
K. law
K. operation
K. procedure
K. rule
K. streak
K. striae
Knapp-Wheeler-Reese operation
knee
Knie's sign
knife, pl. knives
    Agnew canaliculus k.
    Alcon k.
    Bard-Parker k.
    Barkan k.
    Barkan goniotomy k.
    Barraquer k.
    Barraquer keratoplasty k.
    Beard k.
    Beaver k.
    Beaver goniotomy needle k.
    Beer k.
    Beer canaliculus k.
    Beer cataract k.
    Berens cataract k.
    Berens glaucoma k.
    Berens keratoplasty k.
    Berens ptosis k.
    Bishop-Harman k.
    blade k.

knife *(continued)*
    bladebreaker k.
    Castroviejo k.
    Castroviejo discission k.
    Castroviejo twin k.
    cataract k.
    corneal k.
    Cusick goniotomy k.
    Dean iris k.
    Desmarres k.
    Deutschman cataract k.
    diamond k.
    diamond blade k.
    diamond-dusted k.
    discission k.
    dissector k.
    Duredge k.
    Elschnig k.
    Elschnig cataract k.
    Elschnig corneal k.
    Elschnig pterygium k.
    Gill k.
    Gill corneal k.
    Gill-Fine corneal k.
    Gill-Hess k.
    Gills-Welsh k.
    Goldmann serrated k.
    goniopuncture k.
    goniotomy k.
    Graefe k.
    Graefe cataract k.
    Graefe cystitome k.
    Green k.
    Green cataract k.
    Green corneal k.
    Grieshaber k.
    Grieshaber ruby k.
    Grieshaber ultrasharp k.
    k. guard
    Guyton-Lundsgaard k.
    Guyton-Lundsgaard
      cataract k.
    Haab scleral resection k.
    House k.
    House myringotomy k.
    Johnson evisceration k.
    Johnson-Tooke corneal k.
    Keeler-Meyer diamond k.
    Keeler ruby k.
    Kelman k.
    King-Prince k.
    Kirby k.
    Kirby cataract k.
    Knapp k.
    Knapp cataract k.
    KOI k.
    KOI diamond k.
    Lancaster k.
    Lowell glaucoma k.
    Lundsgaard k.
    Martinez k.
    Maumenee goniotomy k.
    McPherson-Wheeler k.
    McPherson-Ziegler k.
    McReynolds k.
    McReynolds pterygium k.
    Meyer k.
    Meyer Swiss diamond
      lancet k.
    Meyer Swiss diamond mini-
      angled k.
    Meyer Swiss diamond
      wedge k.
    Microknife k.
    micrometer k.
    micro surgical k.
    Myocure k.
    k.-needle
    Parker k.
    Parker discission k.
    Paton k.
    Paton corneal k.
    Paufique k.
    Paufique graft k.
    Paufique keratoplasty k.
    ptosis k.
    radial keratotomy k.
    razor blade k.
    Reese ptosis k.
    Rizzuti-Spizziri k.
    Rizzuti-Spizziri cannula k.
    ruby k.
    ruby diamond k.
    sapphire k.
    Sato corneal k.
    scarifier k.
    Scheie k.
    Scheie goniopuncture k.
    Scheie goniotomy k.
    scleral resection k.
    Sharpoint k.
    Sharpoint microsurgical k.
    Sharpoint slit k.
    Short Cut A-OK small-
      incision k.
    Sichel k.

Smith k.
Smith-Fisher k.
Smith-Green k.
Smith-Green cataract k.
Spizziri k.
Spizziri cannula k.
Step-Knife diamond
  blade k.
stiletto k.
stitch-removing k.
Storz cataract k.
Storz-Duredge steel
  cataract k.
Swan k.
Swan discission k.
Tooke k.
Tooke corneal k.
Tooke cornea-splitting k.
Tooke-Johnson corneal k.
Troutman corneal k.
Troutman-Tooke corneal k.
V-lancet k.
von Graefe k.
von Graefe cataract k.
wave-edge k.
Weber k.
Weck k.
Wheeler k.
Wheeler discission k.
Wilder cystitome k.
Ziegler k.

knife-edged lens
Knolle
  K. capsule polisher
  K. capsule scraper
  K. capsule scratcher
  K. lens cortex spatula
  K. lens nucleus spatula
  K. lens speculum
  K. polisher
  K. scraper
Knolle-Kelman cannulated
  cystihtome
Knolle-Pearce irrigating lens loop
Knoll's refraction technique
knot
  bow-tie k.
  partial throw surgeon's k.
  Tripier's operation throw
    square k.
knuckle
  k. of choroid
  k. of loose vitreous

Koby
  K. cataract forceps
  superficial reticular
    degeneration of K.
Koby's cataract
Kocher's sign
Koch-Weeks
  K.-W. bacillus
  K.-W. conjunctivitis
Koeller illumination system
Koenen's tumor
Koeppe
  K. diagnostic lens
  K. goniolens
  K. gonioscopic implant
  K. implant
  K. lens
Koeppe's
  K. disease
  K. nodule
  K. syndrome
Koerber-Salus-Elschnig syndrome
Koffler's operation
KOH
  potassium hydroxide
Köhler illumination
KOI
  KOI diamond knife
  KOI knife
Kollmorgen's elements
Kollner's
  K. law
  K. rule
Kolmer's crystalloid structure
Konoto's tetrad
Korb
  K. contact lens
  K. lens
koroscope
koroscopy
Kowa
  K. camera
  K. Fluorescein System
  K. fundus
  K. hand-held slit lamp
  K. Optimed slit lamp
  K. RC-XV fundus camera
Koyter's muscle
Kozlowski's degeneration
KP
  keratic precipitate

Krabbe's
 K. disease
 K. disease gland
Kraff
 K. capsule polisher
 K. capsule polisher curette
 K. cortex cannula
 K. intraocular utility forceps
 K. lens-inserting forceps
 K. nucleus lens loupe
 K. polisher
 K. suturing forceps
 K. tying forceps
Kraff-Utrata
 K.-U. capsulorrhexis
 K.-U. capsulorrhexis forceps
 K.-U. intraocular utility
 forceps
Kraft forceps
Krakau tonometer
Krasnov lens
Kratz
 K. angled cystitome
 K. capsule scraper
 K. capsule scratcher
 K. diamond-dusted needle
 K. elliptical-style lens
 K. K push-pull iris hook
 K. lens
 K. lens-inserting forceps
 K. lens needle
 K. needle
 K. polisher
 K. polisher/scratcher
 K. posterior chamber
 intraocular lens
 K. scraper
 K. scratcher
 K. "soft" J-loop intraocular
 lens
Kratz-Barraquer wire eye speculum
Kratz-Jensen
 K.-J. polisher/scratcher
 K.-J. scratcher
Kratz-Johnson lens
Kratz-Sinskey
 K.-S. intraocular lens
 K.-S. loop configuration
Kraupa's operation
Krause
 transverse suture of K.
Krause's
 K. gland

 K. lacrimal gland
 K. syndrome
 K. valve
K readings
Kreiger-Spitznas vibrating scissors
Kreiker's operation
Kremer two-point fixation forceps
Krieberg's operation
Kriebig's operation
Krieger
 K. fundus lens
 K. wide-field fundus lens
Krieker's blepharochalasis
Krill's
 K. disease
 K. disk
Krimsky-Prince accommodation rule
Krimsky's
 K. method
 K. prism test
 K. test
Kronfeld
 K. electrode
 K. forceps
 K. refractor
 K. retractor
 K. suturing forceps
Krönlein-Berke operation
Krönlein's
 K. operation
 K. procedure
Krukenberg
 K. pigment spindle forceps
 K. sponge
Krukenberg's
 K. corneal spindle
 K. pigment spindle
 K. spindle
Krupin-Denver long-value implant
Krupin valve
Krwawicz cataract extractor
Krymed Cryopexy Unit
Kryptok
 K. bifocal
 K. implant
 K. lens
krypton
 k. laser
 k. red laser
K-Sol media
K Sol preservation solution

Kufs'
    K. disease
    K. syndrome
Kuglein
    K. irrigating lens
      manipulator
    K. lens manipulator
    K. push/pull
    K. refractor
    K. retractor
Kuglen
    K. hook
    K. manipulating hook
Kuhnt
    K. corneal scarifier
    K. fixation forceps
    K. forceps
Kuhnt-Helmbold operation
Kuhnt-Junius
    K.-J. degeneration
    K.-J. disease
    K.-J. macular degeneration
    K.-J. maculopathy
    K.-J. repair
Kuhnt's
    K. dacryostomy

    K. eyelid operation
    K. illusion
    K. meniscus
    K. operation
    K. postcentral vein
    K. spaces
    K. tarsectomy
Kuhnt-Szymanowski
    K.-S. operation
    K.-S. procedure
Kuhnt-Thorpe operation
Kuler panoramic lens
Kulvin-Kalt forceps
Kurova Shursite lens series
Kurz's syndrome
Kveim
    K. antigen
    K. test
KW
    Keith-Wagener changes
    KW changes
Kwitko conjunctival spreader
Kwitko's operation
Kynex
Kyrle's disease

Laboratories
    Lederal L.
Laboratory
    Bio-Rad L.
laboratory diagnosis
Labrador keratopathy
labyrinth
labyrinthine nystagmus
Lacarrere's operation
lacerate
    l. anterior foramen
    l. foramen
    l. middle foramen
    l. posterior foramen
laceration
    canalicular l.
    central stellate l.
    conjunctival l.
    corneal l.
    corneoscleral l.
    eyebrow l.
    lid margin l.
    tarsal l.
**lacertus musculi recti lateralis
bulbi**
lachrymal (*var. of* lacrimal)
lacquer crack
Lacramore
Lacril
Lacri-Lube NP
Lacri-Lube S.O.P.
lacrimal, lachrymal
    l. abscess
    l. angle duct anomaly
    l. anterior crest
    l. apparatus
    l. artery
    l. awl
    l. bay
    l. bone
    l. calculus
    l. canal
    l. cannula
    l. caruncle
    l. caruncula
    l. conjunctivitis
    l. crest
    l. dilator
    l. drainage
    l. duct

l. ductal cyst
l. duct anlage
l. duct T-tube
duct T-tube l.
l. fistula
l. folds
l. fornix
l. fossa
l. gland
l. gland acinus
l. gland epithelial tumor
l. gland fossa
l. gland gallium uptake
l. gland repair
l. gland tumor
l. groove
l. incisure
l. intubation probe
l. irrigation test
l. lake
l. lens
l. nerve
l. notch
l. nucleus aplasia
l. papilla
l. point
l. posterior crest
l. power
l. probe
l. process
l. pump failure
l. punctal stenosis
l. punctum
l. reflex
l. sac
l. sac bur
l. sac chisel
l. sac fossa
l. sac gouge
l. sac retractor
l. sac rongeur
l. scintillography
l. sound
l. stent
l. stent
l. sulcus
l. sulcus of lacrimal bone
l. sulcus of maxilla
l. surgery
l. syringe

lacrimal *(continued)*
    l. system
    l. trephine
    l. tubercle
    l. vein
lacrimale
    os l.
    punctum l.
lacrimales
    ductus l.
lacrimalin
lacrimalis
    ampulla canaliculi l.
    ampulla ductus l.
    apparatus l.
    canaliculus l.
    caruncula l.
    Föerster's sacci l.
    fornix sacci l.
    fossa glandulae l.
    fossa sacci l.
    glandula l.
    hamulus l.
    incisura l.
    lacus l.
    nervus l.
    pars orbitalis glandulae l.
    pars palpebralis glandulae l.
    plica l.
    rivus l.
    sacculus l.
    saccus l.
    vena l.
lacriman canaliculus
lacrimarum
    stillicidium l.
lacrimase
lacrimation
    excessive l.
    l. reflex
lacrimator
lacrimatory
lacrimoconchalis
    sutura l.
lacrimoconchal suture
lacrimoethmoidal suture
lacrimomaxillaris
    sutura l.
lacrimomaxillary suture
lacrimonasal duct
lacrimotome
lacrimotomy
lacrimoturbinal suture

Lacrisert
Lacrivial
lacteal cataract
lactoferrin
Lactoplate
lacuna, pl. **lacunae**
    Blessig's l.
lacunata
    blepharoconjunctivitis
      Moraxella l.
      Moraxella l.
lacus
    l. lacrimalis
Ladd-Franklin theory
LaForce
    L. knife spud
    L. spud
lag
    dilation l.
    l. dilation
    lid l.
Lagleyze needle
Lagleyze's operation
Lagleyze-Trantas operation
lagophthalmia, lagophthalmos,
  lagophthalmus
    l. conjunctivitis
    spastic l.
lagophthalmic keratitis
Lagrange
    L. scissors
    L. sclerectomy scissors
Lagrange's operation
Laird spatula
laissez-faire lid operation
lake
    lacrimal l.
    tear l.
lambda angle
Lambda Physik EMG 103 laser
Lambert
    L. chalazion forceps
    L. forceps
lambert
lamella, gen. and pl. **lamellae**
    collagen lamellae
    corneal l.
    corneoscleral lamellae
    l. of Fuchs'
    Rabl's lamellae
lamellar
    l. calcification
    l. cataract

l. corneal graft
l. corneal transplant
l. developmental cataract
l. graft
l. groove
l. keratopathy
l. keratoplasty (LKP)
l. refractive keratoplasty
l. separation of lens
l. zonular perinuclear
  cataract
lamellar keratoplasty (LKP)
  superficial l. k.
lamellation
lamina
  anterior limiting l.
  basal l.
  basalis choroideae l.
  basalis corporis ciliaris l.
  Bowman's l.
  l. choriocapillaris
  l. choroidocapillaris
  l. cribrosa
  l. cribrosa sclerae
  l. dots
  l. elastica anterior
  l. elastica posterior
  episcleral l.
  l. fusca eye
  l. fusca sclerae
  l. limitans anterior corneae
  l. limitans posterior corneae
  limiting l.
  orbital l.
  l. orbitalis ossis ethmoidalis
  l. papyracea
  posterior l.
  posterior limiting l.
  l. superficialis musculi
  suprachoroid l.
  l. suprachoroidea
  l. vasculosa choroideae
  l. vitrea
  vitreal l.
  vitreous l.
laminar
  l. flow
  venous l.
laminated
  l. acellular mass
  l. lens
  l. spectacle lens

lamp
  Bausch-Lomb-Thorpe slit l.
  biomicroscope slit l.
  Birch l.
  Birch-Hirschfeld l.
  Burton l.
  Campbell slit l.
  carbon arc l.
  Coburn-Rodenstock l.
  Coburn-Rodenstock slit l.
  Duke-Elder l.
  Eldridge-Green l.
  fluorescent l.
  gas discharge l.
  Gullstrand slit l.
  Haag-Streit slit l.
  Hague cataract l.
  incandescent l.
  infrared slit l.
  Ishihara IV slit l.
  IV slit l.
  Kowa hand-held slit l.
  Kowa Optimed slit l.
  Marco slit l.
  Nikon zoom photo slit l.
  Nitra l.
  Posner slit l.
  Reichert slit l.
  Rodenstock l.
  Rodenstock slit l.
  Specular reflex slit l.
  Thorpe slit l.
  Topcon slit l.
  tungsten-halogen l.
  Universal slit l.
  VG slit l.
  V-slit l.
  Zeiss l.
  Zeiss carbon arc slit l.
  Zeiss-Comberg slit l.
  Zeiss slit l.
Lamprene
Lancaster
  L. Cross
  L. eye magnet
  L. eye speculum
  L. keratome
  L. knife
  L. lid speculum
  L. magnet
  L. red-green projector
Lancaster-O'Connor speculum

Lancaster-Regan
    L.-R. dial 1 chart
    L.-R. dial 2 chart
    L.-R. test
Lancaster's
    L. operation
    L. red-green test
    L. screen test
lance
    Rolf l.
Lancereaux's diabetes
lancet
    Keeler ultrasonic cataract
      removal l.
    Meyer Swiss diamond
      knife l.
    suture l.
    l. suture
    Swan l.
    ultrasonic cataract
      removal l.
Lanchner's operation
Landegger
    L. implant
    L. orbital implant
Landers
    L. biconcave lens
    L. contact lens
    L. irrigating vitrectomy ring
    L. vitrectomy ring
Landers-Foulks temporary
  keratoprosthesis lens
Landolt C
Landolt's
    L. body
    L. broken ring
    L. broken-ring chart
    L. broken-ring test
    L. chart
    L. operation
    L. ring
Landry's ascending paralysis
Landström's muscle
Lane needle
Lange
    L. blade
    L. speculum
Langenbeck's operation
Langer-Giedion
  trichorhinophalangeal syndrome
Langerhans'
    L. cell
    L. granules

Lange's fold
Langhans' giant cells
Lang speculum
lanolin
Lanoxin
lantern test
Larcher's sign
Largactil
large
    l. calorie (C)
    l. kappa angle
    l. physiologic cup
large-angled forceps
large-cell lymphoma
larva
    ocular l.
larval conjunctivitis
larva migrans
    ocular l. m.
    visceral l. m.
Lasag Micropter II laser
lase
Laser
laser
    l. activity
    Aesculap argon
      ophthalmic l.
    Aesculap excimer l.
    Allergan Humphrey l.
    AMO YAG 100 l.
    argon l.
    argon blue l.
    argon-fluoride l.
    argon green l.
    argon-pumped tunable
      dye l.
    Biophysic l.
    Biophysic Medical l.
    Biophysic Medical YAG l.
    blue-green argon l.
    Britt argon l.
    Britt argon/krypton l.
    Britt argon pulsed l.
    Britt BL-12 l.
    Britt krypton l.
    Britt pulsed argon l.
    l. burn
    l. burst
    candela l.
    carbon dioxide l.
    Cardona l.
    Carl Zeiss l.
    Carl Zeiss YAG l.

l. cavity
Cilco argon l.
Cilco Frigitronics l.
Cilco Hoffer Laseridge l.
Cilco krypton l.
Cilco/Lasertek A-K l.
Cilco/Lasertek argon l.
Cilco/Lasertek krypton l.
Cilco YAG l.
CO_2 l.
Coherent 7910 l.
Coherent 900 argon l.
Coherent 920 argon l.
Coherent 920 argon/dye l.
Coherent dye l.
Coherent krypton l.
Coherent Medical YAG l.
Coherent radiation
  argon/krypton l.
Coherent radiation argon
  model 800 l.
continuous l.
continuous-wave argon l.
Cooper l.
Cooper 2000 l.
Cooper 2500 l.
Cooper Laser Sonics l.
CooperVision l.
CooperVision argon l.
CooperVision YAG l.
CO_2 Sharplan l.
l. cyclotherapy
diode l.
dye l.
l. equipment
erbium l.
Evergreen Lasertek l.
excimer l.
Gish micro YAG l.
helium-ion aiming l.
helium-neon aiming l.
HGH l.
HGM argon green l.
HGM intravitreal l.
l. interferometry
intrastromal l.
ion l.
l. ion
l. iridectomy
l. iridotomy
l. keratotomy
krypton l.
krypton red l.

Lambda Physik EMG
  103 l.
Lasag Micropter II l.
laser l.
Lasertek l.
l. lens
liquid organic dye l.
LPK-80 II argon l.
Lumonics l.
l. manipulation
Meditec l.
Merrimac l.
Microlase transpupillary
  diode l.
mode-locked l.
mode-locked Nd:YAG l.
molectron l.
Nanolas Nd:YAG l.
Nanolas neodymium
  YAG l.
Nd:YAG l.
neodymium (Nd) YAG l.
neodymium yttrium
  aluminum garnet l.
Nidek l.
Nidek Laser System l.
OcuLight SL diode l.
oculocutaneous l.
Ophthalas argon l.
Ophthalas argon/krypton l.
Ophthalas krypton l.
orange dye l.
l. photocoagulation
l. photocoagulator
photodisrupting l.
photovaporation l.
photovaporizing l.
Q-switched l.
Q-switched neodymium
  YAG l.
Q-switched ruby l.
l. refractometry
l. ridge
ruby l.
Sharplan argon l.
l. surgery
Takata l.
TE MOO mode beam l.
l. therapy
l. trabeculoplasty
l. tube
tunable dye l.

laser *(continued)*
  twenty/twenty argon-fluoride
    excimer l.
  Visulas argon l.
  Visulas argon C l.
  Visulas argon/YAG l.
  Visulas Nd:YAG l.
  Visulas YAG C l.
  Visulas YAG E l.
  Visulas YAG S l.
  YAG l.
    yttrium-aluminum-garnet
      laser
  yttrium-aluminum-garnet l.
    (YAG laser)
laser-argon device
lasered
laser-filtering surgery
Laserflex
  L. coagulator
  L. lens
Laseridge
  Cilco Hoffer L.
  L. Optics lens
laser-ruby device
Lasertek
  L. laser
lash
  l. abrasion of cornea
  l. margin
  misdirected l.'s
lasing
lastosis
lata
  fascia l.
  Tenon's fascia l.
latency
latent
  l. angle-closure glaucoma
  l. congenital
  l. deviation
  l. diabetes
  l. hyperopia (Hl)
  l. nystagmus
  l. squint
  l. strabismus
late-onset esotropia
lateral
  l. aberration
  l. angle
  l. canthal tendon
  l. canthotomy
  l. canthus

  l. commissure of eyelid
  l. geniculate body (LGB)
  l. geniculate nucleus (LGN)
  l. hemianopsia
  l. horn
  l. illumination
  l. inhibition
  l. margin of orbit
  l. medullary syndrome
  l. nystagmus
  l. oblique conus
  l. orbital decompression
  l. orbital tubercle
  l. orbit tubercle
  l. palpebral ligament
  l. palpebral raphe
  l. palpebral tubercle
  l. phoria
  l. rectus (LR)
  l. rectus extraocular muscles
  l. rectus muscle
  l. rectus palsy
lateralis
  angular oculi l.
  angulus oculi l.
  commissura palpebrarum l.
  raphe palpebralis l.
lateroduction
lateropulsion
laterotorsion
lathe
  l. cutting
  l. lens
lathe-cut contact lens
lathing procedure
lattice
  l. corneal dystrophy
  l. degeneration
  l. degeneration of retina
  l. dystrophy
  l. dystrophy of cornea
  l. keratitis
  l. retinal degeneration
Lauber's disease
laughing gas
Laurence-Biedl syndrome
Laurence-Moon-Bardet-Biedl
  syndrome
Laurence-Moon-Biedl syndrome
Laurence-Moon syndrome
Lauth's canal
lavage

Lavoptik
    L. Eye Wash

aw
    Alexander's l.
    Ångström's l.
    Beer's l.
    Bunsen-Roscoe l.
    Descartes' l.
    Desmarres' l.
    Donders' l.
    Ewald's l.
    Ferry-Porter l.
    Flouren's l.
    Giraud-Teulon l.
    Gullstrand's l.
    Hering's l.
    Horner's l.
    Knapp's l.
    Kollner's l.
    Listing's l.
    Plateau-Talbot l.
    reciprocity l.
    l. of refraction
    Riccò's l.
    Roscoe-Bunsen l.
    Sherrington's l.
    Snell's l.
    Stefan's l.
    Talbot l.
    Weber's l.
    Wundt-Lamansky l.

awford's syndrome
awton corneal scissors
axity
    lid l.
    lower lid l.

ayden infant lens
ayer
    aqueous l.
    aqueous tear l.
    bacillary l.
    basal l.
    Bowman's l.
    Bruch's l.
    Chievitz' l.
    Chievitz' fiber l.
    choriocapillary l.
    columnar l.
    cuticular l.
    epithelial basement l.
    ganglion cell l.
    Haller's l.
    Henle's l.

    Henle's fiber l.
    inner nuclear l.
    inner plexiform l.
    juxtapapillary nerve fiber l.
    limiting l.
    lipid tear l.
    molecular l.
    molecular external l.
    molecular inner l.
    molecular internal l.
    molecular outer l.
    mucous l.
    mucous tear l.
    nerve fiber l. (NFL)
    nerve fiber bundle l.
    nuclear external l.
    nuclear inner l.
    nuclear internal l.
    nuclear outer l.
    outer nuclear l.
    outer plexiform l.
    pigment l.
    plexiform l.
    plexiform external l.
    plexiform inner l.
    plexiform internal l.
    plexiform outer l.
    retinochoroidal l.
    l. of rods and cones
    Sattler's l.
    suprachoroid l.
    tear l.

layered
    l. hyphema
    l. keratoplasty

lazy eye
LC-65
L-Caine
LCAT
    lecithin:cholesterol acyl
      transferase

l-cone
LD+2
LE
    left eye
    lupus erythematosus

lead
    l. citrate stain
    l. incrustation of cornea
    l. poisoning

lead-filled mallet
Leahey's operation

leak
  glue patch l.
  macular l.
leakage
  corneal l.
  juxtapapillary l.
  microaneurysmal l.
Leakey chalazion forceps
leaking
  l. bleb
  l. filtering bleb
leash
least diffusion circle
leaves of capsule
Lebensohn's
  L. chart
  L. reading chart
  L. visual acuity chart
Leber's
  L. amaurosis
  L. aneurysm
  L. atrophy
  L. cell
  L. congenital amaurosis
  L. disease
  L. hereditary optic atrophy
  L. idiopathic stellate
    retinopathy
  L. miliary aneurysm
  L. optic atrophy
  L. syndrome
lecithin:cholesterol acyl transferase
  (LCAT)
lectin
  fluorescein-conjugated l.
Lederal Laboratories
Lefler-Wadsworth-Sidbury foveal
  dystrophy
LeFort classification
left
  l. deorsumvergence
  l. esotropia
  l. exotropia
  l. eye (LE, OS)
  l. gaze
  l. hyperphoria
  l. hypertrophic
  l. hypertropia (LHT)
  l. inferior oblique recession
  l. inferior rectus muscle
  l. superior oblique tuck
  l. superior rectus muscle
  l. sursumvergence

left-beating nystagmus
left-eyed
left-to-right shunting
legal blindness
legally blind
legible
  minimum l.
Le Grand-Geblewics phenomenon
Leigh capsule forceps
Leigh's encephalopathy
leiomyoma
  l. of iris
  l. of uveal tract
leiomyosarcoma
leishmaniasis
  American l.
Leishman's classification
Leiske lens
Leitz microscope
Leland refractor
lema
lemniscus, pl. lemnisci
  optic l.
Lemoine
  L. implant
  L. orbital implant
  L. serrefine
Lemoine-Searcy fixation anchor
  loupe
Lempert-Storz
  L.-S. lens
  L.-S. loupe
Lems lens
length
  axial l.
  chord l.
  focal l.
  temple l.
lengthening
Lens
  L. Clear
  L. Fresh
  L. Lubricant
  L. Mate
  L. Plus
  L. Plus daily cleaner
  L. Plus Oxysept System
  L. Plus rewetting drops
  L. Plus saline
  L. Wet
lens, pl. lenses
  l. aberration
  Abraham iridectomy l.

Abraham iridectomy laser l.
Abraham iridotomy l.
Abraham peripheral button
 iridotomy l.
Abraham YAG laser l.
accommodation of l.
accommodation of
 crystalline l.
Accugel l.
achromatic l.
achromatic spectacle l.
acrylic l.
adherent l.
Airy cylindric l.
Alges bifocal contact l.
Allen-Thorpe l.
all-Perspex CQ l.
all-Perspex Kelman
 Omnifit l.
Amenabar l.
American Medical Optics
 Baron l.
amnifocal l.
AMO intraocular l.
Amsoft l.
anastigmatic l.
angle-fixated l.
angle-supported l.
aniseikonic l.
Anis staple l.
annular bifocal contact l.
anterior l.
anterior chamber l.
AO l.
aphakic l.
aplanatic l.
apochromatic l.
Appolionio l.
Aquaflex l.
Aquaflex contact l.
Aquasight l.
Arlt l.
Arruga l.
artificial l.
aspheric l.
aspherical
 ophthalmoscopic l.
aspheric cataract l.
aspheric contact l.
aspheric spectacle l.
aspheric viewing l.
aspiration of l.
astigmatic l.

auxiliary l.
l. axis
axis of cylindric l. (x)
Azar l.
back surface toric contact l.
Bagolini l.
ballasted contact l.
bandage l.
bandage contact l.
Barkan gonioscopic l.
Barkan goniotomy l.
Baron l.
Barraquer l.
baseball l.
Bausch & Lomb Optima l.
Bayadi l.
Bechert 7mm l.
Beebe l.
beveled-edge l.
bicentric l.
bicentric spectacle l.
biconcave l.
biconcave contact l.
biconvex l.
bicurve contact l.
bicylindrical l.
Bietti l.
bifocal l.
bifocal contact l.
bifocal spectacle l.
Binkhorst l.
Binkhorst four-loop l.
Binkhorst four-loop iris-
 fixated l.
Binkhorst-Fyodorov l.
Binkhorst intraocular l.
Binkhorst iridocapsular l.
Binkhorst two-loop l.
Bi-Soft l.
bispherical l.
bitoric lenses
bitoric contact l.
blooming of l.
blooming spectacle l.
Boberg-Ans l.
Boston contact l.
Boys-Smith laser l.
Brücke's l.
l. capsule
capsule of l.
Cardona fiberoptic
 diagnostic l.
Carl Zeiss l.

lens *(continued)*
  cast resin l.
  cataract l.
  cellulose acetate butyrate
    contact l.
  Centra-Flex l.
  central posterior curve of
    contact l.
  central thickness of
    contact l.
  Charles contact l.
  Charles intraocular l.
  Charles irrigating l.
  Charles irrigating contact l.
  chemically treated l.
  chemically treated
    spectacle l.
  Choyce l.
  Choyce intraocular l.
  Choyce Mark VIII l.
  Cibasoft l.
  Cibasoft contact l.
  Cibathin l.
  Cilco intraocular l.
  Cilco MonoFlex multi-piece
    PMMA intraocular l.
  Cilco-Simcoe II l.
  Cilco-Sonometrics l.
  Clayman l.
  Clayman intraocular l.
  Clayman posterior
    chamber l.
  l. clip
  C-loop posterior chamber l.
  coating of l.
  coating for spectacle l.
  Coburn l.
  Coburn intraocular l.
  collagen bandage l.
  coloboma of l.
  Comberg l.
  Comberg contact l.
  composition of spectacle l.
  compound l.
  concave l.
  concave spectacle l.
  concavoconcave l.
  concavoconvex l.
  condensing l.
  conoid lenses
  conoid l.
  contact l. (CL)
  contact bandage l.

  contact low-vacuum l.
  contour l.
  converging l.
  converging meniscus l.
  convex l.
  convexoconcave l.
  convexoconvex l.
  convex plano l.
  convex spectacle l.
  CooperVision PMMA-ACL
    Flex l.
  Copeland intraocular l.
  Copeland pan chamber l.
  Copeland radial panchamber
    intraocular l.
  Copeland radial panchamber
    UV l.
  coquille plano l.
  corneal l.
  corneal contact l.
  corrected l.
  corrected spectacle l.
  cortex l.
  cortical substance of l.
  cosmetic contact l.
  cosmetic shell contact l.
  CR-39 l.
  crocodile l.
  Crookes l.
  crossed l.
  crown glass l.
  l. crystallina
  crystalline l.
  curvature of l.
  curves of spectacle l.
  cylinder l.
  cylinder lenses
  cylinder spectacle l.
  cylindrical l. (C, cyl.)
  daily-wear lenses
  Darin l.
  decentered l.
  decentration of l.
  diagnostic contact l.
  diagnostic fiberoptic l.
  direct gonioscopic l.
  dislocated l.
  dislocation of l.
  l. dislocation
  dispersing l.
  disposable contact l.
  distortion of l.
  diverging l.

diverging meniscus l.
dot-like l.
double concave l.
double convex l.
double slab-off l.
Doubra l.
l. dressing
Drews l.
dual l.
Dulaney l.
Dura-T l.
edging of l.
edging of spectacle l.
Emery l.
l. epithelium
Epstein collar stud acrylic l.
l. equator
equator of l.
equator of crystalline l.
ERG-Jet disposable
  contact l.
Eschenback Optik l.
l. exchange
executive l.
executive spectacle l.
l. exfoliation glaucoma
l. expressor
extended-wear contact l.
  (EWCL)
eye l.
Fechner intraocular l.
Federov l.
Federov type II
  intraocular l.
Federov type I
  intraocular l.
Feister Dualens l.
l. fiber
fiberoptic diagnostic l.
field l.
finished l.
flat l.
flat contact l.
flat-edge l.
flexible-wear l.
Flexlens l.
flint-glass l.
fluid l.
fluid contact l.
fluidless contact l.
FormFlex l.
four-loop l.
four-mirror goniolens l.

Franklin-style bifocal lenses
Frelex l.
Frenzel l.
Fresnel l.
Friedman hand-held
  Hruby l.
Friedman-Hruby l.
front surface toric contact l.
fundus contact l.
fundus focalizing l.
fundus laser l.
fused bifocal l.
fused multifocal l.
Galin l.
Galin intraocular implant l.
gas-permeable l.
gas-permeable contact l.
generating spectacle l.
Genesis l.
Gill intraocular implant l.
Gilmore l.
Gilmore intraocular
  implant l.
glass l.
l. glide
glued-on hard contact l.
Goldmann l.
Goldmann contact l.
Goldmann diagnostic
  contact l.
Goldmann fundus contact l.
Goldmann macular
  contact l.
Goldmann multi-mirrored l.
Goldmann three-mirror l.
goniofocalizing l.
goniolens l.
gonioscopic l.
Gould intraocular implant l.
Gridley intraocular l.
Gullstrand l.
hand-held Hruby l.
hard contact l. (HCL)
hardened spectacle l.
hardening of l.
Hart pediatric three-
  mirror l.
Hessburg l.
Hidex glass l.
Hoffer-Laseridge
  intraocular l.
honey bee l.
Hruby l.

lens *(continued)*
    Hruby contact l.
    Hunkeler l.
    Hydracon l.
    Hydracon contact l.
    Hydrasoft contact l.
    Hydrocurve l.
    hydrogel l.
    hydrogel contact l.
    Hydron l.
    hydrophilic contact l.
    hydrophobic contact l.
    Hydrosight l.
    immersion l.
    l. implant
    implant l.
    implantation l.
    Implens intraocular l.
    inert material for
      intraocular l.
    infant Karickhoff laser l.
    infant three-mirror laser l.
    Intermedics l.
    Interspace YAG laser l.
    in-the-bag l.
    intraocular l. (IOL)
    IOLAB 108 B l.
    IOLAB intraocular l.
    Ioptex intraocular l.
    Ioptex laser intraocular l.
    Ioptex TabOptic l.
    Irene l.
    iridocapsular l.
    iridocapsular intraocular l.
    iridotomy l.
    iris-fixated l.
    iris-supported l.
    iseikonic l.
    iso-iconic l.
    Jaffe Cilco l.
    J-loop PC l.
    J-loop posterior chamber
      intraocular l.
    Joal l.
    Jung-Schaffer intraocular l.
    Kamerling Capsular 90 l.
    Karickhoff laser l.
    Kearney side-notch l.
    Keeler panoramic l.
    Kelman l.
    Kelman flexible tripod l.
    Kelman Multiflex II l.
    Kelman Omnifit l.

    Kelman Omnifit II
      intraocular l.
    Kelman PC 27LB CapSul l.
    Kelman Quadriflex anterior
      chamber intraocular l.
    Kirby l.
    Kishi l.
    knife-edged l.
    Koeppe l.
    Koeppe diagnostic l.
    Korb l.
    Krasnov l.
    Kratz l.
    Kratz elliptical-style l.
    Kratz-Johnson l.
    Kratz posterior chamber
      intraocular l.
    Kratz-Sinskey intraocular l.
    Kratz "soft" J-loop
      intraocular l.
    Krieger fundus l.
    Krieger wide-field fundus l.
    Kryptok l.
    Kuler panoramic l.
    lacrimal l.
    lamellar separation of l.
    laminated l.
    laminated spectacle l.
    Landers biconcave l.
    Landers contact l.
    Landers-Foulks temporary
      keratoprosthesis l.
    laser l.
    Laserflex l.
    Laseridge Optics l.
    lathe l.
    lathe-cut contact l.
    Layden infant l.
    Leiske l.
    Lempert-Storz l.
    Lems l.
    lenticular l.
    lenticular-cut contact l.
    lenticular spectacle l.
    Lewis l.
    Lieb-Guerry l.
    Lindstrom Centrex l.
    Liteflex l.
    l. localizer
    long-wearing contact l.
    loose l.
    l. loupe
    Lovac gonioscopic l.

luxated l.
luxation of l.
Lynell intraocular l.
Machemer flat l.
Machemer infusion
  contact l.
Machemer magnifying l.
Machemer magnifying
  vitrectomy l.
macular l.
macular contact l.
magnifying l.
Mainster retinal laser l.
l. maker's formula
March laser l.
Mark II magnifocuser l.
Mark IX l.
McCannel l.
McGhan l.
McGhan 3M intraocular l.
McLean l.
McLean prismatic fundus
  laser l.
Medallion l.
Medical Optics PC11 NB
  intraocular l.
Medical Workshop
  intraocular l.
Medicornea Kratz
  intraocular l.
Meditec bandage contact l.
meniscus l.
meniscus concave l.
Meso contact l.
meter l.
microbevel edge l.
microthin l.
mid-coquille l.
minus l.
minus spectacle l.
modified C-loop
  intraocular l.
modified C-loop UV l.
modified J-loop
  intraocular l.
modified J-loop UV l.
mold-injected l.
multicurve contact l.
Multiflex anterior
  chamber l.
multifocal l.
multifocal spectacle l.
Multi-Optics l.

negative meniscus l.
Neolens l.
New Orleans l.
Nokrome bifocal l.
Nova Aid l.
Nova Curve l.
Nova Curve broad C-loop
  posterior chamber l.
Nova Curve Omnicurve l.
Nova Soft II l.
nuclear sclerosis of l.
nucleus of l.
occupational lenses
Oculaid l.
ocular l.
Ocular Gamboscope l.
O'Malley-Pearce-Luma l.
Omnifit intraocular l.
one-piece l.
one-piece multifocal l.
one-plane l.
open l.
Ophtec Co. l.
optical center of l.
optical center of spectacle l.
optical contact l.
Optical Radiation l.
optical zone of contact l.
Optiflex l.
Opti-Vu l.
Opt-Visor l.
Optycryl 60 contact l.
Opus III contact l.
orbital l.
ORC intraocular l.
Orthogon l.
orthoscopic l.
O'Shea l.
Osher l.
panchamber UV l.
Pannu intraocular l.
Pannu type II l.
PanoView Optics l.
Paraperm O2 contact l.
PBII blue loop l.
Pearce posterior chamber
  intraocular l.
pediatric Karickhoff laser l.
pediatric three-mirror
  laser l.
periscopic l.
periscopic concave l.
periscopic convex l.

lens *(continued)*
    Permaflex l.
    Permalens l.
    Perspex CQ-Shearing-Simcoe-
      Sinskey l.
    Petrus single-mirror laser l.
    Peyman l.
    Peyman-Green vitrectomy l.
    Peyman-Tennant-Green l.
    Peyman wide-field l.
    P.F. Lee pediatric
      goniolens l.
    Pharmacia intraocular l.
    Pharmacia Visco J-loop l.
    photobrown lenses
    photochromic l.
    photogray l.
    photosensitive l.
    photosun l.
    piggyback contact l.
    pigmentary deposits on l.
    l. pit
    placode l.
    l. placode
    l. plane
    plano l.
    planoconcave l.
    planoconvex l.
    planoconvex nonridge l.
    Plano T l.
    plastic l.
    Platina l.
    Platina clip l.
    plus l.
    plus spectacle l.
    polycarbonate l.
    Polycon I contact l.
    Polycon II contact l.
    polymethyl methacrylate
      contact l.
    positive meniscus l.
    Posner diagnostic l.
    posterior chamber l.
    posterior chamber
      intraocular l. (PCIOL)
    posterior pole of l.
    l. power
    l. power calculation
    Precision Cosmet l.
    press-on lenses
    press-on Fresnel l.
    primary l.
    prismatic l.

prismatic contact l.
prismatic effect by l.
prismatic gonioscopic l.
prismatic gonioscopy l.
prismatic goniotomy l.
prismatic spectacle l.
prism ballast l.
prism ballasted contact l.
progressive l.
progressive addition l.
progressive multifocal l.
prolonged-wear contact l.
prosthetic l.
protective l.
punctal l.
pupillary l.
radius of l.
Rayner l.
Red Reflex Lens Systems l.
refractive contact l.
l. removal
retroscopic l.
ridge l.
Ridley l.
rigid contact l.
rigid gas-permeable l.
Ritch trabeculoplasty laser l.
RLX l.
Rodenstock l.
Rodenstock panfundus l.
rudiment l.
Ruiz fundus l.
Ruiz fundus contact l.
Ruiz fundus laser l.
safety l.
Saturn II contact lenses
Sauflon l.
Sauflon PW l.
Schachar l.
Scharf l.
Schlegel l.
scleral contact l.
scratch resistant l.
scratch resistant spectacle l.
secondary l.
segmental l.
semifinished l.
semiscleral contact l.
Severin l.
Shearing l.
Shearing intraocular l.
Shearing planar posterior
    chamber intraocular l.

Sheets l.
short C-loop l.
Signet Optical l.
silicone l.
silicone acrylate contact lenses
silicone contact l.
silicone elastomer l.
Silsoft contact l.
Simcoe l.
Simcoe II PC l.
single-cut contact l.
Sinskey l.
Sinskey intraocular l.
l. size
slab-off l.
Slant haptic single-piece intraocular l.
SlimFit ovoid intraocular l.
SlimFit small-incision ovoid l.
Snellen soft contact l.
Soflens l.
soft l.
soft contact l. (SCL)
soft intraocular l.
Soper cone l.
Sovereign bifocal l.
special spectacle l.
spectacle l.
spherical l. (S, sph.)
spherical equivalent l.
spherocylindric l.
spherocylindrical l.
spin-cast l.
l. sponge
l. spoon
Stableflex anterior chamber l.
star l.
l. star
steep contact l.
stigmatic l.
Stokes l.
Strampelli l.
Style S2 clear-loop l.
styrene contact lenses
subluxated l.
subluxation of l.
subluxed l.
substance of l.
Surefit AC 85J l.
Surgidev l.

Surgidev intraocular l.
Surgidev PC BUV 20-24 intraocular l.
Sutherland l.
suture of l.
T l.
telescopic l.
Tennant l.
Tennant Anchorflex AC l.
therapeutic contact l.
thick l.
thin l.
Thorpe four-mirror goniolaser l.
Thorpe four-mirror vitreous fundus laser l.
three-mirror l.
three-mirror contact l.
tight contact l.
Tillyer l.
Tillyer bifocal l.
tilting l.
tinted l.
tinted contact l.
tinting of l.
tinting of spectacle l.
Tolentino prism l.
Tolentino vitrectomy l.
Topcon l.
Topcon aspheric l.
toric l.
toric contact l.
Toric-Optima series l.
toric spectacle l.
toroidal contact l.
trial l.
trial case and l.
tricurve contact lenses
trifocal l.
Trokel l.
Trokel-Peyman laser l.
truncated contact l.
TruVision l.
two-plane l.
Ultex l.
Ultravue l.
uncut l.
uncut spectacle l.
Uniplanar style PC II l.
Univis l.
Urrets-Zavalia retinal surgical l.
UVEX l.

lens *(continued)*
    UV Nova Curve l.
    Varigray l.
    Varilux l.
    vaulting of contact l.
    l. vesicle
    Viscolens l.
    Vision Tech l.
    Volk coronoid l.
    Wang l.
    Weber-Elschnig l.
    Wesley-Jessen l.
    whorl l.
    Wild l.
    Wise iridotomy laser l.
    Wise iridotomy-
      sphincterotomy laser l.
    Woods Concept l.
    Worst goniotomy l.
    Worst Medallion l.
    Worst Platina iris-fixated l.
    X chrom l.
    Yannuzzi l.
    Yannuzzi fundus laser l.
    Youens l.
    Zeiss l.
    Zeiss-Gullstrand l.
    zero power lenses
    l. zonule
lens blank
    blocking of l. b.
Lens Clear
lensectomy
    Charles' l.
    coal-mining l.
Lensept
lenses
Lens-Eze inserter
Lens Fresh
lens-holding forceps
lens-induced
    l.-i. glaucoma
    l.-i. uveitis
lensmeter
    Badal l.
    Nagel l.
Lensometer
    Hardy L.
lensometer
    Allergan l.
    Allergan Humphrey l.
    AO l.
    AO Reichert l.

    AO Reichert Instruments l.
    Carl Zeiss l.
    Coburn l.
    IntraOptics l.
    Marco l.
    Reichert l.
    Topcon l.
    Topcon digital l.
    Topcon LM P5 digital l.
lensopathy
Lens Plus Oxysept
Lensrins
lens-threading forceps
Lens-Wet
lentectomize
lentectomy
lenticonus
lenticula
lenticular
    l. astigmatism
    l. body
    l. bowl
    l. cataract
    l. contact lens
    l. degeneration
    l. fossa
    l. fossa of vitreous body
    l. ganglion
    l. glaucoma
    l. lens
    l. myopia
    l. nucleus
    l. ring
    l. spectacle lens
    l. vesicle
lenticular-cut contact lens
lenticuli
lenticulocapsular
lenticulo-optic
lenticulostriate
lenticulothalamic
lenticulus, pl. **lenticuli**
lentiform
    l. nodule
    nucleus l.
lentigines
lentigines, electrocardiographic conduction abnormalities, ocular hypertelorism, pulmonary stenosis, abnormal genitalia, retardation of growth, and deafness (LEOPARD)
lentiglobus

lentigo maligna
lentis
> apparatus suspensorius l.
> l. articularis
> axis l.
> caligo l.
> capsula l.
> cellulae l.
> cortex l.
> epithelium l.
> equator l.
> equatorial l.
> facies anterior l.
> facies posterior l.
> fibrae l.
> gerontoxon l.
> nucleus l.
> polus anterior l.
> polus posterior l.
> radius of l.
> siderosis l.
> spontaneous ectopia l.
> substantia l.
> substantia corticalis l.
> tunica vasculosa l.
> vortex l.

Lenz's syndrome
LEOPARD
> lentigines, electrocardiographic
> conduction abnormalities,
> ocular hypertelorism,
> pulmonary stenosis, abnormal
> genitalia, retardation of growth,
> and deafness

leopard
> l. fundus
> l. retina

LEOPARD syndrome
leprechaunism
leproma
lepromatous leprosy
leprosa
> keratitis punctata l.

leprosy
> lepromatous l.
> tuberculoid l.

leptomeningeal metastasis
leptomeningitis
Leptospira
> *L. interrogans*

leptospirosis
leptotrichosis conjunctiva

lesion
> boomerang-shaped l.
> bull's eye macular l.
> cervical l.
> choroidal l.
> concentric l.
> conjunctival melanotic l.
> cornea guttate l.
> corneal punctate l.
> dendritic l.
> geographic l.'s
> herpetoid l.
> keratitis l.
> lipocytic l.
> lymphoepithelial l.
> lytic l.'s
> malignant pituitary l.
> melanocytic l.
> melanocytic conjunctival l.
> melanotic l.
> neural l.
> occipital lobe l.
> optic nerve l.
> optic tract l.
> l. of orbit
> osseous l.
> periventricular l.
> pigmented l.'s
> pontine l.'s
> precancerous l.
> pseudocancerous l.
> punched-out l.
> retrogeniculate l.
> satellite l.
> space occupying l.
> sunburst-type l.'s
> unifocal optic nerve l.

L'Esperance erysiphake
lesser
> l. ring
> l. ring of iris

Lester
> L. fixation forceps
> L. lens manipulator

Lester-Burch speculum
Lester-Jones operation
lethal midline granuloma
letter
> l. blindness
> Sloan l.'s
> Snellen l.'s
> l. test

letterbox technique

Letterer-Siwe
  L.-S. disease
  L.-S. syndrome
letter-shaped keratitis
leucitis
leukemia
  granulocytic l.
  hairy-cell l.
  lymphocytic l.
  monocytic l.
leukemic
  l. cells
  l. infiltrate
  l. infiltration
  l. retinitis
  l. retinopathy
leukocoria
leukocyte
  polymorphonuclear l.
leukocytic
leukoderma
  congenital l.
leukodystrophy
  l. dystrophy
  globoid cell l.
  metachromatic l.
  metachromic l.
leukoencephalopathy
  progressive multifocal l.
leukokoria
leukoma
  l. adherens
  adherent l.
leukomalacia
  preventricular l.
leukomas
leukomata
leukomatous
leukopathia, leukopathy
  congenital l.
leukoplakia
leukopsin
leukoscope
leukotomy
  transorbital l.
levallorphan tartrate
levator
  l. aponeurosis disinsertion
  l. aponeurosis repair
  l. injury
  l. muscle
  l. muscle of upper eyelid

l. palpebrae superioris
l. palpebrae superioris
  muscle
l. resection
l. trochlear muscle
level
  acetylcholine receptor
    antibody l.
  fibrinogen l.
  trough l.
Levine spud
Levitt implant
levobunolol hydrochloride
levocabastine
levoclination
levocycloduction
levocycloversion
levoduction
levo-epinephrine
levotorsion
levoversion version
Lewicky
  L. formed cystitome
  L. needle
  L. self-retaining chamber
    maintainer
  L. threaded infusion
    cannula
Lewis
  L. lens
  L. lens loupe
  L. loupe
  L. scoop
Lewy body
Lexan
Lexer's operation
LGB
  lateral geniculate body
LGN
  lateral geniculate nucleus
LHT
  left hypertropia
library temple
Librium
lichenified lid
Lichtenberg corneal trephine
lid
  l. agglutination
  l. block
  Celsus' l.
  l. closure reaction
  l. crease

crusting l.'s
l. crusting
l. droop
l. eversion
l. everter
l. fissure
l. forceps
granular l.
l. lag
l. laxity
lichenified l.
l. loading
l. margin
l. margin laceration
l. notching
l. nystagmus
l. plate
l. reflex
l. retraction
l. scrub
l. speculum
l. thrush
tonic l.'s
l. trephine
lidocaine
l. hydrochloride
l. with epinephrine
Lidoject
Lidoject-1 with epinephrine
lids, lashes, lacrimals, lymphatics (LLLL)
Lieberman
L. fragmentor
L. phaco crusher
Lieberman-Polack double corneal forceps
Lieb-Guerry lens
Liebreich's symptom
Lieppman cystitome
life-belt cataract
ligament
canthal l.
check l.
ciliary l.
cribriform l.
Hueck's l.
hyaloideocapsular l.
lateral palpebral l.
Lockwood's l.
medial canthal l.
medial palpebral l.
palpebral l.
pectinate l.

pectineal l.
suspensory l.
Weigert's l.
Whitnall's l.
Wieger's l.
Zinn's l.
ligamentum, pl. ligamenta
l. anguli iridocornealis
l. pectinatum anguli iridocornealis
l. pectinatum iridis
light
l. adaptation
autokinesis visible l.
axial l.
axial ray of l.
Barkan l.
central l.
l. coagulation
convergent l.
dichromatic l.
l. difference
l. differential threshold
l. discrimination
divergent l.
emergent l.
emergent ray of l.
ether theory of l.
fixation l.
flashes of l.
idioretinal l.
incident l.
incident ray of l.
intrinsic l.
Lumiwand l.
marginal ray of l.
minimum l.
monochromatic l.
near reaction to l.
oblique ray of l.
l. optometer reflex
paraxial ray of l.
l. perception (LP)
peripheral ray of l.
pipe l.
polarized l.
l. projection
l. projection test
reflected l.
l. reflex
refracted l.
l. response of pupil
l. scatter

light *(continued)*
    l. scattering
    l. sensation
    l. sense
    l. sensitivity
    l. stimulus
    l. transmission
    transmitted l.
    ultraviolet l.
    white l.
    Young's theory of l.
light-adapted eye
Lighthouse Low Vision Service
lighting
    paraxial l.
light-near dissociation
lightning
    l. cataract
    l. eye movements
    l. streaks
light-optometer
light-stress test
Lignac-Fanconi syndrome
ligneous
    conjunctivitis l.
    l. conjunctivitis
lilacinus
    Paecilomyces l.
limb
    afferent l.
    black l.
limbal
    l. approach
    l. arcade
    l. compression
    corneal inferior l.
    l. girdle
    l. girdle of Vogt
    l. groove
    l. guttering
    l. incision
    l. luteus retinae
    l. neurofibroma
    l. palpebrales anteriores
    l. palpebrales posteriores
    l. parallel orientation
    l. zone
limbal-based flap
limbi
limbic
    l. keratoconjunctivitis
    l. keratoconjunctivitis
    l. vernal keratoconjunctivitis

limbitis
Limbitrol
limbus, pl. **limbi**
    balding the l.
    congenital dermoid of l.
    conjunctival l.
    l. of cornea
    corneal l.
    cystoid cicatrix of l.
    l. girdle
    l. guttering
    l. mass
    l. parallel orientation
        straddling tattoo mark
    l. of perception
    l. of sclera
limit
    Rayleigh's l.
limitation
    eccentric l.
limiting
    l. angle
    l. lamina
    l. lamina anterior
    l. layer
    l. membrane
limulus lysate test
Lincocin
Lincoff
    L. balloon
    L. balloon catheter
    L. implant
    L. lens sponge
    L. scleral sponge implant
    L. sponge
Lincoff's operation
lincomycin
Lindau's disease
Lindau-von Hippel disease
Linde cryogenic probe
Lindner's
    L. operation
    L. sclerotomy
Lindner spatula
Lindsay's operation
Lindstrom
    L. Centrex lens
    L. lens-insertion forceps
line
    absorption l.'s
    angular l.
    Arlt's l.
    atopic l.

blue l.
corneal l.
corneal iron l.
demarcation l. of retina
l. of direction
Donders' l.
Egger's l.
Ehrlich-Türck l.
face l.
Ferry's l.
fingerprint l.
l. of fixation
Fraunhofer's l.
gray l.
Helmholtz's l.
Hudson's l.
Hudson-Stähli l.
iron l.
iron-ferry l.
iron-Hudson-Stähli l.
iron-stocker l.
Khodadoust l.
mare's hair l.'s
mare's tail l.
Morgan's l.
Paton's l.'s
pigment demarcation l.'s
principal l.
pupillary l.
rejection l.
retinal stress l.'s
Sampoelesi's l.
Schwalbe's l.
l. of sight
Snellen l.
Stähli's l.
Stähli's pigment l.
Stocker's l.
stromal l.
superficial corneal l.
triradiate l.
Turk's l.
l. of vision
visual l.
Vogt l.'s
Zöllner's l.
linea, gen. and pl. **lineae**
l. corneae senilis
l. visus
linear
l. echoes
l. keratopathy
l. perspective

l. scar
l. sebaceous nevus sequence
l. subcutaneous atrophy
l. vision
l. visual acuity test
linkage analysis
Linn-Graefe iris forceps
lip
anterior l.
scleral l.
lipemia
l. retinalis
lipemic
l. retina
l. retinopathy
lipid
l. abnormality
l. accumulation
blood l.'s
l. cell
l. degeneration
l. keratopathy
l. metabolism
l. proteinosis
l. tear layer
lipid-like inclusions
lipidoses
lipidosis
galactosyl ceramide l.
glycolipid l.
glycosphingolipid l.
sphingomyelin l.
lipoatrophic diabetes
lipocyte
lipocytic lesion
lipodermoid
conjunctival l.
lipodystrophy
lipofuscin
lipofuscinosis
Batten's ceroid l.
ceroid l.
neuronal ceroid l.
lipogranuloma
lipogranulomatosis
lipoidosis
l. corneae
lipoid proteinosis
lipoma
orbital l.
lipomatosis
ptosis l.
lipoplethoric diabetes

lipoproteinemia
liposarcoma
Lipo-Tears Forte
lippa
lippitude, lippitudo
Lipschütz inclusion body
lipuric diabetes
liquefaction
    contraction and l.
liquefied vitreous
liquid
    l. organic dye laser
    l. vitreous-aspirating cannula
liquified vitreous
Liquifilm
    Albalon L.
    Bleph-10 L.
    L. forte
    Herplex L.
    HMS L.
    Prefrin L.
    Prefrin Z L.
    P.V. Carpine L.
    L. Tears
    L. Wetting
liquor
    l. corneae
    Morgagni's l.
Lisch nodule
Lister
    L. forceps
    L. lens manipulator
    L. scissors
listeriosis
Listing's
    L. law
    L. plane
    L. reduced eye
    L. schematic eye
Liteflex lens
Lite-Pred
lithiasis
    l. conjunctivae
    conjunctival l.
    l. conjunctivitis
lithium carbonate
lithotriptor
    candela laser l.
Littauer
    L. cilia forceps
    L. dissecting scissors

Littler
    L. dissecting scissors
    L. scissors
Littmann galilean magnification
  changer
LKP
    lamellar keratoplasty
LLLL
    lids, lashes, lacrimals, lymphatics
Llobera fixation forceps
Lloyd stereocampimeter
loa
    Loa l.
loading
    lid l.
loafer temple
Loa loa
lobe
    occipital l.
    palpebral l.
    parietal l.
    temporal l.
    temporoparietal l.
lobotomy
lobulated
lobuli
    coloboma l.
local
    l. anesthetic
    l. tic
localization
    Comberg l.
    spatial l.
localized
    l. albinism
    l. amyloidosis
localizer
    Berman l.
    lens l.
    Roper-Hall l.
    Wildgen-Reck l.
locator
    Berman l.
    Berman foreign body l.
    Bronson-Turner foreign
     body l.
    foreign body l.
    Roper-Hall l.
    Sweet l.
    Wildgren-Reck l.
lock
    Luer cannula l.

locking
mode l.
Lockwood
superior tendon of L.
Lockwood's
L. ligament
L. light reflex
L. tendon
Loctoplate
locus, pl. **loci**
gene l.
retinoblastoma l.
lodoxamide
Loewi's
L. reaction
L. sign
Lofgren's syndrome
log
l. rank
l. units
logadectomy
logarithmic Minimum Angle of Resolution (logMAR)
logMAR
logarithmic Minimum Angle of Resolution
Löhlein's operation
loiasis
Lombert
L. radioscope
L. tonometer
Londermann corneal trephine
Londermann's operation
long
l. ciliary artery
l. ciliary nerve
l. posterior ciliary arteries
l. root of ciliary ganglion
l. sight
longi
nervi ciliares l.
longitudinal
l. aberration
l. axis
l. axis of Fick
l. ciliary muscle
l. fasciculus
l. fiber
l. muscle
long-scale contrast
longsightedness
long-wearing contact lens

Look
L. capsule polisher
L. cortex extractor
L. cystitome
L. I/A coaxial cannula
L. irrigating lens loop
L. irrigating vectis
L. retrobulbar needle
L. suture
looking
forced choice preferential l.
preferential l. (PL)
loop
Axenfeld's l.
Axenfeld's nerve l.
C l.
Clayman-Knolle irrigating lens l.
closed l.
expressor l.
flexible l.
haptic l.
intrascleral nerve l.
J l.
Knolle-Pearce irrigating lens l.
Look irrigating lens l.
Meyer l.
Meyer-Archambault l.
Meyer temporal l.
modified J l.
nerve l.
nylon l.
open l.
Pearce-Knoll irrigating lens l.
prepapillary vascular l.'s
temporal l.
two-angled polypropylene l.
vascular l.
loose
l. contact lens
l. lens
Lopez-Enriquez
L.-E. operation
L.-E. scleral trephine
Lorain's infantilism
Lordan chalazion forceps
lorgnette
Loring ophthalmoscope
loss
axonal l.
blood l.

loss *(continued)*
 field l.
 functional visual l.
 hearing l.
 nonorganic visual l.
 unilateral hearing l.
 l. of vision
 vitreous l.
 l. of vitreous
loteprednol
Lotman Visometer
Lo-Trau
 L.-T. needle
 L.-T. side-cutting needle
Lotze's local signs
louchettes
Louis-Bar syndrome
loupe
 Amenabar l.
 Amenabar lens l.
 angled lens l.
 angled nucleus removal l.
 Arlt l.
 Arlt lens l.
 Atwood l.
 Beebe l.
 Berens lens l.
 binocular l.
 Callahan lens l.
 Castroviejo lens l.
 Elschnig-Weber l.
 FormFlex lens l.
 Gullstrand l.
 Ilg lens l.
 Keeler l.
 Keeler panoramic l.
 Kirby l.
 Kirby intracapsular lens l.
 Kirby intraocular lens l.
 Kirby lens l.
 Kraff nucleus lens l.
 Lemoine-Searcy fixation
  anchor l.
 Lempert-Storz l.
 lens l.
 Lewis l.
 Lewis lens l.
 magnifying l.
 Mark II magnifocuser l.
 New Orleans l.
 New Orleans lens l.
 nucleus delivery l.
 nucleus removal l.

 Ocular Gamboscope l.
 operating l.
 Opt-Visor l.
 panoramic l.
 Simcoe l.
 Simcoe double-end lens l.
 Simcoe II PC nucleus
  delivery l.
 Simcoe nucleus delivery l.
 Simcoe nucleus lens l.
 Snellen lens l.
 Troutman lens l.
 Visitec nucleus removal l.
 Weber-Elschnig l.
 Weber-Elschnig lens l.
 Wilder lens l.
 Zeiss-Gullstrand l.
 Zeiss lens l.
 Zeiss operating field l.
Lovac
 L. fundus contact lens
  implant
 L. gonioscope
 L. gonioscopic lens
 L. six-mirror gonioscopic
  lens implant
 L. six-mirror implant
low
 l. contrast
 l. convex
 l. vision
Lowell glaucoma knife
Löwenstein's operation
lower
 l. eyelid
 l. hemianopsia
 l. lid laxity
 l. lid retractor
 l. lid sling procedure
 l. punctum
 l. retina
Lowe's
 L. oculocerebrorenal
  syndrome
 L. ring
 L. syndrome
Lowe-Terrey-MacLachlan syndrome
low-pressure glaucoma
Lowry's assay
low-tension glaucoma
loxophthalmus
LP
 light perception

LPK-80 II argon laser
LR
    lateral rectus
LSD
    lysergic acid diethylamide
L.T. Jones tear duct tube
Lubricant
    Lens L.
lubricant
    silicone l.
Lubrifair
Lucae dressing forceps
lucency, pl. **lucencies**
lucida
    camera l.
lucidum
    tapetum l.
Lucite
    L. frame
    L. implant
    L. sphere implant
Luedde exophthalmometer
Luedde's
    L. transparent rule
Luer
    L. cannula lock
    L. connections
    L. tube
Luer-Lok
    Yale L.-L.
lues
luetic
    l. chorioretinitis
    l. interstitial keratitis
    l. neuropathy
lumbar puncture
lumbricoides
    Ascaris l.
lumen, pl. **lumina, lumens**
    capillary l.
luminance
luminosity
    l. curve
luminous
    l. flux
    l. intensity (I)
    l. retinoscope
lumirhodopsin
Lumiwand light
Lumonics laser
lunata
    plica l.

Lundsgaard
    L. knife
    L. rasp
    L. sclerotome
Lundsgaard-Burch
    L.-B. corneal rasp
    L.-B. sclerotome
lupus
    l. anticoagulant
    l. erythematosus (LE)
    l. erythematosus cell test
    l. oculopathy
    l. vulgaris
luster
    binocular l.
    corneal l.
    polychromatic l.
lusterless
lustrous central yellow point
lux
luxated lens
luxation
    l. of eyeball
    l. of globe
    l. of lens
Luxo Surgical Illuminator
luxurians
    ectropion l.
Lyda-Ivalon-Lucite implant
Lyell's disease
Lyle's syndrome
Lyme
    L. borreliosis
    L. disease
    L. disease keratitis
lymphadenopathy
lymphangiectasis
lymphangioma
    conjunctival l.
    eyelid l.
lymphatic drainage
lymphatici
lymphatics
    lids, lashes, lacrimals, l.
    (LLLL)
lymphaticus
    nodulus l.
lymphedema
lymphoblast
    reticular l.
lymphoblastic lymphoma

lymphocyte
    B l.
    T l.
lymphocytic
    l. adenohypophysitis
    l. interstitial pneumonitis
    l. leukemia
lymphoepithelial lesion
lymphoepithelioma
lymphogranuloma
    l. venereum
    l. venereum keratitis
lymphoid
    l. follicle
    l. granulomatosis
    l. hyperplasia
    l. infiltration
    l. pseudotumor
    l. tumor
lymphokine
lymphoma
    anterior chamber l.
    Burkitt's l.
    histiocytic l.
    intraocular l.
    large-cell l.
    lymphoblastic l.
    non-Hodgkin's l.

    orbital l.
    porcupine l.
    reticulum cell l.
    signet-ring l.
    T-cell l.
lymphomatoid granulomatosis
lymphomatosis
    ocular l.
lymphophagocytosis
lymphoproliferative
    l. disorder
    l. tumor
lymphoreticulosis
lymphosarcoma
Lynell intraocular lens
Lyon hypothesis
lyophilized
lysed
lysergic
    l. acid
    l. acid diethylamide (LSD)
lysis
    cell l.
lysosomal storage disease
lysosome
lysozyme
Lyteers
lytic lesions

M
blood factor
mega-
morgan
myopia
myopic
3M
3M small aperture Steri-Drape
3M Steri-Drape drape
MacCallan's classification
Macewen's sign
Machek-Blaskovics operation
Machek-Brunswick operation
Machek-Gifford operation
Machek's
M. operation
M. ptosis operation
Machemer
M. calipers
M. cutter
M. diamond dust-coated foreign body forceps
M. flat lens
M. infusion contact lens
M magnifying lens
M. magnifying vitrectomy lens
M. vitreous cutter
machine
CooperVision I/A m.
I/A m.
Stat m.
Stat Scrub handwasher m.
Visual-Tech m.
Mach's band
MacKay-Marg
M.-M. electronic tonometer
M.-M. tonometer
Mack-Brunswick operation
macroadenoma
macroaneurysm
macroblepharia
macrocornea
macrocyst
macrocytic anemia
α₂-macroglobulin
macroglobulinemia
Waldenström's m.
macroperforation

macrophage
macrophthalmia
macrophthalmic
macrophthalmous
macroprolactinoma
macropsia
macroptic
macroreticular dystrophy
macro square-wave jerks
macrostereognosis
macrovessel
macula, pl. maculae
m. adherens
cherry-red m.
cherry-red spot in m.
m. corneae
dragged m.
false m.
m. flava retinae
graying of m.
honeycomb m.
m. lutea
m. lutea retinae
m. retinae
vitelliform degeneration of m.
macular, maculate
m. aplasia
m. area
m. arteriole
m. arteriole occlusion
m. binocular vision
m. choroiditis
m. clusters
m. coloboma
m. contact lens
m. corneal dystrophy
m. degeneration
m. detachment
m. disciform degeneration
m. disease
m. displacement
m. drusen
m. dystrophy
m. ectopia
m. edema
m. evasion
m. graying
m. heredodegeneration
m. hole

macular *(continued)*
    m. holes
    m. hypoplasia
    m. leak
    m. lens
    m. neuroretinopathy
    m. photocoagulation
    m. photostress
    m. pucker
    m. puckering
    m. retinopathy
    m. sparing
    m. splitting
    m. star
    m. stereopsis
    m. suppression
    m. surface wrinkling
    m. venule
maculary
    fasciculus m.
macule
maculocerebral
maculopapillary bundle
maculopapular bundle
maculopathy
    atrophic degenerative m.
    bull's eye m.
    cellophane m.
    cystoid m.
    diabetic m.
    dry senile degenerative m.
    exudative senile m.
    familial
      pseudoinflammatory m.
    Groenouw's type II m.
    heredity m.
    histoplasmosis m.
    Kuhnt-Junius m.
    myopic m.
    niacin m.
    nicotinic acid m.
    pigment epithelial
      detachment m.
    serous detachment m.
    solar m.
    Sorsby's m.
    Stargardt's m.
    toxic m.
    vitelliform m.
maculovesicular
MacVicar double-end strabismus retractor
madarosis

Maddox
    M. prism
    M. rod
Maddox's
    M. rod test
    M. wing test
Madribon
madurae
    Actinomadura m.
Maeder-Danis dystrophy
mafilcon A
Magendie-Hertwig
    M.-H. sign
    M.-H. syndrome
Magendie's
    M. sign
    M. symptom
Magitot's
    M. keratoplasty operation
    M. operation
magnae
    facies orbitalis alae m.
magnesium fluoride
magnet
    Bronson-Magnion m.
    Bronson-Magnion eye m.
    eye m.
    Gruning m.
    Haab m.
    hand-held m.
    hand-held eye m.
    Hirschberg m.
    implant m.
    Lancaster m.
    Lancaster eye m.
    m. operation
    original Sweet m.
    original Sweet eye m.
    rare earth m.
    Schumann giant type m.
    Schumann giant type
      eye m.
    Storz m.
    Storz-Atlas m.
    Storz-Atlas hand m.
    Storz-Atlas hand eye m.
    Storz Microvit m.
    Sweet original m.
magnetic
    m. extraction
    m. implant
    m. operation
    m. resonance angiography

m. resonance imaging
(MRI)
m. resonance imaging scan
magnetism
magnification
relative spectacle m.
magnifier
magnifying
m. glasses
m. lens
m. loupe
m. power
Magnus' operation
Maguire-Harvey
M.-H. cutter
M.-H. vitreous cutter
Maier
sinus of M.
Maier's sinus
main fiber
Mainster retinal laser lens
maintainer
Lewicky self-retaining
chamber m.
Majewsky's operation
major
m. amblyoscope
m. amblyoscope test
annulus iridis m.
m. arcade
m. arterial circle of iris
circulus arteriosus iridis m.
erythema multiforme m.
m. histocompatibility
antigen
m. histocompatibility
complex (MHC)
m. meridian
majoris
facies orbitalis alae m.
Maklakoff tonometer
malabsorption syndrome
Maladie de Graeffe's operation
malalignment
malar eminence
malaria
Malattia-Leventinese
Malbec's operation
Malbran's operation
maleate
naphazoline and
pheniramine m.
pilocarpine and timolol m.

malformation
Arnold-Chiari m.
arteriovenous m.
Chiari's m.
congenital brain m.
dural arteriovenous m.
infratentorial
arteriovenous m.
orbital arteriovenous m.
retinal arteriovenous m.
supratentorial
arteriovenous m.
Malherbe's calcifying epithelioma
maligna
lentigo m.
malignant
m. ciliary epithelioma
m. dyskeratosis
m. epithelial tumor
m. exophthalmos
m. external otitis syndrome
m. glaucoma
m. hypertension
m. hyperthermia
m. melanoma
m. myopia
m. neurilemoma
m. pituitary lesion
m. schwannoma
m. scleritis
m. tumor
malingerer
malingering
Malis
M. Bipolar
Coagulating/Cutting System
M. forceps
Mallazine drops
malleable
mallet
lead-filled m.
mal morado
malnutrition
malprojection
mandible
mandibular dysostosis
mandibulofacial
m. dyostosis
m. dysostosis
m. dystrophy
mandibulo-oculofacial dysmorphia
and dyscephaly

maneuver
Carlo Traverso m. (CTM)
doll's eye m.
doll's head m.
Hallpike m.
notch-and-roll m.
Nylen-Barany m.
oculocephalic m.
Valsalva's m.
wall push m.
Manhattan
M. Eye & Ear probe
M. Eye & Ear spatula
M. Eye & Ear suturing
forceps
M. forceps
manifest
m. deviation
m. hyperopia (Hm)
m. latent nystagmus
m. refraction
m. strabismus
manifestation
neuro-ophthalmic m.
manipulation
cervical m.
laser m.
pharmacologic m.
physical m.
manipulator
angled Vico m.
button-tip m.
Judson-Smith m.
Kuglein irrigating lens m.
Kuglein lens m.
Lester lens m.
Lister lens m.
McIntyre irrigating iris m.
Visitec vico m.
manner
McLean's m.
Mannis
M. probe
M. suture
mannitol salts agar medium
mannosidosis
Mann's sign
manometer
Honan m.
Tycos m.
manometry
manoptoscope

Manson-Aebli corneal section scissors
Manson double-ended strabismus hook
Manz's gland
map-dot
m.-d. corneal dystrophy
m.-d. dystrophy
map-dot-fingerprint
m.-d.-f. corneal epithelial dystrophy
m.-d.-f. dystrophy
map pattern
mapping
chromosome m.
deletion m.
visually evoked potential m.
marble bone disease
marbleization
Marcaine
M. HCl
M. HCl with epinephrine
marcescens
Serratia m.
March
M. laser lens
M. laser sclerostomy needle
M. needle
Marchesani's syndrome
Marco
M. chart projector
M. lensometer
M. radius gauge
M. refractor
M. slit lamp
M. SurgiScope
Marco's perimeter
Marcus
M. Gunn (MG)
M. Gunn afferent defect
M. Gunn dot
M. Gunn jaw-winking syndrome
M. Gunn phenomenon
M. Gunn pupil (MG)
M. Gunn pupillary sign
M. Gunn relative afferent defect
M. Gunn sign
M. Gunn syndrome
mare's
m. hair lines
m. tail line

Marfan's
  M. disease
  M. syndrome
margin
  ciliary m.
  eyelid m.
  fimbriated m.
  infraorbital m.
  lash m.
  lid m.
  orbital m.
marginal
  m. blepharitis
  m. catarrhal ulcer
  m. chalazion forceps
  m. corneal degeneration
  m. corneal ulcer
  m. crystalline dystrophy
  m. degeneration
  m. degeneration of cornea
  m. dystrophy
  m. entropion
  m. furrow
  m. furrow degeneration
  m. keratitis
  m. melt
  m. myotomy
  m. ray of light
  m. rays
  m. ring ulcer of cornea
  m. tear strip
  m. ulcer
marginoplasty
margo, pl. margines
  m. ciliaris iridis
  m. infraorbitalis orbitae
  m. lacrimalis maxillae
  m. lateralis orbitae
  m. medialis orbitae
  m. orbitalis
  m. palpebra
  m. pupillaris iridis
  m. supraorbitalis orbitae
  m. supraorbitalis ossis
    frontalis
Marie's ataxia
Marie-Strümpell disease
Marinesco-Sjögren syndrome
Mariotte
  blind spot of M.
Mariotte's
  M. blind spot

  M. experiment
  M. spot
Maritima
  Succus Cineraria M.
Mark
  M. II magnifocuser lens
  M. II magnifocuser loupe
  M. IX lens
mark
  limbus parallel orientation
    straddling tattoo m.
marker
  Amsler m.
  Amsler scleral m.
  biprong muscle m.
  Bores axis m.
  Castroviejo corneal
    transplant m.
  Castroviejo scleral m.
  corneal transplant m.
  Desmarres m.
  Feldman RK optical
    center m.
  Fink biprong m.
  Fink muscle m.
  Gass scleral m.
  Gonin m.
  Gonin-Amsler m.
  Green corneal m.
  Green-Kenyon corneal m.
  Hoffer optical center m.
  Hoopes corneal m.
  Neumann-Shepard
    corneal m.
  Neumann-Shepard oval
    optical center m.
  O'Brien m.
  O'Connor m.
  ocular m.
  optical zone m.
  Osher-Neumann corneal m.
  radial keratotomy m.
  RK m.
  Ruiz-Nordan trapezoidal m.
  scleral m.
  Shepard optical center m.
  Simcoe corneal m.
  Thornton optical center m.
  Visitec RK zone m.
  m.'s for zone
marking pen
Marlex mesh
Marlin Salt System II

Marlow's test
Marmor
　　pattern dystrophy of
　　　pigment epithelium of
　　　Byers and M.
Maroteaux-Lamy syndrome
Marquez-Gomez
　　M.-G. conjunctival graft
　　M.-G. operation
Marshall syndrome
martegiani
　　area m.
Martinez
　　M. corneal transplant
　　　centering ring
　　M. corneal trephine blade
　　M. disposable corneal
　　　trephine
　　M. dissector
　　M. keratome
　　M. knife
Martin Surefit lens pusher
mascara particle inclusions
Masciuli silicone sponge
maser
masked diabetes
masque biliaire
masquerade
　　m. syndrome
　　m. technique
mass
　　cicatricial m.
　　hyaline m.
　　laminated acellular m.
　　limbus m.
　　mulberry-shaped m.
　　mycelial m.
　　ochre m.
　　ovoid m.
Massachusetts
　　M. Vision Kit (MVK)
　　M. XII Vitrectomy System
　　　(MVS)
Masselon
　　M. glasses
　　M. spectacles
massive
　　m. granuloma of sclera
　　m. periretinal proliferation
　　　(MPP)
mast cell
master-dominant eye

master eye
Masuda-Kitahara disease
Mate
　　Lens M.
　　Soft M.
material
　　alloplastic donor m.
　　autogenous donor m.
　　coating m.
　　contrast m.
　　cyanographic contrast m.
　　cyanographin contrast m.
　　donor m.
　　fibrillar m.
　　gallium citrate contrast m.
　　gelatinous m.
　　heterogeneous donor m.
　　heterogenous donor m.
　　homogeneous donor m.
　　homogenous donor m.
　　hyaline m.
materials primary dye
matrix
　　extracellular m.
　　stromal m.
matter
　　particulate m.
mattering
Mattis
　　M. corneal scissors
　　M. scissors
mattress suture
maturation
　　delayed visual m.
mature
　　m. cataphoria
　　m. cataract
maturity-onset diabetes
Mauksch-Maumenee-Goldberg
　　operation
Mauksch's operation
Maumenee
　　M. capsule forceps
　　M. corneal forceps
　　M. erysiphake
　　M. forceps
　　M. goniotomy knife
　　M. goniotomy knife cannula
　　M. iris hook
　　M. knife goniotomy cannula
　　M. needle
　　M. Suregrip forceps

M. vitreous aspirating
  needle
M. vitreous sweep spatula
Maumenee-Colibri corneal forceps
Maumenee-Goldberg operation
Maumenee-Park
  M.-P. eye speculum
  M.-P. speculum
Maunoir iris scissors
Mauthner's test
Max
  M. Fine forceps
  M. Fine scissors
Maxidex
maxilla, gen. **maxillae**, pl. **maxillae**
  incisura maxillae
  infraorbital margin of m.
  infraorbital sulcus of m.
  lacrimal sulcus of m.
  margo lacrimalis maxillae
  processus zygomaticus
    maxillae
  sulcus infraorbitalis maxillae
  zygomatico-orbital process of
    the m.
maxillaris
  nervus m.
maxillary
  m. bone
  m. nerve
  m. osteomyelitis
  m. sinusitis
maximum tolerated medical
  therapy (MTMT)
Maxitrol
Maxwell-Lyons sign
Maxwell's
  M. ring
  M. spot
Mayo
  M. scissors
  M. stand
May's sign
Mazzotti's reaction
M band
McCannel
  M. implant
  M. lens
  M. suture
McCannell ocular pressure reducer
McCarey-Kaufman (M-K)
  M.-K. media

M.-K. medium (M-K
  medium)
M.-K. transport medium
McCarthy's reflex
McClure iris scissors
McCool capsule retractor
McCullough
  M. forceps
  M. suturing forceps
McDonald expressor
M cells
McGannon
  M. refractor
  M. retractor
McGavic's operation
McGhan
  M. implant
  M. lens
  M. 3M intraocular lens
McGregor conjunctival forceps
McGuire
  M. conformer
  M. corneal scissors
  M. forceps
  M. I/A system
  M. marginal chalazion
    forceps
  M. scissors
McGuire's operation
McIntyre
  M. coaxial cannula
  M. coaxial irrigating-
    aspirating system
  M. fish-hook needle holder
  M. I/A needle
  M. I/A system
  M. infusion set
  M. irrigating/aspirating unit
  M. irrigating hook
  M. irrigating iris
    manipulator
  M. irrigation/aspiration
    needle
  M. irrigation/aspiration
    system
  M. needle
  M. nylon cannula connector
  M. reverse cystitome
  M. spatula
  M. truncated cone
McIntyre-Binkhorst irrigating
  cannula
McKee speculum

McKinney
    M. eye speculum
    M. fixation ring
McLaughlin's operation
McLean
    M. capsule forceps
    M. capsulotomy scissors
    M. classification of
    melanoma
    M. forceps
    M. lens
    M. muscle recession forceps
    M. prismatic fundus laser
    lens
    M. scissors
    M. suture
    M. tonometer
McLean's
    M. fashion
    M. manner
    M. operation
    M. technique
McNeill-Goldmann
    M.-G. blepharostat
    M.-G. ring
m-cone
McPherson
    M. angled forceps
    M. bent forceps
    M. corneal forceps
    M. corneal section scissors
    M. forceps
    M. irrigating forceps
    M. micro iris forceps
    M. micro suture forceps
    M. needle holder
    M. scissors
    M. spatula
    M. speculum
    M. trabeculotome
    M. tying forceps
    M. tying iris forceps
McPherson-Castroviejo
    M.-C. corneal section
    scissors
    M.-C. scissors
McPherson-Vannas
    M.-V. micro iris scissors
    M.-V. scissors
McPherson-Westcott
    M.-W. conjunctival scissors
    M.-W. stitch scissors

McPherson-Wheeler
    M.-W. blade
    M.-W. knife
McPherson-Ziegler knife
McQueen vitreous forceps
McReynolds
    M. hook
    M. keratome
    M. knife
    M. lid retracting hook
    M. pterygium knife
    M. pterygium scissors
    M. scissors
    M. spatula
McReynolds'
    M. operation
    M. pterygium transplant
    M. technique
M-delphine
Means' sign
measles
    German m.
measurement
    box m.
    criterion-free m.
    diurnal intraocular
    pressure m.
    prism cover m.
    Rushton's ocular m.'s
    Stenstrom's ocular m.'s
measuring
meatus
mecamylamine
mechanical
    m. acquired ptosis
    m. ectropion
    m. ptosis
    m. strabismus
mechanics
    fluid m.
mechanism
    m. of action
    cholinergic m.
    Hering's after-image m.
    immune m.
    oculogyric m.
    pursuit m.
    trigger m.
mechanized scissors
Mecholyl test
Meckel-Gruber syndrome
MED
    minimal effective diameter

Medallion lens
media
> chondroitin sulfate m.
> contrast m.
> dioptric m.
> Kaufman's m.
> K-Sol m.
> McCarey-Kaufman m.
> ocular m.
> opaque m.
> otitis m.
> refracting m.
> refractive m.
> Sabouraud's m.

medial
> m. angle
> m. angle of eye
> m. arteriole of retina
> m. canthal ligament
> m. canthal repair
> m. canthal tendon
> m. canthus
> m. commissure of eyelid
> m. ectropion
> m. horn
> m. longitudinal fasciculus (MLF)
> m. palpebral ligament
> m. rectus (MR)
> m. rectus extraocular muscles
> m. rectus muscle
> m. rectus palsy
> m. venulae of retina

medialis
> angular oculi m.
> angulus oculi m.
> commissura palpebrarum m.
> venula retinae m.

median
> m. longitudinal fasciculus
mediaometer
mediator
> inflammatory m.

Medical
> M. Optics PC11 NB intraocular lens
> M. Optics PC11NB intraocular lens implant
> M. Workshop intraocular lens
> M. Workshop intraocular lens implant

medical
> m. adenomectomy
> m. ophthalmoscopy
medicamentosus
Medicornea
> M. Kratz intraocular lens
> M. Kratz intraocular lens implant

Meditec
> M. bandage contact lens
> M. laser
Mediterranean anemia
medium, pl. **media**
> anaerobic m.
> culture media
> gram-negative media
> Kaufman m.
> mannitol salts agar m.
> McCarey-Kaufman m. (M-K medium)
> McCarey-Kaufman transport m.
> M-K m.
>> McCarey-Kaufman medium
medium/solution
Medrol
medroxyprogesterone acetate
Medrysone
medrysone
medullary
> m. cystic disease
> m. optic disease
> m. ray
medullated nerve fiber
medulloblastoma tumor
medulloepithelioma
> adult m.
> embryonal m.
> orbital m.
Medusa head
Meek's operation
Meesman's
> M. dystrophy
> M. epithelial corneal dystrophy
> M. epithelial dystrophy
> M. juvenile epithelial dystrophy
mega- (M)
megalocornea
megalopapilla

megalophthalmus
  anterior m.
megalopsia, megalopia
meglumine/sodium
  iothalamate m.
megophthalmus
meibomian
  m. blepharitis
  m. conjunctivitis
  m. cyst
  m. duct
  m. gland
  m. gland carcinoma
  m. gland expressor
  m. sty
meibomianitis
meibomitis
Meigs' syndrome
melanin
melanocyte
melanocytic
  m. conjunctival lesion
  m. hamartoma
  m. lesion
  m. nevus
melanocytoma
melanocytosis
  congenital m.
  congenital ocular m.
  congenital oculodermal m.
  ocular m.
  oculodermal m.
melanogenesis
melanokeratosis
  striate m.
melanoma
  choroidal m.
  Cloudman mouse m.
  conjunctival m.
  cutaneous m.
  m. of eyelid
  intraocular m.
  m. of iris
  juvenile m.
  malignant m.
  McLean classification of m.
  nodular m.
  ocular m.
  orbital m.
  pagetoid m.
  posterior uveal m.
  spindle A m.
  spindle B m.

  tapioca m.
  tapioca iris m.
  uveal m.
melanomalytic glaucoma
melanomata
melanophage
melanosis
  acquired m.
  m. bulbi
  diabetic m.
  m. iridis
  m. oculi
  oculodermal m.
  presenile m.
  primary acquired m.
  m. sclerae
melanosome
melanotic
  m. lesion
  m. progonoma
  m. sarcoma
Melauskas
  M. acrylic implant
  M. orbital implant
Melkersson-Rosenthal syndrome
Melkersson's syndrome
Mellaril
Meller
  M. lacrimal sac retractor
  M. refractor
Meller's operation
Mellinger speculum
mellitus
  diabetes m.
  gestational diabetes m.
  insulin-dependent
    diabetes m. (IDDM)
  non-insulin-dependent
    diabetes m. (NIDDM)
Melsman's
  M. corneal dystrophy
  M. dystrophy
melt
  corneal m.
  corneoscleral m.
  marginal m.
  sterile m.
  stromal m.
membrana, gen. and pl. **membranae**
  m. capsularis lentis
    posterior
  m. choriocapillaris
  m. epipapillaris

m. fusca
m. granulosa externa
m. granulosa interna
m. hyaloidea
m. limitans externa
m. limitans interna
m. nictitans
m. pupillaris
m. ruyschiana
m. vitrea
membranacea
cataracta congenita m.
membrane
anterior hyaloid m. (AHM)
Barkan's m.
basement m.
bilaminar m.
Bowman's m.
Bruch's m.
choroidal m.
choroidal neovascular m.
conjunctival m.
connective tissue m.
contraction of cyclitic m.
cyclitic m.
Demours' m.
Descemet's m.
Duddell's m.
endothelial cell basement m.
epipapillary m.
epiretinal m.
epithelial basement m.
external limiting m.
fibroproliferative m.
Fresnel m.
glassy m.
gliotic m.
Haller's m.
Henle's m.
Hovius' m.
hyaline m.
hyalitis anterior m.
hyaloid m.
hyaloid posterior m.
idiopathic preretinal m.
inner limiting m.
intermuscular m.
internal limiting m.
Jacob's m.
limiting m.
m. lipid cell
mucous m.
neovascular m.

nictitating m.
onion skin-like m.
outer limiting m.
m. peeler-cutter
m. peeling
periorbital m.
posterior hyaloid m. (PHM)
preretinal m.
pupillary m.
purpurogenous m.
Reichert's m.
retrocorneal m.
ruyschiana m.
Ruysch's m.
secondary m.
serous m.
stripping m.
subretinal m. (SRM)
subretinal neovascular m.
tarsal m.
Tenon's m.
trabecular m.
vitreal m.
vitreous m.
Wachendorf's m.
wrinkling m.
Zinn's m.
membranectomy
membranous
m. cataract
m. conjunctivitis
m. rhinitis
memory
immunologic m.
mendelian disorder
Mendez
M. astigmatism dial
M. cystitome
Menière's syndrome
meningeal
m. carcinomatosis
m. cells
m. hemangiopericytoma
m. hydrops
meninges
meningioma
angioblastic m.
fibroblastic m.
nerve sheath m.
ocular m.
optic nerve m.
orbital m.
perioptic m.

meningioma *(continued)*
 perioptic sheath m.
 sphenoid m.
 sphenoid wing m.
 suprasellar m.
meningitidis
 Neisseria m.
meningitis
meningocele
meningococcosis
meningococcus conjunctivitis
meningocutaneous angiomatosis
meniscus, pl. **menisci**
 m. concave lens
 converging m.
 diverging m.
 m. floater
 Kuhnt's m.
 m. lens
 negative m.
 periscopic m.
 positive m.
 tear of m.
Menkes' syndrome
Mentanium vitreoretinal instrument set
Mentor
 M. BVAT II Video Acuity
 M. Exeter ophthalmoscope
 M. fine-focus microscope
 M. microscope
 M. pre-cut drain
 M. wet-field cautery
 M. wet-field electrocautery
 M. wet-field eraser
Mentor-Maumenee Suregrip forceps
meperidine hydrochloride
mepivacaine
meprobamate
mercurial
 organic m.
mercurialentis
mercury (Hg)
 millimeters of m. (mmHg)
 m. pressure
meridian
 m. of cornea
 corneal m.
 equatorial m.
 m. of eyeball
 horizontal m.
 major m.

steepest m.
 vertical m.
meridiani bulbi oculi
meridianus
meridional
 m. aberration
 m. amblyopia
 m. balance
 m. ciliary muscle fiber
 m. fibers of ciliary muscle
 m. fold
 m. implant
 m. refractometer
Merkel's cell neoplasm
Merocel
 M. sponge
 M. surgical spear
meropia
Merrimac laser
Mersilene suture
merthiolate
Mesco
mesectoderm
mesenchymal
 m. cells
 m. ridge
 m. tumor
mesenchyme
 hemocytic m.
 neurogenic m.
 orbital m.
mesenchymoma
mesh
 Marlex m.
 tantalum m.
meshing
meshwork
 trabecular m. (TM)
mesiris
mesochoroidea
Meso contact lens
mesocornea
mesoderm
mesodermal dysgenesis
mesodermalis
 primary dysgenesis m.
mesophryon
mesopia
mesopic perimetry
mesoretina
mesoridazine
mesoropter

metabolic
  m. cataract
  m. disorder
  m. storage disease
  m. syndrome cataract
metabolic-toxic
metabolism
  amino acid m.
  carbohydrate m.
  copper m.
  glycolipid m.
  inborn error of m.
  lipid m.
  mineral m.
  uric acid m.
metachromatic leukodystrophy
metachromic leukodystrophy
metacontrast
metaherpetic
  m. keratitis
  m. ulcer
metakeratitis
  herpetic m.
metal
  aluminum m.
metameric color
metamorphopsia
  m. varians
metaplastic epithelial cells
metarhodopsin
metastasis, pl. metastases
  chiasmal m.
  hematopoietic m.
  leptomeningeal m.
  orbital m.
  tumor m.
  m. of tumor
  uveal m.
metastatic
  m. carcinoma
  m. choroiditis
  m. endophthalmitis
  m. ophthalmia
  m. retinitis
  m. tumor
Fletcher speculum
Metenier's sign
Meter
  Guyton-Minkowski Potential
    Acuity M.
  Potential Acuity M. (PAM)
  Vuero M.

meter
  m. angle
  footcandle m.
  m. lens
meter-candle
methacholine
  m. chloride
methacrylate
  methyl m.
  polymethyl m. (PMMA)
methacycline
methamphetamine
methanol
methaqualone
MethaSite
methazolamide
methicillin
method
  Barraquer's m.
  confrontation m.
  Con-Lish polishing m.
  contact m.
  Crawford's m.
  Credé's m.
  Cuignet's m.
  direct m.
  gradient m.
  Hirschberg's m.
  Holmgren m.
  immersion m.
  immunodiagnostic m.
  Krimsky's m.
  modified band lid m.
  Mueller's m.
  optical density m.
  Pfeiffer-Komberg m.
  rag-wheel m.
  Sweet's m.
  twirling m.
  Westergren m.
  Wheeler m.
  Wolfe's m.
methohexital
Methopto
methosulfate
  trimethidium m.
methotrexate
methoxsalen
methoxyflurane
Methulose
methyl
  m. alcohol
  m. cyanoacrylate glue

methyl *(continued)*
    m. methacrylate
    m. methacrylate implant
    m. salicylate
methylcellulose
    hydroxypropyl m.
methyldopa
methylene
    m. blue
    m. blue dye test
methylergonovine
methylmethacrylate
methylparaben
methylpentynol
methylphenidate
    cocaine m.
methylprednisolone
methysergide
Metico forceps
Metimyd
metipranolol
metoprolol
Metreton
metric
    m. ophthalmoscope
    m. ophthalmoscopy
metrizamide
metronoscope
metubine iodide
Metycaine
MEWDS
    multiple evanescent white dot
    syndrome
Meyer
    M. knife
    M. loop
    M. Swiss diamond knife
    lancet
    M. Swiss diamond lancet
    knife
    M. Swiss diamond mini-
    angled knife
    M. Swiss diamond wedge
    knife
    M. temporal loop
Meyer-Archambault loop
Meyer-Schwickerath
    M.-S. coagulator
    M.-S. light coagulation
    M.-S. operation

Meyhoeffer
    M. chalazion curette
    M. curette
Meyhoeffer's chalazion
Meynert's
    M. commissure
    superior commissura of M.
MF
    mutton fat
MG
    Marcus Gunn
    Marcus Gunn pupil
MHA-TP test
    microhemaglutination test for
    Treponema pallidum
MHC
    major histocompatibility
    complex
mica spectacles
micelles in vitreous
Michaelson's
    M. counter pressure
    M. operation
Michel
    M. pick
    M. spur
miconazole
Micra double-edged diamond blade
micro
    m. Colibri forceps
    m. eye movement
    m. movement
    m. movements of eye
    m. round-tip needle
    m. sponge
    m. surgical knife
microadenoma
microaneurysm
microaneurysmal leakage
microangiography
microbevel edge lens
microbial keratitis
microbiallergic conjunctivitis
microblepharia, microblepharism,
    microblepharon, microblephary
microcautery unit
microcephaly
microcoria
microcornea
microcyst
    Blessig-Iwanoff m.
    epithelial m.
    punctate epithelial m.

microcystic
    m. corneal dystrophy
    m. dystrophy
    m. edema
    m. epithelial dystrophy
microcytic anemia
microdrift
microembolism, pl. microemboli
    retinal m.
microfilaria
microglia
microgonioscope
microhemagglutination test
microhemaglutination test for
    Treponema pallidium (MHA-TP
    test)
microinfarction
microkeratome
    Barraquer m.
Microknife knife
Microlase transpupillary diode
    laser
Micro-Lite
Micromatic ophthalmometer
micromegalopsia
micrometer
    m. disk
    m. knife
    Tolman m.
    ultrasonic m.
micromovement
micronystagmus
micropannus
microperforation
microphakia
microphotography
microphthalmia, microphthalmos
    colobomatous m.
    cystic m.
microphthalmoscope
microphthalmus
Micropigmentation System
micropigmentation system
micropins
    Pischel m.
micropoint
    m. needle
    m. suture
microproliferation
micropsia
microptic
microsaccades

microscissors
    Keeler m.
microscope
    Beckerscope binocular m.
    Bio-Optics specular m.
    Bitumi monobjective m.
    Cohan-Barraquer m.
    CooperVision m.
    corneal m.
    Czapski m.
    electron m.
    Fiberlite m.
    Heyer-Schulte m.
    Keeler specular m.
    Leitz m.
    Mentor m.
    Mentor fine-focus m.
    Moller m.
    OM 2000 operation m.
    operating m.
    OpMi m.
    PRO CEM-4 m.
    Pro-Koester wide-field
      SCM m.
    slit-lamp m.
    specular m.
    Storz m.
    Topcon m.
    video specular m.
    Weck m.
    Wild M 690 m.
    Wild operating m.
    Zeiss m.
    Zeiss-Barraquer cine m.
    Zeiss-Barraquer surgical m.
    Zeiss operating m.
microscopic hyphema
microscopy
    electron m.
    fundus m.
    scanning electron m.
    specular m.
microsomia
    hemifacial m.
microspectroscope
microspherometer
microspherophakia
Microsponge
    Alcon M.
    M. Teardrop sponge
microstrabismic amblyopia
microstrabismus

microsurgery
    Grieshaber's ultrasharp m.
microthin
    m. contact lens
    m. lens
Microtonometer
    Computon M.
microtremor
    unilateral m.
microtropia
microtropic syndrome
microtubule
microvascular abnormality
microvilli
microvillus
Microvit
    M. probe
    M. Probe System
    M. vitrector
microvitrector
microvitreoretinal (MVR)
    m. blade
    m. spatula
microwave
    m. radiation injury
micro Westcott scissors
midazolam
midbrain reticular formation
mid-coquille lens
middle cerebral artery
midfacial fracture
midline
    m. granuloma
    m. position
    m. position of gaze
midperiphery
Mieten's syndrome
MIF
    migration inhibition factor
migraine
    m. equivalent
    m. headache
    ophthalmic m.
    m. ophthalmoplegia
    ophthalmoplegic m.
    retinal m.
migrainous ophthalmoplegia
migrans
    erythema chronicum m.
    visceral larva m.
migration
    implant m.
    m. inhibition factor (MIF)

    pigmentary m.
    m. theory
migratory ophthalmia
Mikulicz's
    M. disease
    M. syndrome
Mild
    Inflamase M.
    Pred M.
mild chromic suture
milia
    eyelid m.
miliary aneurysm
milk-alkali syndrome
milky cataract
Millard-Gubler syndrome
Miller-Fisher syndrome
Miller-Nadler glare tester
Miller's syndrome
Milles' syndrome
millet seed nodule
Millex filter
millijoule (mJ)
millilambert
millimeters of mercury (mmHg)
millimicron (mu)
Millipore filter
Milroy Artificial Tears
Milroy's disease
mimicking
    finger m.
mind blindness
mineral metabolism
mineralocorticoids
miner's
    m. blindness
    m. disease
    m. nystagmus
miniature
    m. blade
    m. forceps
minify
mini-keratoplasty
    Castroviejo's m.-k.
    m.-k. stitch scissors
minimal
    m. amplitude nystagmus
    m. brain dysfunction
    m. effective diameter
    (MED)
minimum
    m. cognoscibile
    m. deviation

m. legible
m. light
m. light threshold
m. perceptible acuity
m. separable
m. separable acuity
m. separable angle
m. visible
m. visible angle
m. visual angle
mini ophthalmic drape
minocycline
minor
    annulus iridis m.
    circulus arteriosus iridis m.
minoxidil
Minsky's
    M. circle
    M. intramarginal splitting
    M. operation
minus
    m. carrier
    m. carrier contact lens
    m. cyclophoria
    cyclophoria m.
    cyclotropia m.
    m. cyclotropia
    m. cylinder
    m. lens
    m. spectacle lens
Miocel
Miochol solution
miosis
    irritative m.
    paralytic m.
    pupil m.
    pupillary m.
    senescent m.
    senile m.
    spastic m.
    spinal m.
    traumatic pupillary m.
Miostat
miotic
    m. pupil
    m. therapy
Mira
    M. AGL-400
    M. cautery
    M. diathermy
    M. diathermy unit
    M. electrocautery
    M. endovitreal cryopencil

    M. photocoagulator
    M. unit
mirabile
    rete m.
Miracon
MiraFlow
MiraFlow Extra-Strength
MiraSept System
MiraSol
mire
mires
    image of m.
    keratometer m.
    m. of ophthalmometer
mirror
    m. area
    m. coating
    concave m.
    convex m.
    m. haploscope
    head m.
    m. image
misdirected lashes
misdirection phenomenon
misty vision
mitochondria
mitochondrial
    m. cytopathy
    m. myopathy
mitomycin
mitosis
mitotic
mitral valve prolapse
Mittendorf dot
Mitzuo's phenomenon
mixed
    m. astigmatism
    m. cataract
    m. esotropia
    m. strabismus
    m. tumor
mixing
    color m.
mJ
    millijoule
M-K
    McCarey-Kaufman
    M.-K. medium
MK
    M. IV ophthalmoscope
MLF
    medial longitudinal fasciculus

mmHg
    millimeters of mercury
Möbius', Moebius'
    M. disease
    M. sign
    M. syndrome
Möbius-von Graefe-Stellway sign
modality
Modane
mode
    m. of action
    free running m.
    m. locking
    pulse m.
model
    Bohr's m.
    ICR rat m.
    reduced eye m.
mode-locked
    m.-l. laser
    m.-l. Nd:YAG laser
modification
    Deller's m.
    Smith's m.
    Van Herick's m.
modified
    m. band lid method
    m. C-loop intraocular lens
    m. C-loop UV lens
    m. J loop
    m. J-loop intraocular lens
    m. J-loop UV lens
    m. monovision
    m. Van Lint block
    m. Van Lint's anesthesia
    m. Wies procedure
modulation transfer function
Moebius' (*var. of* Möbius')
Moehle
    M. cannula
    M. corneal forceps
    M. forceps
Mohs' microsurgical resection
Moiré's fringe
moistened fine mesh gauze
    dressing
Moisture drops
molded
    m. frame
    m. pressing
molding
    cast m.

compression m.
    injection m.
mold-injected lens
molectron laser
molecular
    m. dissociation theory
    m. external layer
    m. genetics
    m. inner layer
    m. internal layer
    m. layer
    m. outer layer
Moller microscope
Moll's gland
molluscum
    conjunctivitis m.
    m. conjunctivitis
    m. contagiosum
Molteno
    M. episcleral explant
    M. implant
Monakow's syndrome
Moncrieff cannula
Moncrieff's
    M. discission
    M. operation
mongolian
    m. fold
    m. spot
mongolism
mongoloid slant
moniliasis
monitor
    cardiac m.
monitoring
monoblepsia
monochroic
monochromacy
    cone m.
monochromasia
monochromasy
    blue cone m.
    rod m.
monochromat
    cone m.'s
    rod m.
monochromatic
    m. aberration
    m. cone
    m. eye
    m. green
    m. light
    m. rays

monochromatism
blue cone m.
cone m.
rod m.
X-linked blue cone m.
monochromic
monocle
monoclonal antibody
monocular
m. aphakia
m. bandage
m. confrontation visual
· field test
m. depth perception
m. diplopia
m. dressing
m. field defect
m. fixation
m. glaucoma
m. heterochromia
m. indirect ophthalmoscope
m. oscillopsia
m. patch
m. strabismus
m. telescope
m. temporal crescent
m. vision
monoculus
monocyte
monocytic leukemia
monodiplopia
monofilament nylon suture
monofixational phoria
monofixation syndrome
monolateral strabismus
mononuclear
m. cell infiltration
m. reaction
m. response
mononucleosis
infectious m.
monophosphate
adenosine m. (AMP)
cyclic adenosine m. (cAMP)
cyclic guanosine m.
monophthalmica
polyopia m.
monophthalmos
monopia
monosomy
m. G syndrome
monostearate
glyceryl m.

monovision
modified m.
monoxide
carbon m.
moon
m. blindness
m. circulated
Moore
M. lens forceps
M. lens-inserting forceps
Mooren's
M. corneal ulcer
M. ulcer
Moore's lightning streak
Moore-Troutman corneal scissors
Moran's
M. operation
M. proptosis
Morax-Axenfeld conjunctivitis
Moraxella
M. lacunata
Morax's
M. keratoplasty
M. operation
Morck's
M. cement
M. cement bifocal
Morel-Fatio-Lalardie operation
morgagnian
m. cataract
m. globule
Morgagni's
M. cataract
M. globule
M. liquor
M. spheres
morgan (M)
Morgan's
M. dot
M. line
Moria
M. obturator
M. one-piece speculum
M. trephine
Moria-France
dacryocystorhinostomy clamp
morning
m. glory
m. glory anomaly
m. glory disk
m. glory optic atrophy
m. glory optic disk
anomaly

morning *(continued)*
    m. glory retinal detachment
    m. glory syndrome
    m. ptosis
morphine
Morquio-Brailsford syndrome
Morquio's syndrome
mosaic
    m. pattern
    trisomy 9 m.
mosaicism
Mosher's operation
Mosher-Toti operation
Mosler's diabetes
mosquito
    m. clamp
    m. hemostatic forceps
Moss'
    M. operation
    M. traction
Motais' operation
motile scotoma
motility
    m. implant
    ocular m.
motion
    against m.
    hand m. (HM)
    m. parallax
    m. vision
    with m.
motor
    m. function
    m. fusion
    m. nerve
    m. oculi
    m. root
    m. root of ciliary ganglion
    m. tic
    Visuscope m.
motor-output disability
Motrin
Mot-R-Pak vitrectomy system
mottled appearance
mottling
    early receptor potential m.
    (ERPM)
    m. of fundus
Moulton lacrimal duct tube
mounds
    pearl white m.

mount
    unstained wet m.
    wet m.
by mouth (p.o.)
movement
    cardinal ocular m.'s
    cogwheel m.
    cogwheel ocular m.'s
    cogwheel pursuit m.
    conjugate m.
    conjugate m. of eyes
    conjugate ocular m.'s
    corrective m.
    disjugate m.
    disjugate m. of eyes
    disjunctive m.
    drift m.'s
    extraocular m.'s (EOM)
    eye m.'s
    fixational ocular m.
    flick m.'s
    following m.
    fusional m.
    gaze m.
    hand m. (HM)
    lightning eye m.'s
    micro m.
    micro eye m.
    nonoptic reflex eye m.'s
    non-rapid eye m.
    nystagmoid m.'s
    ocular m.
    paradoxical m. of eyelids
    perverted ocular m.
    pursuit m.
    rapid eye m.'s (REM)
    saccadic m.
    saccadic eye m.
    scissors m.
    synkinetic m.
    torsional m.
    vergence eye m.'s (VEM)
    vermiform m.
    version m.
    vertical m.'s
    voluntary eye m.
    yoke m.
mover
    primary m.
MPC automated intravitreal scissors
MPP
    massive periretinal proliferation

**MP Video endoscopic lens
  attachment**
MR
  medial rectus
MRI
  magnetic resonance imaging
  MRI scan
M-Rinse
M-TEC 2000 Surgical System
MTL trial frame
MTMT
  maximum tolerated medical
  therapy
mu
  millimicron
mucicarmine stain
mucin
  m. strands
  m. of tcar
mucinous adenocarcinoma tumor
mucocele
  sinus m.
mucocutaneous
  m. candidiasis
  m. junction
mucoepidermoid
mucolipidosis, pl. **mucolipidoses**
  m. IV
mucomycosis
Mucomyst
mucopolysaccharide
  stromal m.
mucopolysaccharidoses
mucopolysaccharidosis
mucopurulent conjunctivitis
mucopyocele
mucormycosis
mucosae
  hyalinosis cutis et m.
mucosal
  m. neuroma
  m. pemphigoid
mucotome
  Castroviejo m.
mucous
  m. assay
  m. discharge
  m. layer
  m. membrane
  m. membrane graft
  m. ophthalmia
  m. tear layer
  m. thread

mucous-like strands
mucoviscidosis
mucus
  ropy m.
Mueller
  M. cautery
  M. electric corneal trephine
  M. electrocautery
  M. electronic tonometer
  M. eye shield
  M. implant
  M. lacrimal sac retractor
  M. refractor
  M. shield
  M. speculum
  M. trephine
Mueller
  cells of M.
  radial cells of M.
Mueller's
  M. cell
  M. fiber
  M. gland
  M. method
  M. muscle
  M. operation
  M. trigone
Muhlberger orbital implant
mulberry-shaped mass
mulberry-type papilloma
Muldoon lacrimal dilator
Mules
  M. implant
  M. scoop
  M. sphere
  M. vitreous sphere
Mules' operation
Mulibrey nanism
multicellular
multicentric
multicurve contact lens
multifactorial disease
Multiflex anterior chamber lens
multifocal
  m. chorioretinal disease
  m. choroiditis
  m. fibrosclerosis
  m. hemorrhagic sarcoma
  m. lens
  Nokrome fused m.'s
  m. spectacle lens

multiforme
    erythema m.
    glioblastoma m.
multilaminar
multilobar
multilocular vesicle
Multilux
multimode
multinucleated
    m. epithelial cell
    m. giant cell
    m. giant epithelial cell
Multi-Optics lens
multiple
    m. endocrine neoplasia
    m. evanescent white dot
      syndrome (MEWDS)
    m. lentigines syndrome
    m. myeloma
    m. sclerosis
    m. vision
Multi-Purpose
    ReNu M.-P.
multivesicular bodies
mumps
    m. keratitis
Munsell's color
Munson's sign
mural cell
muramidase
Murdock eye speculum
Murdock-Wiener eye speculum
Murdoon eye speculum
Murine
    M. Plus
    M. sterile saline
Muro 128
Murocel
Murocoll-2
Muro Opcon
Muro Opcon A
Muro Tears
musca, pl. muscae
    muscae volitantes
muscegenetic
muscle
    abducens m.
    abductor m.'s
    adductor m.'s
    agonist m.
    belly of m.
    m. belly
    bound-down m.

Bowman's m.
Brücke's m.
ciliaris m.
ciliary m.
circular ciliary m.
m. clamp
m. cone
m. contraction headache
cyclovertical m.
m. depressor
m. dilator
dilator m.
disinserted m.
elevator m.
extraocular m. (EOM)
extrinsic m.'s
m. of eye
eyelid m.
m. force
m. forceps
frontalis m.
m. hook
Horner's m.
inferior m.
inferior oblique m.
inferior oblique
    extraocular m.'s
inferior rectus m.
inferior rectus
    extraocular m.'s
inferior tarsal m.
intraocular m. (IOM)
intrinsic m.
intrinsic ocular m.
iridic m.
Koyter's m.
Landström's m.
lateral rectus m.
lateral rectus
    extraocular m.'s
left inferior rectus m.
left superior rectus m.
levator m.
levator palpebrae
    superioris m.
levator trochlear m.
longitudinal m.
longitudinal ciliary m.
medial rectus m.
medial rectus
    extraocular m.'s
meridional fibers of
    ciliary m.

Mueller's m.
oblique m.
ocular m.
oculorotatory m.
orbicularis m.
orbicularis oculi m.
orbicularis oris m.
orbital m.
palpebrae superioris m.
palsies of m.
m. paretic nystagmus
preseptal orbicularis m.
pupillary sphincter m.
radial dilator m.
recession of m.
rectus m.
rectus lateralis m.
rectus medialis m.
m. relaxant
m. resection
resection of m.
Riolan's m.
Rouget's m.
m. sheath
sphincter m.
superciliary m.
superior m.
superior oblique m.
superior oblique
  extraocular m.'s
superior rectus m.
superior rectus
  extraocular m.'s
superior tarsal m.
tarsal m.
temporalis m.
m. transposition
trochlear m.
trochlea of superior
  oblique m.
yoked m.
muscular
  m. asthenopia
  m. balance
  m. dystrophy
  m. fascia
  m. funnel
  m. insufficiency
  m. strabismus
  m. vein
musculus, gen. and pl. **musculi**
  musculi bulbi
  m. ciliaris

m. corrugator supercilii
m. depressor supercilii
m. dilator pupilla
lamina superficialis musculi
m. levator palpebrae
  superioris
m. obliquus inferior bulbi
m. obliquus inferior oculi
m. obliquus superior bulbi
m. obliquus superior oculi
musculi oculi
m. orbicularis
m. orbicularis oculi
m. orbiculris oculi
m. orbitalis
m. procerus
m. rectus inferior bulbi
m. rectus inferior oculi
m. rectus lateralis bulbi
m. rectus lateralis oculi
m. rectus medialis bulbi
m. rectus medialis oculi
m. sphincter pupilla
m. tarsalis inferior
m. tarsalis superior
mushroom
  corneal m.
  m. corneal graft
  m. graft
Mustarde
  M. awl
  M. rotational cheek flap
Mustarde's
  M. graft
  M. operation
mustard gas
mutation
  point m.
mutton fat (MF)
mutton-fat keratic precipitate
MVB blade
MVK
  Massachusetts Vision Kit
MVR
  microvitreoretinal
  MVR blade
MVS
  Massachusetts XII Vitrectomy
  System
Myambutol
myasthenia
  m. gravis
  m. syndrome

myasthenia-like syndrome
myasthenic nystagmus
mycelia
mycelial mass
Mycitracin
mycobacteria
    atypical m.
mycobacterial disease
Mycobacterium
    M. africanum
    M. bovis
    M. chelonei
    M. fortuitum
    M. tuberculosis
mycosis fungoides
Mycostatin
mycotic
    m. infection
    m. keratitis
    m. snowball opacities
mycotoxicity
Mydfrin
Mydramide
Mydrapred
Mydriacyl
Mydriafair
mydriasis
    accidental m.
    alternating m.
    amaurotic m.
    bounding m.
    factitious m.
    fixed m.
    paralytic m.
    spasmodic m.
    spastic m.
    spinal m.
    springing m.
    traumatic m.
mydriatic
    m. provocative test
    m. rigidity
    m. test
    m. test for angle-closure
      glaucoma
    m. test for glaucoma
mydriatic-cycloplegic therapy
Mydrilate
myectomy operation
myelinated
    m. fiber
    m. nerve fiber
myelinating

myelination
myelin disorder
myelitis
myeloidin
myeloma
    multiple m.
    osteosclerotic m.
myelomatosis
    disseminated
      nonosteolytic m.
myelo-optic neuropathy
myiasis
    cutaneous m.
    ocular m.
myoblastoma
    granular cell m.
myocardial infarction
Myochrysine
myoclonal
myoclonus
    m. nystagmus
    ocular m.
    startle m.
myoculator
Myocure
    M. blade
    M. blade scalpel
    M. knife
    M. phacoblade
    M. scalpel
myodesopsia
myodiopter
myoepithelial cells
myofibril
myofibroblast
myofibromatosis
myogenic
    m. acquired ptosis
    m. ptosis
myoid visual cell
myokymia
    eyelid m.
    superior m.
    superior oblique m.
myoneural
myopathy
    mitochondrial m.
    ocular m.
    visceral m.
myope
myopia (M)
    axial m.
    choroiditis m.

chromic m.
crescent m.
curvature m.
degenerative m.
high m.
index m.
m. index
lenticular m.
malignant m.
night m.
pathologic m.
pernicious m.
physiologic m.
prematurity m.
primary m.
prodromal m.
progressive m.
refractive m.
school m.
senile lenticular m.
simple m.
space m.
transient m.
myopic (M)
m. anisometropia
m. astigmatism (As.M.)
m. choroidal atrophy
m. choroidopathy
m. conus
m. crescent

m. degeneration
m. keratomileusis
m. maculopathy
m. reflex
myorhythmia
oculomasticatory m.
myoscope
myosin filament
myosis
myositis
orbital m.
myotomy
marginal m.
m. operation
Z m.
myotonia
m. congenita
m. dystrophica
myotonic
m. cataract
m. dystrophy
m. dystrophy cataract
m. pupil
myringotomy blade
Mysoline
Mytrate
myxedema
myxoid
myxoma

N

N
nasal
n
index of refraction
nano-
N_2O cryosurgical unit
NA
numerical aperture
naboctate
naboctate HCl
Nadbath
N. block
N. facial block
Nadbath's
N. akinesia
Nadler superior radial scissors
nadolol
Naegeli's syndrome
Nafazair
nafcillin
Naffziger's operation
NAG
narrow-angle glaucoma
Nagel
N. anomaloscope
N. lensmeter
Nagel's test
Nager's syndrome
nail-patella syndrome
Nairobi's eye
naked vision (Nv.)
nalidixic acid
nalorphine
naloxone
nana
Hymenolepsis n.
nanism
Mulibrey n.
nano- (n)
Nanolas
N. Nd:YAG laser
N. neodymium YAG laser
nanometer (nm)
nanophthalmia, nanophthalmos
nanosecond (nsec)
naphazoline
n. and antazoline phosphate
n. HCl
n. and pheniramine maleate
Naphcon-A
Naphcon Forte
naphthalinic cataract
naproxen sodium
narrow-angle glaucoma (NAG)
narrowing
arteriolar n.
n. of arteriole
n. of retinal arteriole
narrow-slit illumination
nasal (N)
n. architecture
n. arteriole of retina
n. border of optic disk
n. canal
n. duct
n. fundus ectasia
n. hemianopsia
n. hemorrhage
n. isopter
n. mucosal identification
n. packs
n. periphery
n. polyp
n. retina
n. step
n. step defect
n. venule of retina
nasalis
commissura palpebrarum n.
nasalization
nasal-tip dressing
nasi
cancrum n.
inferior meatus n.
nasion
nasoantritis
nasociliaris
nervus n.
nasociliary
n. nerve
n. neuralgia
nasofrontalis
vena n.
nasofrontal vein
nasojugal fold
nasolabial fold
nasolacrimal
n. canal
n. duct
n. duct obstruction

nasolacrimal *(continued)*
    n. duct probe
    n. gland
    n. groove
    n. obstruction
    n. reflex
    n. sac
nasolacrimalis
    ductus n.
naso-orbital fracture
nasopharyngeal fibroangioma
nasopharynx
nasoseptitis
nasosinusitis
Natacyn
natamycin
Naturale
    Duratears N.
    Tears N.
Natural Tears
Nd
    neodymium
Nd:YAG
    N. cyclophotocoagulation
    N. laser
near
    n. acuity testing
    distance and n. (D&N)
    n. esotropia (ET′)
    n. fixation
    n. fixation position of gaze
    n. gaze
    n. point absolute
    n. point of accommodation
      (NPA)
    n. point of convergence
      (NPC)
    n. reaction
    n. reaction to light
    n. reflex
    n. response
    n. sight
    n. triad
    n. vision
    n. vision test
    n. vision testing
    n. visual acuity (NVA)
    n. visual point (NVP)
near-point relative
near-reflex spasm
nearsighted

nearsightedness
nebula, pl. **nebulae**
    corneal n.
necrobiotic xanthogranuloma
necrogranulomatous keratitis
necrolysis
    epidermal n.
    toxic epidermal n. (TEN)
necrosis
    anterior segment n.
    aseptic bone n.
    caseous n.
    conjunctival n.
    fibrinoid n.
    retinal n.
    stromal n.
    white retinal n.
necroticans
    scleritis n.
necrotic infectious conjunctivitis
necrotizing
    n. nodular scleritis
    n. papillitis
    n. scleritis
needle
    ACS n.
    Agnew tattooing n.
    Agrikola tattooing n.
    Alcon CU-15 4-mil n.
    Alcon irrigating n.
    Alcon reverse cutting n.
    Alcon spatula n.
    Alcon taper cut n.
    Alcon taper point n.
    Amsler n.
    Amsler aqueous
      transplant n.
    aqueous transplant n.
    Atkinson n.
    Atkinson retrobulbar n.
    Atkinson single-bevel blunt-
      tip n.
    Atkinson tip peribulbar n.
    Barraquer n.
    Barraquer-Vogt n.
    B-D n.
    bent blunt n.
    bent 22-gauge n.
    blunt n.
    Bowman n.
    Bowman cataract n.
    Bowman stop n.
    Burr butterfly n.

butterfly n.
BV100 n.
Calhoun n.
Calhoun-Hagler n.
Calhoun-Hagler lens n.
Calhoun-Merz n.
Castroviejo vitreous
  aspirating n.
cataract n.
cataract aspirating n.
CD-5 n.
Charles n.
Charles Flute n.
Charles vacuuming n.
Chiba eye n.
Cibis n.
Cibis ski n.
Cleasby spatulated n.
CooperVision irrigating n.
CooperVision spatulated n.
corneal n.
couching n.
Crawford n.
CU-8 n.
CUA n.
Curran knife n.
Dailey cataract n.
Davis knife n.
Dean n.
Dean knife n.
discission n.
Drews cataract n.
DS-9 n.
Ellis foreign body n.
Elschnig extrusion n.
Ethicon n.
extended round n.
extrusion n.
Fisher eye n.
flute n.
foreign body n.
Fritz vitreous transplant n.
30-gauge n.
Geuder keratoplasty n.
Girard anterior chamber n.
Girard cataract aspirating n.
Girard phacofragmatome n.
Girard-Swan knife-n.
Graefe n.
Grieshaber n.
Grieshaber ophthalmic n.
GS-9 n.
Gueder keratoplasty n.

Haab n.
Haab knife n.
Hessburg lacrimal n.
Heyner n.
Heyner double n.
n. holder
Ilg n.
Iliff-Wright n.
Iliff-Wright fascia n.
illuminated suction n.
Iocare titanium n.
IOLAB n.
IOLAB irrigating n.
IOLAB taper-cut n.
IOLAB taper-point n.
IOLAB titanium n.
iris knife n.
Kalt corneal n.
Kara cataract n.
Knapp n.
Knapp knife-n.
Kratz n.
Kratz diamond-dusted n.
Kratz lens n.
Lagleyze n.
Lane n.
Lewicky n.
Look retrobulbar n.
Lo-Trau n.
Lo-Trau side-cutting n.
March n.
March laser sclerostomy n.
Maumenee n.
Maumenee vitreous
  aspirating n.
McIntyre n.
McIntyre I/A n.
McIntyre
  irrigation/aspiration n.
micropoint n.
micro round-tip n.
Oaks n.
Oaks double n.
peribulbar n.
probe n.
n. probe
puncture n.
puncture-tip n.
razor n.
razor-tip n.
retrobulbar n.
Reverdin suture n.
reverse-cutting n.

needle *(continued)*
    Riedel n.
    Sabreloc n.
    Sato cataract n.
    Scheie n.
    Scheie cataract-aspirating n.
    sclerostomy n.
    side-cutting spatulated n.
    Simcoe n.
    Simcoe aspirating n.
    Simcoe II PC aspirating n.
    Simcoe suture n.
    SITE n.
    SITE irrigating/aspirating n.
    SITE macrobore n.
    SITE macrobore plus n.
    SITE Phaco I/A n.
    ski n.
    n. spatula
    spatulated n.
    n. spoon
    spoon n.
    n. spud
    spud n.
    n. stick
    Stocker n.
    Subco n.
    subconjunctival n.
    Surgicraft suture n.
    suturing n.
    Swan n.
    taper-cut n.
    taper-point n.
    tattooing n.
    tax double n.
    TG-140 n.
    titanium n.
    triple-facet-tip n.
    ultrasonic cataract-removal
      lancet n.
    Ultrasonic lancet n.
    Viers n.
    vitreous aspirating n.
    vitreous transplant n.
    Vogt-Barraquer corneal n.
    Vogt-Barraquer eye n.
    von Graefe knife n.
    Weeks n.
    Wergeland n.
    Wergeland double n.
    Wooten n.
    Worst n.
    Wright n.

    Wright fascia n.
    Wright ophthalmic n.
    Yale Luer-Lok n.
    Ziegler iris knife-n.
    Ziegler knife-n.

needling

negative
    n. accommodation
    n. afterimage
    n. convergence
    cyclophoria n.
    cyclotropia n.
    n. eyepiece
    n. image
    n. meniscus
    n. meniscus lens
    n. scotoma
    n. vertical divergence
    n. vertical vergence

Neher's operation

Nehra-Mack operation

Neisseria
    N. gonorrhoeae
    N. meningitidis

neisserial conjunctivitis

nematodiasis

Nembutal

Neocidin

Neo-Cobefrin

Neo-Cortef

NeoDecadron

Neo Dexair

neodymium (Nd)
    n. (Nd) YAG laser
    n. yttrium aluminum garnet
      laser

Neo-Flow

neoformans
    Cryptococcus n.

Neo-Hydeltrasol

NeoKnife cautery

Neolens lens

Neo-Medrol

Neomixin

neomycin
    n. and dexamethasone
    n., polymixin B, and
      dexamethasone
    n., polymixin B, and
      gramicidin
    n., polymyxin B, and
      hydrocortisone
    n. sulfate

Neomycin-Dex
Neonatal
neonatal
    n. adrenoleukodystrophy
    n. adrenoleukodystrophy
      dystrophy
    n. conjunctivitis
    n. gliosis
    n. herpes
    n. hypoglycemia
    n. inclusion blennorrhea
    n. inclusion conjunctivitis
    n. jaundice
neonate
neonatorum
    blennorrhea n.
    ophthalmia n.
neoplasia
    endocrine n.
    intraepithelial n.
    multiple endocrine n.
neoplasm
    choroidal n.
    Merkel's cell n.
    secondary malignant n.
neoplastic angioendotheliomatosis
Neo-Polycin
Neosporin
neostigmine test
Neo-Synephrine
    N.-S. Cocaine mixture 50:50
    N.-S. Hydrochloride
    N.-S. Viscous
Neo-Tears
Neotricin
neovascular
    n. angle-closure glaucoma
    n. glaucoma (NVG)
    n. membrane
    n. net
    n. tuft
neovascularization
    choroidal n. (CNV)
    corneal n.
    disk n.
    n. of disk
    disseminated asymptomatic
      unilateral n.
    interstitial n.
    n. of new vessels elsewhere
      (NVE)
    preretinal n.
    n. of retina

    retinal n.
    retinal quadrant n.
    stromal n.
    subretinal n. (SRNV)
    vitreous n.
nephritica
    retinitis n.
nephritis, pl. nephritides
nephroblastoma
nephrogenic diabetes insipidus
nephropathic
    n. cystine storage disease
    n. cystinosis
nephrophthisis
nephrosis
nephrotic syndrome
Neptazane
Nernst glower
nerve
    abducens n.
    abducent n. (N.VI)
    aberrant degeneration of
      third n.
    aberrant regeneration of n.
    acoustic n.
    afferent n.
    block n.
    n. block
    n. bundle
    ciliary n.
    n. core
    corneal n.
    cranial n. (CN)
    n. cross section
    cupping of optic n.
    efferent n.
    eighth cranial n.
    facial n.
    n. fiber
    n. fiber axons
    n. fiber bundle
    n. fiber bundle defect
    n. fiber bundle layer
    n. fiber layer (NFL)
    n. fiber layer dropout
    fifth cranial n.
    fourth cranial n.
    frontal n.
    ganglionic layer of optic n.
    ganglionic stratum of
      optic n.
    ganglion layer of optic n.
    ganglion stratum of optic n.

nerve *(continued)*
   n. head angioma
   n. head drusen
   infraepitrochlear n.
   infraorbital n.
   infratrochlear n.
   n. input
   input n.
   intermedius n.
   intervaginal space of
     optic n.
   lacrimal n.
   n. layer of retina
   long ciliary n.
   n. loop
   maxillary n.
   motor n.
   nasociliary n.
   oculomotor n. (N.III)
   ophthalmic n.
   optic n. (N.II)
   output n.
   n. palsy
   peripheral n.
   petrosal n.
   second cranial n.
   sensory n.
   seventh cranial n.
   n. sheath
   n. sheath meningioma
   short ciliary n.'s
   sixth cranial n.
   supraorbital n.
   supratrochlear n.
   tentorial n.
   third cranial n.
   trigeminal n. (N.V)
   trochlear n. (N.IV)
   vascular circle of optic n.
   vidian n.
   zygomatic n.
nervea
   tunica n.
Nervocaine
   N. with epinephrine
nervosa
   anorexia n.
nervous asthenopia
nervus, pl. nervi
   nervi ciliares breves
   nervi ciliares longi
   n. infraorbitalis
   n. lacrimalis

   n. maxillaris
   n. nasociliaris
   n. oculomotorius
   n. ophthalmicus
   n. opticus
   n. supraorbitalis
   n. trigeminus
   n. trochlearis
   n. zygomaticus
Nesacaine
nests and strands of cells
net
   neovascular n.
Nettleship-Falls X-linked ocular albinism
Nettleship iris repositor
Nettleship-Wilder dilator
network
   peritarsal n.
   trabecular n.
   vascular n.
Neubauer forceps
Neumann razor blade fragment holder
Neumann-Shepard
   N.-S. corneal marker
   N.-S. oval optical center marker
neural
   n. crest
   n. crest cell
   n. lesion
   n. rim
   n. tube
neuralgia
   nasociliary n.
   postherpetic n.
   supraorbital n.
   trifacial n.
   trigeminal n.
   vidian n.
neurasthenic asthenopia
neurectomy
   opticociliary n.
neurilemma
neurilemmitis
neurilemmosarcoma
neurilemoma
   ameloblastic n.
   eyelid n.
   malignant n.
neurinoma
neurinomatosis

neurite
neuritic atrophy
neuritis, pl. neuritides
    anterior ischemic optic n.
     (AION)
    atherosclerotic ischemic n.
    intraocular n.
    intraocular optic n.
    n. nodosa
    optic n.
    optic demyelinating n.
    orbital n.
    paraneoplastic optic n.
    postocular n.
    retrobulbar n.
    retrobulbar optic n.
neuroanatomy
neurobiology
neuroblast
neuroblastic
neuroblastoma
neurochorioretinitis
neurochoroiditis
neurodealgia
neurodeatrophia
neurodegenerative syndrome
neuroectoderm
neuroepithelial layer of retina
neuroepithelioma
    orbital n.
neuroepithelium
neurofibroma
    eyelid n.
    iris n.
    limbal n.
    orbital n.
    plexiform n.
    uveal n.
neurofibromatosis
neurogenic
    n. acquired ptosis
    n. iris atrophy
    n. mesenchyme
    n. ptosis
    n. tumor
neuroglia
    immature n.
neurohumoral
neurohypophysis
neuroimaging
neuroleptic malignant syndrome

neurologic
    n. examination
    n. syndrome
neuroma
    acoustic n.
    facial n.
    mucosal n.
    orbital n.
    plexiform n.
neuromatosis
    elephantiasis n.
neurometrics
neuromyelitis
    n. optica
neuromyotonia
    ocular n.
neuron
    abducens internuclear n.'s
    Golgi n.'s
    Golgi I n.
    Golgi II n.
    retinal n.'s
neuronal ceroid lipofuscinosis
neuro-ophthalmic manifestation
neuro-ophthalmologic
    n.-o. case history
    n.-o. diagnosis
    n.-o. examination
neuro-ophthalmology
neuropapillitis
neuroparalytic
    n. keratitis
    n. keratopathy
    n. ophthalmia
neuropathy
    anterior ischemic optic n.
     (AION)
    arteriosclerotic ischemic
     optic n.
    arteritic ischemic optic n.
    dysthyroid optic n.
    giant axonal n.
    hypertrophic interstitial n.
    inflammatory optic n.
    ischemic optic n. (ION)
    Jamaican optic n.
    luetic n.
    myelo-optic n.
    nonarteritic anterior
     ischemic optic n.
    onion bulb n.
    optic n.
    parainfectious optic n.

neuropathy *(continued)*
    peripheral n.
    radiation-induced optic n.
    toxic optic n.
    uremic optic n.
neurophakomatosis
neurophthalmological investigation
neurophthalmology
neuroradiologic
neuroretinal rim
neuroretinitis
    diffuse unilateral n.
    diffuse unilateral
      subacute n. (DUSN)
neuroretinopathy
    acute macular n.
    hypertensive n.
    macular n.
neurospongium
neurosurgical
neurosyphilis
neurosyphilitic
neurotomy
    opticociliary n.
neurotonic pupil
neurotrophic
    n. keratitis
    n. keratopathy
neurotropic
neutral
    n. density filter
    n. density filter test
    n. filter
    n. point
    n. zone
neutrality
neutralization
neutralize
neutralizing
neutrophil
neutrophils
nevi
nevocyte
nevoid
nevoxanthoendothelioma
    juvenile n.
nevus, pl. **nevi**
    basal cell n.
    blue n.
    choroidal n.
    compound n.
    conjunctival n.
    conjunctival pigmented n.

    dermal n.
    episcleral n.
    epithelial n.
    eyelid n.
    n. flammeus
    intradermal n.
    junctional n.
    melanocytic n.
    n. of osteoma Ota
    n. of Ota
    Ota's n.
    n. sebaceus of Jodassohn
    Spitz's n.
    strawberry n.
    subepithelial n.
    uveal n.
Nevyas
    N. double sharp cystitome
    N. lens forceps
    N. retractor
New
    N. Orleans Eye & Ear
      fixation forceps
    N. Orleans lens
    N. Orleans lens loupe
    N. Orleans loupe
    N. York erysiphake
    N. York Eye & Ear
      Hospital fixation forceps
newborn conjunctivitis
Newcastle
    N. disease
    N. disease virus
newtonian aberration
Newton's disk
new vessels disk
Nezelof syndrome
NFL
    nerve fiber layer
NI
    no improvement
niacinamide
niacin maculopathy
nialamide
nicking
    arteriolar n.
    arteriovenous n.
    AV n.
    n. of retinal vein
Nicolas-Favre disease
Nicol prism
nicotinate
    aluminum n.

nicotinic
    n. acid
    n. acid maculopathy
nicotinyl alcohol
nictation
nictitans
    membrana n.
nictitating
    n. membrane
    n. spasm
nictitation
Nida's
    N. nicking operation
    N. operation
NIDDM
    non-insulin-dependent diabetes
    mellitus
Nidek
    N. AR-2000 Objective
    Automatic refractor
    N. Auto Refractometer NR-
    1000F
    EchoScan by N.
    N. laser
    N. Laser System laser
Nieden's syndrome
Niemann-Pick
    N.-P. disease
    N.-P. type C disease
nifedipine
niger
    Hyoscyamus n.
night
    n. blindness
    n. myopia
    n. sight
    n. vision
night-vision goggle
nigra
    cataract n.
nigricans
    acanthosis n.
    pseudoacanthosis n.
nigroid body
nigrum
    tapetum n.
N.II
    optic nerve
N.III
    oculomotor nerve
Nikolsky's sign

Nikon
    N. Auto Refractometer NR-
    1000F
    N. Retinopan fundus
    camera
    N. zoom photo slit lamp
nimodipine
niphablepsia
niphotyphlosis
nipper
    House-Dieter n.
nit
Nitra lamp
nitrate
    cellulose n.
    phenylmercuric n.
    pilocarpine n.
    silver n.
nitrite
    amyl n.
nitrofurantoin
nitroglycerin
nitrosourea
nitrous oxide
N.IV
    trochlear nerve
Nizetic's operation
Nizoral
NLP
    no light perception
nm
    nanometer
NMR
    nuclear magnetic resonance
no
    n. faci
    n. improvement (NI)
    n. light perception (NLP)
Noble forceps
Nocardia
    N. asteroides
    N. brasiliensis
    N. caviae
nocardiosis
    ocular n.
Nocito
    N. eye implant
    N. implant
nocturnal amblyopia
nodal
    n. plane
    n. point

node
>preauricular n.'s
>Rosenmüller's n.

nodosa
>conjunctivitis n.
>iritis n.
>neuritis n.
>periarteritis n. (PAN, PN)
>polyarteritis n.

nodosum
>erythema n.

nodular
>n. conjunctivitis
>n. degeneration
>n. episcleritis
>n. fasciitis
>n. iritis
>n. melanoma
>n. scleritis

nodular scleritis
>necrotizing n. s.

nodule
>n.'s in actinomycosis
>Busacca's n.
>conjunctival n.
>Dalen-Fuchs n.
>epibulbar Fordyce n.'s
>episcleral n.
>episcleral rheumatic n.
>Fordyce's n.
>iris n.
>Koeppe's n.
>lentiform n.
>Lisch n.
>millet seed n.
>pseudorheumatoid n.'s
>rheumatic n.
>n.'s in schistosomiasis
>n.'s in sparganosis

nodulus
>n. conjunctivalis
>n. lymphaticus

Nokrome
>N. bifocal
>N. bifocal lens
>N. fused multifocals

Nolvadex

nomogram
>Harrison-Stein n.
>n. system

nonabsorbable suture

nonaccommodation

nonaccommodative
>n. esodeviation
>n. esophoria
>n. esotropia

nonarteritic anterior ischemic optic neuropathy

nonatopic allergic conjunctivitis

noncicatricial entropion

noncomitant
>n. heterotropia
>n. squint
>n. strabismus

nonconcomitant strabismus

noncongestive glaucoma

noncontact tonometer

nondepolarizing muscle relaxant

nondescript

nondisjunction

nonepithelial tumor

nonexudative

nongranulomatous
>n. choroiditis
>n. uveitis

non-Hodgkin's lymphoma

noninfiltrative

non-insulin-dependent
>n.-i.-d. diabetes mellitus (NIDDM)

noninvasive corneal redox fluorometry

nonionic surfactant

nonleaking bleb

nonophthalmos

nonoptic reflex eye movements

nonorganic visual loss

Nonoxynol

nonparalytic strabismus

nonpenetrant gene

nonpenetrating keratoplasty

nonperfusion
>capillary n.

nonpigmented ciliary epithelium

nonproliferative
>n. diabetic retinopathy (NPDR)
>n. retinopathy

non-rapid eye movement

nonrefractive accommodative esotropia

nonrhegmatogenous
n. detachment
n. retinal detachment
nonsteroidal anti-inflammatory drug (NSAID)
nonulcerative
n. blepharitis
n. interstitial keratitis
Noonan's syndrome
norepinephrine
norfloxacin
normal
n. correspondence
n. distribution
n. fundus
n. retinal correspondence (NRC)
normal-finger tension
Norman-Wood syndrome
normocytic
n. anemia
n. hypochromic anemia
Normol
Norrie's disease
North American blastomycosis
Northern
Tracor N.
nortriptyline
notation
standard n.
notch
cerebellar n.
n. of iris
lacrimal n.
supraorbital n.
notch-and-roll maneuver
notching
lid n.
note blindness
Nothnagel's syndrome
Nova
N. Aid lens
N. Curve broad C-loop posterior chamber lens
N. Curve lens
N. Curve Omnicurve lens
Dioptron N.
N. Soft II lens
novobiocin
Novocain
Novus 2000 ophthalmoscope
novyi
Borrelia n.

Noyes
N. forceps
N. iridectomy scissors
N. iris scissors
NP-207
NPA
near point of accommodation
NPC
near point of convergence
NPDR
nonproliferative diabetic retinopathy
NRC
normal retinal correspondence
NR-1000F
Nidek Auto Refractometer N.
Nikon Auto Refractometer N.
NS
nuclear sclerosis
NSAID
nonsteroidal anti-inflammatory drug
nsec
nanosecond
N[sub]2[n]O cryosurgical unit
nubbin
nubecula
Nuck
canal of N.
nuclear
n. antigen
n. arc
n. bronzing
n. cataract
n. changes
n. chromatin
n. cytoplasmic ratio
n. developmental cataract
n. expression
n. external layer
n. inner layer
n. internal layer
n. magnetic resonance (NMR)
n. ophthalmoplegia
n. outer layer
n. palsy
n. sclerosis (NS)
n. sclerosis of lens
n. tissue
n. zone

nuclear ophthalmoplegia
    progressive n. o.
nuclei
nucleocapsids
nucleolar
nucleoli
nucleoplasm
nucleotide
    cyclic n.
nucleus, pl. nuclei
    accessory n.
    n. delivery loupe
    dense brunescent n.
    Edinger-Westphal n.
    n. expressor
    geniculate n.
    lateral geniculate n. (LGN)
    n. of lens
    lenticular n.
    n. lentiform
    n. lentis
    Perlia's n.
    pretectal n.
    pyknotic nuclei
    n. removal loupe
    rostral interstitial n.
nudge test
Nugent
    N. aspirator
    N. fixation forceps
    N. forceps
    N. hook
    N. rectus forceps
    N. soft cataract aspirator
    N. superior rectus forceps
Nugent-Gradle scissors
Nugent-Green-Dimitry erysiphake
Nulicaine
null
    n. condition
    n. point
    n. zone
numerical aperture (NA)
nummular keratitis
Nurulon suture
nutans
    spasm n.
NutraTear
nutrient
nutritional
    n. amblyopia
    n. blindness
    n. deficiency cataract

N.V
    trigeminal nerve
Nv.
    naked vision
NVA
    near visual acuity
NVE
    neovascularization of new
      vessels elsewhere
NVG
    neovascular glaucoma
N.VI
    abducent nerve
NVP
    near visual point
nyctalope
nyctalopia
    n. with congenital myopia
Nylen-Barany maneuver
nylon
    n. frame
    n. loop
    n. suture
    n. 66 suture
nystagmic
nystagmiform
nystagmogram
nystagmograph
nystagmography
nystagmoid-like oscillation
nystagmoid movements
nystagmus
    acquired jerk n.
    acquired pendular n.
    after-n.
    ageotrophic n.
    amaurosis n.
    amaurotic n.
    ataxic n.
    aural n.
    Baer's n.
    Bekhterev's n.
    blockage n.
    n. blockage syndrome
    caloric n.
    caloric-induced n.
    central n.
    cervical n.
    Cheyne's n.
    circular n.
    compressive n.
    congenital n.
    conjugate n.

constant n.
convergence n.
convergence-evoked n.
convergence retraction n.
deviational n.
disjunctive n.
dissociated n.
downbeat n.
drug-induced n.
elliptic n.
elliptical n.
end-gaze n.
end-point n.
end-position n.
epileptic n.
fatigue n.
fixation n.
galvanic n.
gaze n.
gaze-evoked n.
gaze paretic n.
horizontal n.
hysterical n.
incongruent n.
irregular n.
Jensen's jerk n.
jerk n.
labyrinthine n.
latent n.
lateral n.
left-beating n.
lid n.
manifest latent n.
miner's n.
minimal amplitude n.

muscle paretic n.
myasthenic n.
myoclonus n.
oblique n.
ocular n.
opticokinetic n.
optokinetic n. (OKN)
oscillating n.
paretic n.
pendular n.
periodic alternating n.
perverted n.
physiologic n.
positional n.
railroad n.
rebound n.
retraction n.
right-beating n.
rotary n.
rotation n.
rotational n.
rotatory n.
see-saw n.
sensory deprivation n.
strabismic n.
n. test
torsional n.
undulatory n.
upbeat n.
vertical n.
vestibular n.
vibratory n.
voluntary n.

nystatin

O
oxygen
OAG
open-angle glaucoma
Oaks
O. double needle
O. double straight cannula
O. needle
O. straight cannula
Oasis feather micro scalpel
obcecation
object
Berens test o.
o. blindness
o. displacement
o. distance
fixation o.
o. of regard
o. size
o. space
test o.
object/image
o./i. conjugacy
o./i. relationship
objective
achromatic o.
apochromatic o.
o. optometer
o. perimetry
o. refractor
o. test
o. vertigo
object-space focus
obligatory suppression
oblique
o. aberration
o. astigmatism
o. fiber
o. illumination
inferior o. (IO)
o. muscle
o. muscle hook
o. nystagmus
o. palsy
o. prism
o. prism device
o. ray of light
superior o. (SO)

obliterans
endarteritis o.
thromboangiitis o.
obliterated
O'Brien
O. block
O. fixation forceps
O. forceps
O. lid block
O. marker
O. spud
O. stitch scissors
O'Brien-Elschnig fixation forceps
O'Brien's
O. akinesia technique
O. anesthesia
O. cataract
O. technique
obscura
camera o.
obscuration
transient visual o.
obscure vision
Obstbaum
O. lens spatula
O. synechia spatula
obstruction
carotid o.
congenital nasolacrimal
duct o.
nasolacrimal o.
nasolacrimal duct o.
outflow o.
primary acquired
nasolacrimal duct o.
(PANDO)
obstructive
o. glaucoma
o. hydrocephalus
o. retinal vasculitis
obturator
Moria o.
occipital
o. apoplexy
o. cortex
o. lobe
o. lobe lesion
occipitofrontalis
venter frontalis musculi o.

occipitothalamica
   radiatio o.
occipitothalamic radiation
occluded pupil
occludens
   zonula o.
occluder
   eye o.
   Halberg trial clip o.
   Pram o.
   thumb o.
occlusion
   branch retinal artery o.
      (BRAO)
   branch retinal vein o.
      (BRVO)
   o. of branch vein
   branch vein o.
   carotid artery o.
   central retinal artery o.
      (CRAO)
   central retinal vein o.
      (CRVO)
   choroidal vascular o.
   macular arteriole o.
   punctal o.
   o. of pupil
   retinal arterial o.
   retinal artery o.
   retinal vascular o.
   retinal vein o.
   o. of retinal vein
   retinal venous o.
   o. therapy
   vascular o.
   o. of vein
occlusive
   o. disease
   o. vascular disease
occlusor
   Elastoplast eye o.
Occucoat solution
**occult temporal arteritis of
   Simmons**
occupational
   o. lenses
   o. ophthalmology
ochre
   o. hemorrhage
   o. mass
ochre-colored whorls

ochronosis
   exogenous o.
   ocular o.
Ochsner
   O. cartilage forceps
   O. forceps
   O. hook
   O. tissue/cartilage forceps
   O. tissue forceps
O'Connor
   O. depressor
   O. flat hook
   O. iris forceps
   O. lid forceps
   O. marker
   O. sharp hook
   O. sponge forceps
   O. tenotomy hook
O'Connor-Elschnig fixation forceps
O'Connor-Peter operation
O'Connor's
O'Connor's operation
octofluoropropane gas
Octopus
   O. automated perimetry
   O. 500 EZ
   O. perimeter
   O. 201 perimeter
   O. 201 perimeter test
   O. perimetry
   O. test
Ocu-Bath
Ocu-Caine
Ocu-Carpine
Ocu-Chlor
Ocuclear
Ocu-Cort
Ocu-Dex
Ocudose
   Timoptic in O.
   Timoptic O.
Ocu-Drop
Ocufen
ocufilcon
Ocugestrin
Oculab Tono-Pen
Oculaid lens
Ocular
   O. Gamboscope lens
   O. Gamboscope loupe
ocular
   o. adnexa
   o. adnexal tumor

o. albinism
o. alignment
o. angle
o. ataxia
o. axis
o. ballottement
o. barrier
o. bobbing
o. capsule
o. cicatricial pemphigoid
o. cone
o. crisis
o. cul-de-sac
o. cup
o. dipping
o. disease
o. dominance
o. dominance columns
o. dysmetria
o. effect
o. flora
o. flutter
o. gymnastics
o. herpes
o. histoplasmosis
o. histoplasmosis syndrome
o. humor
o. hypertelorism
o. hypertension (OHT)
o. hypertension glaucoma
o. hypertensive glaucoma
o. hypotelorism
o. hypotony
o. image
o. immunology
o. inflammation
o. injury
o. ischemic syndrome
o. larva
o. larva migrans
o. lens
o. lymphomatosis
o. marker
o. media
o. melanocytosis
o. melanoma
o. meningioma
o. motility
o. motility test
o. movement
o. muscle
o. muscle palsy
o. muscle paralysis

o. muscle transplant
o. myiasis
o. myoclonus
o. myopathy
o. neuromyotonia
o. nocardiosis
o. nystagmus
o. ochronosis
o. onchocerciasis
o. oscillation
o. palsy
o. paralysis
o. pathology
o. pemphigoid
o. pemphigus
o. phthisis
o. plastic
o. pressure reducer
o. prosthesis
Putterman-Chaflin o.
o. refraction
o. region
o. rigidity
o. saccade
o. siderosis
o. sign
o. sparganosis
o. spectrum
o. syphilis
o. syphilitic disease
o. tension (Tn)
o. tilt reaction
o. torticollis
o. toxicity
o. toxocariasis
o. toxoplasmosis
o. trauma
o. tumor
o. vaccinia conjunctivitis
o. vertigo
o. vesicle
ocularis
    angor o.
    vitrina o.
ocularist
ocular melanocytosis
    congenital o. m.
ocularmucous membrane syndrome
oculentum
oculi
    adnexa o.
    albuginea o.
    aqua o.

oculi *(continued)*
　bulbus o.
　camera o.
　congenital melanosis o.
　deprimens o.
　elephantiasis o.
　endothelium o.
　equator bulbi o.
　fascia lata musculares o.
　fascia musculares o.
　fiber orbicularis o.
　fibers of orbicularis o.
　fundus o.
　hypertonia o.
　hypotonia o.
　melanosis o.
　meridiani bulbi o.
　motor o.
　musculi o.
　musculus obliquus
　　inferior o.
　musculus obliquus
　　superior o.
　musculus orbicularis o.
　musculus orbicularis o.
　musculus rectus inferior o.
　musculus rectus lateralis o.
　musculus rectus medialis o.
　pars caeca o.
　pars lacrimalis musculi
　　orbicularis o.
　pars orbitalis musculi
　　orbicularis o.
　pars palpebralis musculi
　　orbicularis o.
　polus anterior bulbi o.
　polus posterior bulbi o.
　pseudotumor o.
　sphincter o.
　tapetum o.
　tendo o.
　trochlea musculi obliqui
　　superioris o.
　tunica adnata o.
　tunica albuginea o.
　tunica conjunctiva bulbi o.
　tunica fibrosa o.
　tunica nervosa o.
　tunica vascularis o.
　tunica vasculosa o.
　tutamina o.
　o. uterque
　vaginae o.

　vena choroideae o.
　vitrina o.
　white tunica fibrosa o.
OcuLight SL diode laser
Oculinum
oculist
oculistics
oculi unitas (both eyes) (OU)
oculi uterque (each eye) (OU)
oculoauricular dysplasia
oculoauriculovertebral dysplasia
oculobuccogenital syndrome
oculocalorie response
oculocardiac reflex
oculocephalic
　o. anomaly
　o. maneuver
　o. reflex
　o. vascular anomaly
oculocephalogyric reflex
oculocerebral syndrome
oculocerebromucomycosis
oculocerebrorenal
　o. dystrophy
　o. syndrome
oculocerebrovasculometer
oculocutaneous
　o. albinism
　o. albinoidism
　o. laser
　o. syndrome
oculodentodigital dysplasia
oculodermal
　o. disorder
　o. melanocytosis
　o. melanosis
oculodigital
　o. reflex
　o. sign of Franchesseti
oculofacial paralysis
oculoglandular
　o. conjunctivitis
　o. disease
　o. syndrome
　o. tularemia
oculography
　photoelectric o.
　photosensor o.
oculogravic illusion
oculogyral illusion
oculogyration
oculogyria

oculogyric
    o. auricular reflex
    o. crisis
    o. mechanism
oculomandibulodyscephaly
oculomandibulofacial dyscephaly
oculomasticatory myorhythmia
oculometer
oculometroscope
oculomigraine
oculomotor
    o. apraxia
    o. cranial nerve palsy
    o. decussation
    o. nerve (N.III)
    o. palsy
    o. root
    o. root of ciliary ganglion
    o. synkinesis
    o. system
oculomotorius
    nervus o.
oculomycosis
oculonasal
Ocu-Lone
oculopathy
    hypertensive o.
    lupus o.
    pituitarigenic o.
oculopharyngeal
    o. dystrophy
    o. reflex
    o. syndrome
oculoplastic
oculoplasty corneal protector
oculopneumoplethysmography (OPG)
oculopupillary reflex
oculoreaction
oculorenal syndrome
oculorespiratory reflex
oculorotatory muscle
oculosensory
    o. cell reflex
    o. reflex
oculospinal
oculosympathetic
    o. dysfunction
    o. paresis
oculotoxic
oculovertebral dysplasia
oculozygomatic

Ocu-Lube
oculus, pl. oculi
    visio o.
oculus dexter (right eye) (OD)
oculus sinister (left eye) (OS)
ocumeter
Ocu-Mycin
Ocu-Pentolate
Ocu-Phrin
Ocu-Pred A
Ocu-Pred Forte
Ocuscan
    O. A-scan biometric
      ultrasound
    Sonometric O.
    O. 400 Transducer
Ocusert
    O. device
    O. Pilo-20
    O. Pilo-40
Ocusil
Ocusoft scrub
Ocu-Sol
Ocu-Spor B
Ocu-Spor G
Ocusporin
Ocu-Sul 10
Ocu-Sul 15
Ocu-Sul 30
Ocu-Tears
Ocutome
    O. II Fragmentation System
    O. probe
    O. vitrectomy unit
ocutome
    Berkeley Bioengineering o.
    CooperVision o.
    disposable o.
Ocutricin
Ocutricin HC
Ocu-Trol
Ocu-Tropic
Ocu-Tropine
Ocuvite
OCuZIN
Ocu-Zoline
OCVM system
OD
    oculus dexter (right eye)
    right eye
ODN
    ophthalmodynamometry
O'Donoghue angled DCR probe

Odyssey phacoemulsification system
ofloxacin
O'Gawa
    O. cataract-aspirating
      cannula
    O. suture-fixation forceps
    O. two-way aspirating
      cannula
Ogston-Luc operation
Oguchi's disease
Ogura
    O. cartilage forceps
    O. operation
    O. tissue/cartilage forceps
    O. tissue forceps
OHT
    ocular hypertension
oil
    silicone o.
oily secretion
ointment
    ophthalmic o.
Okamura's technique
Oklahoma iris wire retractor
OKN
    optokinetic nystagmus
old
    o. eye
    o. sight
oligodendrocyte
Olivella-Garrigosa photocoagulator
Olk
    O. vitreoretinal pick
    O. vitreoretinal spatula
Olympus fundus camera
OM
    OM 2000 operation
      microscope
    OM 4 ophthalmometer
O'Malley
    O. implant
    O. self-adhering lens
      implant
O'Malley-Heintz
    O.-H. cutter
    O.-H. infusion cannula
    O.-H. vitreous cutter
O'Malley-Pearce-Luma lens
OMM
    ophthalmomandibulomelic
    OMM dysplasia
    OMM syndrome
Omnifit intraocular lens

Omni-Park speculum
OMS
    OMS Empac
      Irrigation/Aspiration Unit
    OMS Machemer/Parel VISC
Onchocerca
    O. caecutiens
    O. volvulus
onchocerciasis
    ocular o.
onchocercosis
onchodermatitis
oncocytoma
one and one-half syndrome
one-piece
    o.-p. bifocal
    o.-p. lens
    o.-p. multifocal lens
one-plane lens
one-snip
    o.-s. operation
    o.-s. punctum
    o.-s. punctum operation
One Solution
onion
    o. bulb neuropathy
    o. skin-like membrane
onyx
opaca
    cornea o.
opacification
    corneal o.
    cortical o.
opacified cuff
opacity, pl. **opacities**
    calcium-containing opacities
    Caspar ring o.
    congenital lens opacities
    corneal o.
    corneal deep o.
    deep corneal stromal
      opacities
    dense opacities
    disciform o.
    dust-like opacities
    early lens opacities
    facetted avascular
      disciform o.
    interface o.
    mycotic snowball opacities
    snowball o.
    spotty corneal opacities
    striate opacities

stromal opacities
vitreous o.
opalescent cornea
opaque
    o. arcus
    o. media
Opcon
    Muro O.
Opcon-A
OP-D005
open
    o. lens
    o. loop
open-angle glaucoma (OAG)
open-funnel detachment
opening
    orbital o.
    o. of orbital cavity
    palpebral o.
    punctal o.'s
open-sky
    o.-s. cryoextraction
    o.-s. cryoextraction operation
    o.-s. technique
    o.-s. trephination
    o.-s. vitrectomy
operating
    o. loupe
    o. microscope
operation
    ab externo filtering o.
    Adams' o.
    Adams' o. for ectropion
    Adler's o.
    Agnew's o.
    Agrikola's o.
    Allen's o.
    Allport's o.
    Alsus' o.
    Alsus-Knapp o.
    Alvis' o.
    Ammon's o.
    Amsler's o.
    Anagnostakis' o.
    Anel's o.
    Angelucci's o.
    annular corneal graft o.
    Argyll-Robertson o.
    Arion's o.
    Arlt-Jaesche o.
    Arlt's o.
    Arrowhead's o.
    Arroyo's o.

    Arruga-Berens o.
    Arruga's o.
    Badal's o.
    Bangerter's pterygium o.
    Bardelli's lid ptosis o.
    Barkan-Cordes linear
      cataract o.
    Barkan's o.
    Barkan's double
      cyclodialysis o.
    Barkan's goniotomy o.
    Barraquer's o.
    Barraquer's enzymatic
      zonulolysis o.
    Barraquer's keratomileusis o.
    Barrie-Jones
      canaliculodacryorhinos-
      tomy o.
    Barrio's o.
    Basterra's o.
    Beard-Cutler o.
    Beard's o.
    Beer's o.
    Benedict's o.
    Benedict's orbit o.
    Berens' o.
    Berens' pterygium
      transplant o.
    Berens' sclerectomy o.
    Berens-Smith o.
    Berke-Motais o.
    Berke's o.
    Bethke's o.
    Bielschowsky's o.
    Birch-Hirschfeld
      entropion o.
    Blair's o.
    Blasius' lid flap o.
    Blaskovics' o.
    Blaskovics' canthoplasty o.
    Blaskovics' dacryostomy o.
    Blaskovics' inversion of
      tarsus o.
    Blaskovics' lid o.
    Blatt's o.
    Böhm's o.
    Bonaccolto-Flieringa o.
    Bonaccolto-Flieringa scleral
      ring o.
    Bonaccolto-Flieringa
      vitreous o.
    Bonnet's o.
    Bonnet's enucleation o.

operation *(continued)*
    Bonzel's o.
    Borthen's iridotasis o.
    Bossalino's blepharoplasty o.
    Bowman's o.
    Boyd's o.
    Brailey's o.
    bridge pedicle flap o.
    Bridge's o.
    Briggs' strabismus o.
    Bromley's foreign body o.
    Bronson's foreign body
      removal o.
    Budinger's blepharoplasty o.
    Burch's evisceration o.
    Burch's eye evisceration o.
    Burow's flap o.
    Buzzi's o.
    Byron Smith's o.
    Byron Smith's ectropion o.
    Cairn's o.
    Caldwell-Luc o.
    Calhoun-Hagler o.
    Calhoun-Hagler lens
      extraction o.
    Callahan's o.
    Campodonico's o.
    Carter's o.
    Casanellas' lacrimal o.
    Casey's o.
    Castroviejo's o.
    Castroviejo-Scheie
      cyclodiathermy o.
    cataract extraction o.
    cautery o.
    Celsus' o.
    Celsus-Hotz o.
    Celsus' spasmodic
      entropion o.
    cerclage o.
    Chandler's o.
    Chandler's vitreous o.
    Chandler-Verhoeff o.
    Cibis' o.
    cinching o.
    Cleasby's o.
    Cleasby's iridectomy o.
    Collin-Beard o.
    Comberg's foreign body o.
    Conrad's o.
    Conrad's orbital blowout
      fracture o.
    Cooper's o.

    corneal graft o.
    Crawford's sling o.
    crescent o.
    Critchett's o.
    Crock's o.
    Crock's encircling o.
    cryoextraction o.
    cryotherapy o.
    Csapody's orbital repair o.
    Cupper-Faden o.
    Cusick's o.
    Cusick-Sarrail ptosis o.
    Custodis' o.
    Cutler-Beard o.
    Cutler's o.
    cyclodiathermy o.
    Czermak's pterygium o.
    dacryoadenectomy o.
    dacryocystectomy o.
    dacryocystorhinotomy o.
    dacryocystostomy o.
    dacryocystotomy o.
    Dailey's o.
    Dalgleish's o.
    Daviel's o.
    decompression of orbit o.
    de Grandmont's o.
    Deiter's o.
    De Klair's o.
    de Lapersonne's o.
    Del Toro's o.
    Derby's o.
    Desmarres' o.
    de Vincentiis o.
    de Wecker's o.
    Dianoux's o.
    diathermy o.
    Dickey-Fox o.
    Dickey's o.
    Dickson-Wright o.
    Dieffenbach's o.
    dilation of punctum o.
    discission of lens o.
    D'ombrain's o.
    drainage of lacrimal
      gland o.
    drainage of lacrimal sac o.
    Duke-Elder o.
    Dunnington's o.
    Dupuy-Dutemps o.
    Durr's o.
    Duverger-Velter o.
    Elliot's o.

Elschnig's o.
Elschnig's canthorrhaphy o.
Ely's o.
encircling of globe o.
encircling of scleral
  buckle o.
enucleation of eyeball o.
equilibrating o.
Erbakan's inferior fornix o.
Escapini's cataract o.
Esser's inlay o.
Eversbusch's o.
evisceration o.
Ewing's o.
excision of lacrimal
  gland o.
excision of lacrimal sac o.
exenteration of orbital
  contents o.
extracapsular cataract
  extraction o.
Faden's o.
Fanta's cataract o.
Fasanella's o.
Fasanella-Servat ptosis o.
fascia lata sling for
  ptosis o.
Fergus' o.
Filatov-Marzinkowsky o.
Filatov's o.
filtering o.
Fink's o.
Flajani's o.
Foerster's o.
Fould's entropion o.
Fox's o.
Franceschetti's o.
Franceschetti's coreoplasty o.
Franceschetti's corepraxy o.
Franceschetti's deviation o.
Franceschetti's
  keratoplasty o.
Franceschetti's pupil
  deviation o.
Fricke's o.
Friedenwald-Guyton o.
Friedenwald's o.
Friede's o.
Frost-Lang o.
Fuchs' o.
Fuchs' canthorrhaphy o.
Fuchs' iris bombe
  transfixation o.

Fukala's o.
Gayet's o.
Georgariou's cyclodialysis o.
Gifford's o.
Gifford's delimiting
  keratotomy o.
Gillies' o.
Gillies' scar correction o.
Girard's keratoprosthesis o.
Goldmann-Larson foreign
  body o.
Gomez-Marquez lacrimal o.
Gonin's o.
Gonin's cautery o.
goniotomy o.
Gradle o.
Gradle's keratoplasty o.
Graefe's o.
Greaves' o.
Grimsdale's o.
Grossmann's o.
Gutzeit's dacryostomy o.
Guyton's o.
Guyton's ptosis o.
Halpin's o.
Harman's o.
Harms-Dannheim
  trabeculotomy o.
Hasner's o.
Heine's o.
Heisrath's o.
Herbert's o.
Hess' o.
Hess' eyelid o.
Hess' ptosis o.
Hiff's o.
Hill's o.
Hippel's o.
Hogan's o.
Holth's o.
Horay's o.
Horvath's o.
Hotz-Anagnostakis o.
Hotz entropion o.
Hughes' o.
Hummelsheim's o.
Hunt-Transley o.
Iliff-Haus o.
Iliff's o.
Imre's o.
Imre's lateral
  canthoplasty o.
indentation o.

operation *(continued)*

intracapsular cataract
  extraction o.
iridectomy o.
iridencleisis o.
iridodialysis o.
iridotasis o.
iridotomy o.
Irvine's o.
Jaesche-Arlt o.
Jaesche's o.
Jaime's o.
Jaime's lacrimal o.
Jameson's o.
Jensen's o.
Johnson's o.
Jones' o.
Katzin's o.
Kelman's o.
keratectomy o.
keratocentesis o.
keratomileusis o.
keratoplasty o.
keratotomy o.
Key's o.
King's o.
Kirby's o.
Knapp-Imre o.
Knapp's o.
Knapp-Wheeler-Reese o.
Koffler's o.
Kraupa's o.
Kreiker's o.
Krieberg's o.
Krönlein-Berke o.
Krönlein's o.
Kuhnt-Helmbold o.
Kuhnt's o.
Kuhnt's eyelid o.
Kuhnt-Szymanowski o.
Kuhnt-Thorpe o.
Kwitko's o.
Lacarrere's o.
Lagleyze's o.
Lagleyze-Trantas o.
Lagrange's o.
laissez-faire lid o.
Lancaster's o.
Lanchner's o.
Landolt's o.
Langenbeck's o.
Leahey's o.
Lester-Jones o.

Lexer's o.
Lincoff's o.
Lindner's o.
Lindsay's o.
Löhlein's o.
Londermann's o.
Lopez-Enriquez o.
Löwenstein's o.
Machek-Blaskovics o.
Machek-Brunswick o.
Machek-Gifford o.
Machek's o.
Machek's ptosis o.
Mack-Brunswick o.
Magitot's o.
Magitot's keratoplasty o.
magnet o.
magnetic o.
Magnus' o.
Majewsky's o.
Maladie de Graeffe's o.
Malbec's o.
Malbran's o.
Marquez-Gomez o.
Mauksch-Maumenee-
  Goldberg o.
Mauksch's o.
Maumenee-Goldberg o.
McGavic's o.
McGuire's o.
McLaughlin's o.
McLean's o.
McReynolds' o.
Meek's o.
Meller's o.
Meyer-Schwickerath o.
Michaelson's o.
Minsky's o.
Moncrieff's o.
Moran's o.
Morax's o.
Morel-Fatio-Lalardie o.
Mosher's o.
Mosher-Toti o.
Moss' o.
Motais' o.
Mueller's o.
Mules' o.
Mustarde's o.
myectomy o.
myotomy o.
Naffziger's o.
Neher's o.

Nehra-Mack o.
Nida's o.
Nida's nicking o.
Nizetic's o.
O'Connor-Peter o.
O'Connor's o.
Ogston-Luc o.
Ogura o.
one-snip o.
one-snip punctum o.
open-sky cryoextraction o.
optical iridectomy o.
orbital implant o.
Pagenstecher's o.
Panas' o.
pars plana o.
pattern cut corneal graft o.
Paufique's o.
peripheral iridectomy o.
Peter's o.
Physick's o.
Pico's o.
plombage o.
pocket o.
Polyak's o.
Poulard's o.
Power's o.
Preziosi's o.
probing lacrimonasal
  duct o.
Putenney's o.
Quaglino's o.
Raverdino's o.
Ray-Brunswick Mack o.
Ray-McLean o.
reattachment of choroid o.
reattachment of retina o.
recession of ocular
  muscle o.
Redmond-Smith o.
Reese-Cleasby o.
Reese-Jones-Cooper o.
Reese's o.
Reese's ptosis o.
removal of foreign body o.
Richet's o.
Rosenburg's o.
Rosengren's o.
Roveda's o.
Rowbotham's o.
Rowinski's o.
Rubbrecht's o.
Ruedemann's o.

Rycroft's o.
Saemisch's o.
Safar's o.
Sanders' o.
Sato's o.
Savin's o.
Sayoc's o.
Scheie's o.
Schepens o.
Schimek's o.
Schirmer's o.
Schmalz's o.
scleral buckling o.
scleral fistulectomy o.
scleral shortening o.
scleroplasty o.
sclerotomy o.
sector iridectomy o.
Selinger's o.
seton o.
Shaffer's o.
Shugrue's o.
Sichi's o.
Silva-Costa o.
Silver-Hildreth o.
slant o.
slant muscle o.
Smith-Indian o.
Smith-Kuhnt-Szymanowski o.
Smith's o.
Smith's eyelid o.
Snellen's o.
Snellen's ptosis o.
Soriano's o.
Soria's o.
Sourdille's keratoplasty o.
Sourdille's ptosis o.
Spaeth's cystic bleb o.
Spaeth's ptosis o.
Speas' o.
Spencer-Watson o.
Spencer-Watson Z-plasty o.
splitting lacrimal papilla o.
Stallard-Liegard o.
Stallard's eyelid o.
Stallard's flap o.
step graft o.
Stocker's o.
Stock's o.
Straith's o.
Straith's eyelid o.
Strampelli-Valvo o.
Streatfield-Fox o.

operation *(continued)*
    Streatfield's o.
    Streatfield-Snellen o.
    Suarez-Villafranca o.
    Summerskill's o.
    suture of cornea o.
    suture of eyeball o.
    suture of iris o.
    suture of muscle o.
    suture of sclera o.
    Szymanowski-Kuhnt o.
    Szymanowski's o.
    Tansley's o.
    Tasia's o.
    tattoo of cornea o.
    Teale-Knapp o.
    tenotomy o.
    Terson's o.
    Tessier's o.
    Thomas' o.
    three-snip o.
    three-snip punctum o.
    Tillett's o.
    Toti-Mosher o.
    Toti's o.
    Townley-Paton o.
    trabeculectomy o.
    Trainor-Nida o.
    Trainor's o.
    transfixion of iris o.
    transplantation of muscle o.
    Trantas' o.
    trapdoor scleral buckle o.
    Tripier's o.
    Troutman's o.
    Truc's o.
    Tudor-Thomas o.
    tumbling technique o.
    Ulloa's o.
    Uyemura's o.
    Van Milligen's o.
    Verhoeff-Chandler o.
    Verhoeff's o.
    Verwey's o.
    Verwey's eyelid o.
    Viers' o.
    Vogt's o.
    Von Ammon's o.
    von Blaskovics-Doyen o.
    von Graefe's o.
    von Hippel's o.
    Waldhauer's o.
    Walter Reed o.
    Watzke's o.
    Weeker's o.
    Weeks' o.
    Weisinger's o.
    Wendell Hughes o.
    Werb's o.
    West's o.
    Weve's o.
    Wharton-Jones o.
    Wheeler-Reese o.
    Wheeler's o.
    Whitnall's o.
    Whitnall's sling o.
    Wicherkiewicz's o.
    Wicherkiewicz's eyelid o.
    Wiener's o.
    Wies' o.
    Wilmer's o.
    Wolfe's o.
    Wolfe's ptosis o.
    Worst's o.
    Worth's o.
    Worth's ptosis o.
    Wright's o.
    Young's o.
    Ziegler's o.
    Zylik's o.

opercula

operculated tear

operculum, gen. **operculi**,
  pl. **opercula**

OPG
  oculopneumoplethysmography

Ophacet

ophryogene
    ulerythema o.'s

Ophtec Co. lens

Ophthacet

Ophthaine

Ophthalas
    O. argon/krypton laser
    O. argon laser
    O. krypton laser

Ophthalgan

ophthalmagra

ophthalmalgia

ophthalmatrophia

ophthalmectomy

ophthalmencephalon

Ophthalmetron
    Safir O.

ophthalmia
    actinic ray o.

Brazilian o.
catarrhal o.
caterpillar o.
caterpillar-hair o.
o. eczematosa
Egyptian o.
electric o.
o. electrica
flash o.
gonorrheal o.
granular o.
o. hepatica
hivialis o.
jequirity o.
o. lenta
metastatic o.
migratory o.
mucous o.
o. neonatorum
o. neonatorum
neuroparalytic o.
o. nivalis
o. nodosa
periodic o.
phlyctenular o.
pseudotuberculous o.
purulent o.
reaper's o.
scrofulous o.
spring o.
strumous o.
sympathetic o.
transferred o.
ultraviolet ray o.
varicose o.
vegetable o.
ophthalmiatrics
ophthalmic
    o. artery
    o. artery aneurysm
    o. cautery
    o. cul-de-sac
    o. cup
    o. disorder
    o. drug
    o. electrocautery
    o. examination
    o. ganglion
    o. hook
    o. hyperthyroidism
    o. migraine
    o. nerve

    o. ointment
    o. plexus
    o. reaction
    o. solution
    o. sponge
    o. test
    o. vein
    o. vesicle
ophthalmica
    vesicula o.
Ophthalmic Moldite Powder
ophthalmicus
    caliculus o.
    herpes o.
    nervus o.
    varicella-zoster o.
    zoster o.
ophthalmitic
ophthalmitis
ophthalmoblennorrhea
ophthalmocarcinoma
ophthalmocele
ophthalmocopia
ophthalmodesmitis
ophthalmodiagnosis
ophthalmodiaphanoscope
ophthalmodiastimeter
ophthalmodonesis
ophthalmodynamometer
    Bailliart o.
    Reichert o.
    suction o.
ophthalmodynamometry (ODN)
ophthalmodynia
ophthalmoeikonometer
ophthalmofunduscope
ophthalmogram
ophthalmograph
ophthalmography
ophthalmogyric
ophthalmoleukoscope
ophthalmolith
ophthalmologic
ophthalmologist
Ophthalmology
    Association of Technical
      Personnel in O. (ATPO)
    Joint Commission on Allied
      Health Personnel in O.
      (JCAHPO)
ophthalmology
    occupational o.

ophthalmomalacia
ophthalmomandibulomelic (OMM)
    o. dysplasia
ophthalmomelanosis
ophthalmomeningea
    vena o.
ophthalmomeningeal vein
ophthalmometer
    American Optical o.
    Javal o.
    Javal-Schiotz o.
    Micromatic o.
    mires of o.
    OM 4 o.
ophthalmometroscope
ophthalmometry
ophthalmomycosis
ophthalmomyiasis
ophthalmomyitis
ophthalmomyositis
ophthalmomyotomy
ophthalmoneuritis
ophthalmoneuromyelitis
ophthalmopathy
    endocrine o.
    external o.
    Graves' o.
    internal o.
    thyroid o.
ophthalmophacometer
ophthalmophantom
ophthalmophlebotomy
ophthalmophthisis
ophthalmoplasty
ophthalmoplegia
    basal o.
    chronic progressive o.
    chronic progressive
      external o. (CPEO)
    exophthalmic o.
    o. externa
    external o.
    fascicular o.
    infectious o.
    o. interna
    internal o.
    internuclear o. (INO)
    o. internuclearis
    migraine o.
    migrainous o.
    nuclear o.
    orbital o.
    painful o.

    Parinaud's o.
    partial o.
    o. partialis
    o. progressiva
    progressive o.
    progressive external o.
      (PEO)
    pseudointernuclear o.
    Sauvineau's o.
    thyrotoxicosis o.
    total o.
    o. totalis
ophthalmoplegic
    o. exophthalmos
    o. migraine
    o. muscular dystrophy
ophthalmoptosis
ophthalmoreaction
    Calmette's o.
ophthalmorrhagia
ophthalmorrhea
ophthalmorrhexis
ophthalmoscope
    Alcon indirect o.
    AO binocular indirect o.
    AO Reichert Instruments
      binocular indirect o.
    Bailliart o.
    binocular o.
    binocular indirect o.
    cordless monocular
      indirect o.
    demonstration o.
    direct o.
    Exeter o.
    Fison indirect binocular o.
    Friedenwald o.
    Ful-Vue o.
    ghost o.
    Gullstrand o.
    Halberg indirect o.
    halogen o.
    Helmholtz o.
    indirect o.
    Keeler o.
    Loring o.
    Mentor Exeter o.
    metric o.
    MK IV o.
    monocular indirect o.
    Novus 2000 o.
    polarizing o.
    Polle pod attachment for o.

Propper-Heine o.
Reichert binocular
  indirect o.
Reichert Ful-Vue o.
Reichert Ful-Vue
  binocular o.
Schepens o.
Schepens binocular
  indirect o.
Schepens-Pomerantzeff o.
Visuscope o.
Welch-Allyn o.
Zeiss o.
ophthalmoscopic
ophthalmoscopy
binocular indirect o.
direct o.
indirect o.
medical o.
metric o.
slit-lamp o.
o. with reflected light
ophthalmospectroscope
ophthalmospectroscopy
ophthalmostasis
ophthalmostat
ophthalmostatometer
ophthalmosteresis
ophthalmosynchysis
ophthalmothermometer
ophthalmotomy
ophthalmotonometer
ophthalmotonometry
ophthalmotoxin
ophthalmotrope
ophthalmotropometer
ophthalmotropometry
ophthalmovascular
ophthalmoxerosis
ophthalmoxyster
Ophthalon suture
Ophtha P/S
Ophthascan
Ophthas subjective optometer
Ophthel
Ophthetic
Ophthochlor
Ophthocort
OpMi microscope
opponent
o. color
o. colors theory
Opraflex drape

opsin
cone o.
opsinosis
opsiometer
opsoclonia
opsoclonus
Optacon
Optacryl
Opt-Ease
Optef
Op-Temp
O.-T. cautery
O.-T. disposable cautery
O.-T. disposable
  electrocautery
optesthesia
Op-Thal-Zin
Optho
RO O.
Opti-Bon
optic
o. agnosia
o. angle
o. aphasia
o. artery
o. atrophy
o. canal
o. center
o. chiasm
o. coloboma
o. commissure
o. cul-de-sac
o. cup
o. cupping
o. cup-to-disk ratio
o. decussation
o. demyelinating neuritis
o. disk
o. disk cupping
o. disk drusen
o. disk drusen calcification
o. evagination
o. foramen
o. foramina
o. ganglion
o. glioma
o. groove
o. hyperesthesia
o. implant
o. iridectomy
o. keratoplasty
o. lemniscus
o. muscle recession

optic *(continued)*
    o. nerve (N.II)
    o. nerve atrophy
    o. nerve coloboma
    o. nerve disease
    o. nerve drusen
    o. nerve dysplasia
    o. nerve fiber
    o. nerve glioma
    o. nerve head
    o. nerve hypoplasia
    o. nerve lesion
    o. nerve meningioma
    o. nerve pit
    o. nerve sheath
    o. nerve tumor
    o. neuritis
    o. neuropathy
    o. papilla (p)
    o. papilla cavity
    o. perineuritis
    o. pits
    o. primordium
    o. radiation
    o. recess
    o. stalk
    o. sulcus
    o. thalamus
    o. tract
    o. tract lesion
    o. tract syndrome
    o. vesicle
optica
    radiatio o.
opticae
    commissurae o.
optical
    o. aberration
    o. alexia
    o. allachesthesia
    o. axis
    o. bench
    o. blur
    o. breakdown
    o. center
    o. centering instrument
    o. center of lens
    o. center of spectacle lens
    o. clarity
    o. contact lens
    o. correction
    o. cross
    o. density method

    o. fossa
    o. frame
    o. glass
    o. illusion
    o. image
    o. iridectomy
    o. iridectomy operation
    o. keratoplasty
    o. nodal point
    o. pachymeter
    o. power
    o. rehabilitation
    o. system
    o. zone
    o. zone of contact lens
    o. zone marker
optically empty
Optical Radiation lens
optic disk
    choked o. d.
    cupping of o. d.
    pallor of o. d. *(var. of*
      pallor of o. d.)
optici
    circulus vasculosus nervi o.
    discus nervi o.
    evulsio nervi o.
    excavatio papillae nervi o.
    radix lateralis tractus o.
    radix medialis tractus o.
    vaginae externa nervi o.
    vaginae interna nervi o.
    vaginae nervi o.
optician
opticianry
opticist
Opti-Clean
Opti-Clean II
optic nerve (N.II)
    aplasia of o. n.
    atrophy of o. n.
    tumor of o. n.
opticochiasmatic, optochiasmic
    o. arachnoiditis
opticociliary, optociliary
    o. neurectomy
    o. neurotomy
    o. shunt vessels
    o. vessels
opticocinerea
opticofacial
    o. reflex
    o. winking reflex

opticokinetic nystagmus
opticomyelitis
opticonasion
opticopupillary
Opticrom
Opticrom 4%
Optics
    Allergan Medical O. (AMO)
    American Medical O.
optics
    Fresnel o.
    geometric o.
    o. of intraocular lens
    physical o.
    physiologic o.
    reverse o.
opticum
    chiasma o.
    foramen o.
opticus
    axis o.
    canaliculus infraorbitalis o.
    canalis o.
    discus o.
    nervus o.
    porus o.
    recessus o.
Optiflex lens
Opti-Free
Optigene
Optik
Optimmune
optimum
Optimyd
OptiPranolol
Optipress
Opti-Pure System
Optised
Optisoap
Opti-Soft
optist
Opti-Tears
Opti-Vu lens
Opti-Zyme enzymatic cleaner
optoblast
optogram
optokinesis
optokinetic
    o. drum
    o. nystagmus (OKN)
    o. reflex
    o. stimulus
    o. tape

Optokinetic stimulator
optomeninx
optometer
    automatic infrared o.
    objective o.
    Ophthas subjective o.
optometrist
optometry
optomotor reflex
optomyometer
optophone
optostriate
optotype
Optrex
Opt-Visor
    O.-V. lens
    O.-V. loupe
Optycryl 60 contact lens
Optyl frame
Opus III contact lens
ora
    o. globule
    o. serrata
    o. serrata retinae
oral
    o. administration
    o. contraceptive
orange
    o. dye laser
    o. punctate pigmentation
Oratrol
orbiculare
    os o.
orbiculare
    Pityrosporum o.
orbicularis
    alopecia o.
    o. ciliaris
    o. muscle
    musculus o.
    musculus o. oculi
    o. oculi muscle
    o. oris muscle
    o. phenomenon
    o. pupillary reflex
    o. reaction
    o. reflex
    o. sign
orbicular muscle of eye
orbiculoanterocapsular fiber
orbiculociliary fiber
orbiculoposterocapsular fiber

orbit
aneurysm of o.
blow-out fracture of o.
contusion of o.
dermoid of o.
emphysema of o.
fracture of o.
o. hamartoma
intraorbital margin of o.
lateral margin of o.
lesion of o.
roof of o.
supraorbital margin of o.

orbitae
aditus o.
corpus adiposum o.
exenteratio o.
margo infraorbitalis o.
margo lateralis o.
margo medialis o.
margo supraorbitalis o.
paries interior o.
paries lateralis o.
paries medialis o.
paries superior o.

orbital
o. abscess
o. adipose tissue
o. akinesia
o. amyloidosis
o. anesthesia
o. aneurysm
o. angiography
o. angioma
o. angiosarcoma
o. aperture
o. apex
o. apex syndrome
o. arch
o. arch of frontal bone
o. arteriovenous
malformation
o. axis
o. blow-out fracture
o. bone
o. border of sphenoid bone
o. canal
o. cavity
o. cellulitis
o. compressor
o. content
o. crest
o. cyst

o. decompression
o. depressor
o. dermoid
o. dystopia
o. echography
o. emphysema
o. encephalocele
o. enlargement
o. enucleation compressor
o. exenteration
o. extension
o. fascia
o. fasciitis
o. fat
o. fat pad
o. fibroma
o. fibromatosis
o. fibrosarcoma
o. fissure
o. floor
o. floor fracture
o. floor implant
o. floor prosthesis
o. fracture
o. ganglion
o. glioma
o. granuloma
o. hamartoma
o. height
o. hemangioendothelioma
o. hemangioma
o. hemangiopericytoma
o. hematoma
o. hernia
o. hypertelorism
o. hypotelorism
o. hypoxia
o. implant
o. implant operation
o. inferior rim
o. lamina
o. lens
o. lipoma
o. lymphoma
o. margin
o. medulloepithelioma
o. melanoma
o. meningioma
o. mesenchyme
o. metastasis
o. muscle
o. myositis
o. neuritis

o. neuroepithelioma
o. neurofibroma
o. neuroma
o. opening
o. ophthalmoplegia
o. palsy
o. pathology
o. periosteum
o. periostitis
o. pit
o. plane
o. plane of frontal bone
o. plate of ethmoid bone
o. plate of frontal bone
o. portion of eyelid
o. prosthesis
o. pseudotumor
o. radiology
o. region
o. resilience
o. rhabdomyosarcoma
o. rim
o. rim fracture
o. roentgenogram
o. roof
o. section
o. septum
o. sulci of frontal bone
o. sulcus
o. superior fissure
o. surgery
o. syndrome
o. tomography
o. trauma
o. tumor
o. varix
o. vasculitis
o. venography
o. vessel
o. wall fracture
o. width
o. wing of sphenoid bone
orbitale
planum o.
septum o.
orbitales
fasciae o.
orbitalia
cribra o.
orbitalis
margo o.
musculus o.
orbitocranial trauma

orbitography
Graves' o.
orbitomalar foramen
orbitonasal
orbitonometer
orbitonometry
orbitopathy
thyroid o.
orbitorhinomucormycosis
orbitostat
orbitotemporal
orbitotomy
Berke-Krönlein o.
ORC intraocular lens
ordered array
ordering
Dyer nomogram system of
lens o.
orf
organ
o. transplantation
o. of vision
visual o.
organelle
cytoplasmic o.'s
organic
o. amblyopia
o. mercurial
organism
coliform o.
organized vitreous
organogenesis
organum
o. visuale
o. visus
orientation
limbal parallel o.
oriented
radially o.
original
o. Sweet eye magnet
o. Sweet magnet
oris
pars marginalis musculi
orbicularis o.
sphincter o.
ornithine
o. decarboxylation
o. tolerance test
orodigitofacial dysplasia
orthofusor
Orthogon lens
orthokeratology

Ortho-Lite
orthometer
Ortho-Novum
orthophoria
orthophoric
orthopia
orthoposition
orthoptic
orthoptist
orthoptoscope
Ortho-Rater
orthoscope
orthoscopic
    o. lens
    o. spectacles
orthoscopy
orthotropia
orthotropic
Or-Toptic M
OS
   left eye
   oculus sinister (left eye)
os
    o. lacrimale
    o. orbiculare
    o. palatinum
    o. planum
    o. unguis
oscillating
    o. nystagmus
    o. vision
oscillation
    nystagmoid-like o.
    ocular o.
oscillatory potential
oscillopsia
    monocular o.
O'Shea lens
Osher
    O. foreign body forceps
    O. hook
    O. lens
Osher-Neumann corneal marker
Osler-Rendu-Weber syndrome
Osmitrol
Osmoglyn
osmolarity
osmotherapy
    hypertonic o.
osmotic
    o. cataract
    o. pressure

ossea
    bulla o.
osseous
    o. anomaly
    o. choristoma
    o. lesion
    o. system
osseus
    tarsus o.
ossification
ossis
    bulla ethmoidalis o.
ossium
    fragilitas o.
osteitis deformans
osteoblastoma
osteoclastoma
osteocyte
osteodystrophy
osteogenesis imperfecta
osteoma
    o. Ota
    uveal o.
osteomyelitis
    maxillary o.
osteo-onychodysplasia
osteopetrosis
osteosclerotic myeloma
osteosynthesis
osteotomy
ostium
    internal o.
Ota
    nevus of O.
    nevus of osteoma O.
    osteoma O.
Ota's
    O. nevus
    O. nevus syndrome
otitis media
otolith
otomandibular dysostosis
OU
   both eyes
   oculi unitas (both eyes)
   oculi uterque (each eye)
ouabain
outer
    o. canthus
    o. limiting membrane
    o. nuclear layer
    o. plexiform layer

o. retina
o. segment
outflow
  aqueous o.
  coefficient of o.
  coefficient of facility of o.
  conventional o.
  o. disorder
  facility of o.
  o. obstruction
  o. resistance
  trabecular o.
  unconventional o.
  uveoscleral o.
outpouching
output nerve
oval
  o. cornea
  o. cup erysiphake
  o. eye
  o. eyepatch
ovale
  Pityrosporum o.
oval-shaped vernal ulcer
overaction
  inferior oblique o.
overcorrection
overrefraction
overflow diabetes
overlap
overriding
overripe cataract
overt diabetes
overwear syndrome (OWS)
ovoid mass

ovum
OWS
  overwear syndrome
oxacillin
oxidation
  o. of solution
oxide
  ethylene o.
  nitrous o.
  yellow mercuric o.
oxidopamine
oximeter
  pulse o.
oxprenolol
Oxsoralen
oxyblepsia
oxycephaly
oxygen (O)
  o. flow
  o. flux
  hyperbaric o.
  o. performance
  o. permeability
  o. toxicity
  o. transmissibility
oxymetazoline
oxymorphone hydrochloride
oxyopia
oxyopter
oxyphenbutazone
oxytetracycline
oyster shuckers' keratitis
ozena
ozenous
ozone

p
    optic papilla
    pico-
    pupil
P2 prolongation
PAB
    p-aminobenzoic acid
PABA
    p-aminobenzoic acid
pachometer
    corneal p.
    Humphrey ultrasonic p.
    Packo pars plana
    cannula p.
Pach-Pen tonometer
pachyblepharon
pachyblepharosis
pachymeter
    optical p.
    Villasensor ultrasonic p.
pachymetry
Pack
    Barrier Phaco
    Extracapsular P.
Packer tunnel silicone sponge
Packo
    P. pars plana cannula
    P. pars plana cannula
    pachometer
packs
    nasal p.
pad
    eye p.
    felt p.
    orbital fat p.
    Pro-Ophtha eye p.
    spectacle frame p.
    Telfa p.
paddle temple
paddy keratitis
Paecilomyces lilacinus
Pagenstecher's operation
pagetoid melanoma
Paget's disease
pain
    atypical facial p.
    facial p.
    jaw muscle p.
    p. reaction
painful ophthalmoplegia

palatine bone
palatini
    processus orbitalis ossis p.
palatinum
    os p.
palatoethmoidalis
    sutura p.
palatomaxillaris
    sutura p.
palatomaxillary suture
palinopsia
palisading orbital granuloma
pallidum
    Treponema p.
Pallin lens spatula
Pallister-Hall syndrome
pallor
    disk p.
    p. of disk
    horizontal band p.
    p. of optic disk
    sector p.
    temporal artery p.
palmoplantaris
    dyskeratosis p.
    keratosis p.
    recessive keratosis p.
palpebral
    p. adipose bags
    p. cartilage
    p. commissure
    p. conjunctiva
    p. fascia
    p. fissure
    p. fold
    p. furrow
    p. gland
    p. ligament
    p. lobe
    p. oculogyric reflex
    p. opening
    p. raphe
    p. slant
    p. vein
palpebrales
    venae p.
palpebralis
palpebrarum
    facies anterior p.
    facies posterior p.

palpebrarum *(continued)*
    pediculosis p.
    raphe p.
    rima p.
    tendo p.
    xanthoma p.
palpebrate
palpebration
palpebritis
palpebronasal fold
palsy, pl. **palsies**
    abducens p.
    accommodative p.
    Bell's p.
    brachial plexus p.
    cerebral p.
    congenital abducens
     nerve p.
    congenital oculomotor
     nerve p.
    cranial nerve p.
    double elevator p.
    elevator p.
    external p.
    facial p.
    Féréol-Graux p.
    fourth nerve p.
    gaze p.
    inhibitional p.
    internal p.
    ischemic oculomotor p.
    lateral rectus p.
    medial rectus p.
    palsies of muscle
    nerve p.
    nuclear p.
    oblique p.
    ocular p.
    ocular muscle p.
    oculomotor p.
    oculomotor cranial nerve p.
    orbital p.
    progressive supranuclear p.
    (PSP)
    pseudoabducens p.
    pseudobulbar p.
    saccade p.
    sector p.
    seventh nerve p.
    sixth cranial nerve p.
    sixth nerve p.
    stem p.
    superior p.

    superior oblique p.
    supranuclear ocular p.
    third nerve p.
    twelfth nerve p.
PAM
    Potential Acuity Meter
    PAM procedure
pamoate
    hydroxyzine p.
PAN
    periarteritis nodosa
Panas' operation
panchamber UV lens
Pancoast
    P. superior sulcus syndrome
    P. syndrome
    P. tumor
pancreatic
    p. diabetes
    p. disease
pancuronium bromide
PANDO
    primary acquired nasolacrimal
    duct obstruction
panencephalitis
    subacute sclerosing p.
    (SSPE)
panfundoscope
    Rodenstock p.
panfundus
Panmycin
Pannu
    P. intraocular lens
    P. type II lens
pannus, pl. **panni**
    allergic p.
    p. carnosus
    corneal p.
    p. crassus
    degenerative p.
    p. degenerativus
    p. eczematosus
    eczematous p.
    glaucomatous p.
    phlyctenular p.
    p. siccus
    p. tenuis
    p. trachomatosus
    trachomatous p.
panophthalmia, panophthalmitis
Panoptic bifocal
Panoptik
panoramic loupe

PanoView Optics lens
panphotocoagulation
panretinal
    p. ablation
    p. argon laser
      photocoagulation
    p. photocoagulation (PRP)
pansinusitis
pantachromatic
pantankyloblepharon
pantoscope
    Keeler's p.
pantoscopic
    p. angle
    p. angling
    p. effect
    p. spectacles
    p. tilt
Panum's fusion area
panuveitis
    herpes p.
Papanicolaou technique
paper
    p. plate
    Schirmer filter p.
papilla, pl. papillae
    p. of Bergmeister
    Bergmeister's p.
    cobblestone p.
    conjunctival p.
    drusen of optic p.
    giant papillae
    lacrimal p.
    optic p. (μ)
    splitting of lacrimal p.
papillary
    p. area
    p. conjunctivitis
    p. stasis
papillary hypertrophy
    giant p. h. (GPH)
papilledema
papilliform tumor
papillitis
    ischemic p.
    necrotizing p.
papilloma
    caruncular p.
    conjunctival p.
    eyelid p.
    mulberry-type p.
    pedunculated p.
    sessile p.

papillomacular
    p. bundle
    p. nerve fiber bundle
papillomatosis
papillopathy
    ischemic p.
papillophlebitis
papilloretinitis
papillovitreal
papule
papulosa
    iritis p.
papulosis
papyracea
    lamina p.
PAR
    posterior apical radius
parablepsia
paracentesis
    anterior chamber p.
    aqueous p.
paracentral
    p. defect
    p. nerve fiber bundle
    p. scotoma
paracentric
parachroia
parachroma
parachromatism
parachromatopsia
paradoxical
    p. diplopia
    p. movement of eyelids
    p. pupil
    p. pupillary phenomenon
    p. pupillary reflex
paraequilibrium
parafovea
parafoveal halo
parafoveolar
paraganglioma
parainfectious optic neuropathy
parakeratosis
parakinesis
parakinetic
paraldehyde
parallactic
parallax
    binocular p.
    crossed p.
    direct p.
    heteronymous p.
    homonymous p.

parallax *(continued)*
    motion p.
    stereoscopic p.
    p. test
    vertical p.
parallel
    p. interface
    p. rays
parallelism of gaze
paralysis, pl. **paralyses**
    abducens p.
    abducens facial p.
    p. of accommodation
    amaurotic pupillary p.
    bulbar p.
    congenital abducens
      facial p.
    congenital bulbar p.
    congenital oculofacial p.
    conjugate p.
    convergence p.
    divergence p.
    facial p.
    p. of gaze
    internuclear p.
    Klumpke's p.
    Landry's ascending p.
    ocular p.
    ocular muscle p.
    oculofacial p.
    periodic p.
    psychogenic p.
    pupillary p.
    Todd's p.
    Weber's p.
paralytic
    p. ectropion
    p. heterotropia
    p. miosis
    p. mydriasis
    p. strabismus
paralyticum
    ectropion p.
paramacular
paramedian pontine reticular
  formation (PPRF)
parameter
paramethadione
paramethasone
paranasal
    p. sinus
    p. sinusitis
paraneoplastic optic neuritis

Paraperm O2 contact lens
paraphimosis
    p. palpebrae
paraproteinemia
parasellar syndrome
parasitic
    p. blepharitis
    p. uveitis
paraspinal
paraspinous
parastriate
    p. area
    p. visual cortex
parasympathetic
    p. nerve system
    p. pathway
parasympatholytic agent
parasympathomimetic agent
parathyroid
    p. adenoma
    p. disorder
parathyroidism
paratrachoma
paravenous
paraxial
    p. lighting
    p. ray of light
    p. rays
Paredrine test
Parel-Crock
    P.-C. cutter
    P.-C. vitreous cutter
parenchyma
parenchymatosus
    xerosis p.
parenchymatous
    p. corneal dystrophy
    p. dystrophy
    p. keratitis
parenteral administration
paresis
    oculosympathetic p.
paretic nystagmus
parfocal
paries
    p. interior orbitae
    p. lateralis orbitae
    p. medialis orbitae
    p. superior orbitae
parietal
    p. eye
    p. lobe
    p. lobe field defect

parieto-occipital artery
parieto-occipitalis
    arcus p.-o.
parieto-occipital-temporal junction
Parinaud-plus syndrome
Parinaud's
    P. conjunctivitis
    P. oculoglandular
      conjunctivitis
    P. oculoglandular syndrome
    P. ophthalmoplegia
    P. syndrome
Parker
    P. discission knife
    P. knife
Parker-Heath
    P.-H. anterior chamber
      syringe
    P.-H. cautery
    P.-H. electrocautery
    P.-H. piggyback probe
Park-Guyton-Callahan speculum
Park-Guyton-Maumenee speculum
Park-Guyton speculum
parkinsonism
Park-Maumenee speculum
Parks-Bielschowsky three-step
  head-tilt test
Park speculum
p arm
parophthalmia
parophthalmoncus
paropsia, paropsis
paroxysm
paroxysmal
Parrot's sign
Parry-Romberg syndrome
Parry's disease
pars
    p. caeca oculi
    p. caeca retinae
    p. ciliaris retinae
    p. corneoscleralis
    p. iridica retinae
    p. lacrimalis musculi
      orbicularis oculi
    p. marginalis musculi
      orbicularis oris
    p. nervosa retinae
    p. optica hypothalami
    p. optica retinae
    p. orbitalis glandulae
      lacrimalis

    p. orbitalis gyri frontalis
      inferioris
    p. orbitalis musculi
      orbicularis oculi
    p. orbitalis ossis frontalis
    p. palpebralis glandulae
      lacrimalis
    p. palpebralis musculi
      orbicularis oculi
    p. pigmentosa retinae
    p. plana
    p. plana approach
    p. plana corporis ciliaris
    p. plana operation
    p. plana vitrectomy
    p. planitis
    p. plicata
    p. plicata corporis ciliaris
    p. scleralis
    p. uvealis
partial
    p. albinism
    p. cataract
    p. keratoplasty
    p. ophthalmoplegia
    p. sclerectasia
    p. throw surgeon's knot
    p. trisomy 10q
partially sighted
particulate
    p. matter
    p. retinopathy
PAS
    periodic-acid Schiff
    peripheral anterior synechia
Pascheff's conjunctivitis
passant
    boutons en p.
passive
    p. duction
    p. forced duction test
    p. illusion
paster
past-pointing
PAT
    prism adaptation test
Patau's syndrome
patch
    binocular eye p.
    Bitot's p.'s
    cotton-wool p.'s
    Donaldson eye p.
    p. eye

patch *(continued)*
    glue p.
    p. graft
    histoacryl glue p.
    Hutchinson's p.
    monocular p.
    salmon p.
    scopolamine p.
    scopolamine ear p.
    Snugfit eye p.
    venous sheath p.
    wicking p.
    wicking glue p.
patching
patchy window defects
patellar fossa
patency
    tear duct p.
patent iridectomy
pathogen
pathogenesis
pathognomonic
pathologic, pathological
    p. cupping
    p. myopia
pathological
pathology
    ocular p.
    orbital p.
pathway
    anterior visual p.
    canalicular p.
    infranuclear p.
    parasympathetic p.
    retrochiasmal p.
    sensory visual p.
    supranuclear p.
    sympathetic p.
    visual p.
patient
    pediatric p.
    straight-eyed p.
Paton
    P. anterior chamber lens
      implant forceps
    P. capsule forceps
    P. corneal knife
    P. corneal transplant forceps
    P. corneal trephine
    P. double spatula
    P. eye shield
    P. knife
    P. needle holder

    P. shield
    P. single spatula
    P. single speculum
    P. suturing forceps
    P. transplant spatula
    P. transplant speculum
    P. trephine
    P. tying/stitch removal
      forceps
Paton's lines
pattern
    A p.
    Antoni p.'s
    p. arborization
    arborization p.
    arteriovenous p.'s
    AV p.'s
    blur p.
    comedo p.
    contiguous p.
    p. cut corneal graft
      operation
    p. dystrophy
    p. dystrophy of pigment
      epithelium of Byers and
      Marmor
    p. electroretinogram
    Harrington-Flocks
      multiple p.
    map p.
    mosaic p.
    peau d'orange p.
    scatter p.
    shagreen p.
    V p.
    vortex p.
    Zellballen p.
pattern-cut corneal graft
pattern-evoked electroretinogram
    (PERG)
pauciarticular disease
paucity
Paufique
    P. graft knife
    P. keratoplasty knife
    P. knife
    P. suturing forceps
    P. trephine
Paufique's
    P. keratoplasty
    P. operation
    P. synechiotomy
Paul lacrimal sac retractor

paving-stone degeneration
Pavlo-Colibri corneal forceps
Payne retractor
PBII blue loop lens
PC
    posterior chamber
P&C
    prism and cover test
PCC
    posterior central curve
PCF
    pharyngoconjunctival fever
PCIOL
    posterior chamber intraocular
      lens
PCLI
    posterior chamber lens implant
PD
    prism diopter
    pupillary distance
PDR
    proliferative diabetic retinopathy
PE
    pigment epithelium
peaking
peanut implant
pear cataract
Pearce
    P. coaxial
      irrigating/aspirating cannula
    P. posterior chamber
      intraocular lens
Pearce-Knoll irrigating lens loop
pearl
    p. cyst
    p. diver's keratopathy
    Elschnig's p.
    iris p.
    string of p.
    p. white mounds
pear-shaped pupil
peau
    p. de chagrin
    p. d'orange pattern
pectinate
    p. ligament
    p. ligament of iris
    p. villi
pectineal ligament
Peczon
    P. I/A cannula
    P. I/A unit
    P. I/A vectis

PED
    pigment epithelial detachment
pediatric
    p. Karickhoff laser lens
    p. ocular sarcoidosis
    p. patient
    p. speculum
    p. three-mirror laser lens
pedicle
    p. cone
    p. flap
pediculosis palpebrarum
pediculous blepharitis
pedigree
    p. analysis
    p. chart
pedunculated
    p. papilloma
peek sign
peeler-cutter
    membrane p.-c.
peeling
    membrane p.
pefloxacin
PEG
    polyethylene glycol
PEK
    punctate epithelial keratopathy
Pel-Ebstein fever
pellagra
Pelli-Robson chart
pellucid
    corneal p.
    p. degeneration
    p. marginal corneal
      degeneration
    p. marginal degeneration
    p. marginal retinal
      degeneration
pellucidum
    septum cavum p.
Pel's crisis
pemphigoid
    benign mucosal p.
    bullous p.
    Cibis' p.
    cicatricial p.
    mucosal p.
    ocular p.
    ocular cicatricial p.
pemphigus
    ocular p.
    p. vulgaris

pen
    gentian violet marking p.
    marking p.
    skin marking p.
    surgical marking p.
penalization
Penbriten
pencil
    cataract p.
    p. cautery
    glaucoma p.
    retinal detachment p.
    vitreous p.
    Wallach cryosurgical p.
pendular nystagmus
penetrance
penetrant gene
penetrating
    p. corneal graft
    p. corneal transplant
    p. full-thickness corneal
      graft
    p. graft
    p. injury
    p. keratoplasty (PK, PKP)
penetration
penicillamine
penicillin
    acid-resistant p.
    synthetic p.
penicillinase
penicillin G
Penicillium
penlight
Penn-Anderson
    P.-A. fixation forceps
    P.-A. scleral fixation forceps
Penrose drain
pentachromic
pentafilcon A
pentagonal block excision
Penthrane
pentigetide
pentobarbital sodium
Pentolair
pentolinium
Pentothal
Pentyde
penumbra
PEO
    progressive external
      ophthalmoplegia
pepper and salt fundus

Pepper Visual Skills for Reading Test
percentile
perceptible acuity
perception
    binocular depth p.
    color p.
    depth p.
    facial p.
    light p. (LP)
    limbus of p.
    monocular depth p.
    no light p. (NLP)
    simultaneous p.
    simultaneous foveal p.
     (SFP)
    simultaneous macular p.
     (SMP)
    visual p.
perfilcon A
perfluorocarbon
perfluorodecalin
perfluoropropane gas
perforans
    scleromalacia p.
perforating keratoplasty
perforation
    corneal p.
performance
    equivalent oxygen p. (EOP)
    oxygen p.
perfringens
    Clostridium p.
perfusion
PERG
    pattern-evoked
    electroretinogram
periaqueductal syndrome
periarteritis nodosa (PAN, PN)
peribulbar
    p. injection
    p. needle
pericanalicular connective tissue
pericentral
    p. rod-cone dystrophy
    p. scotoma
perichiasmal
perichoroidal, perichorioidal
    p. space
perichoroideale
    spatium p.
periconchitis
pericorneal plexus

pericyte
peridectomy
perifoveolar
perikeratic
perilenticular
perilimbal
    p. suction
    p. suction cup
perimeter
    Allergan Humphrey p.
    arc p.
    arc and bowl p.'s
    automated p.
    automated hemisphere p.
    Brombach's p.
    Canon's p.
    Cilco p.
    CooperVision p.
    CooperVision imaging p.
    p. corneal reflex test
    Digilab p.
    Ferree-Rand p.
    Goldmann's p.
    Humphrey's p.
    kinetic p.
    Marco's p.
    Octopus p.
    Octopus 201 p.
    p. projection
    projection p.
    Schweigger's p.
    Schweigger's hand p.
    static p.'s
    Topcon p.
    Tübinger p.
perimetric
perimetry
    achromatic p.
    arc p.
    automated p.
    automated static
      threshold p.
    binocular p.
    chromatic p.
    color p.
    computed p.
    flicker p.
    Goldmann's p.
    Goldmann's kinetic p.
    hemisphere projection p.
    kinetic p.
    mesopic p.
    objective p.

    Octopus p.
    Octopus automated p.
    profile p.
    quantitative p.
    quantitative threshold p.
    scotopic p.
    static p.
perineural cell
perineuritis
    optic p.
    syphilitic optic p.
perinuclear
    p. cataract
periocular
    p. drug sensitivity
    p. injection
periodic
    p. alternating nystagmus
    p. esotropia
    p. exotropia
    p. ophthalmia
    p. paralysis
    p. strabismus
periodic-acid Schiff (PAS)
periophthalmia
periophthalmic
periophthalmitis
perioptic
    p. meningioma
    p. sheath meningioma
perioptometry
periorbit
periorbital
    p. cellulitis
    p. edema
    p. fat atrophy
    p. membrane
periorbitis
periosteum
    orbital p.
periostitis
    orbital p.
peripapillary
    p. choroidal atrophy
    p. coloboma
    p. scar
    p. sclerosis
    p. scotoma
periphacitis
periphakitis
peripheral
    p. anterior synechia (PAS)
    p. cataract

peripheral *(continued)*
>   p. chorioretinal atrophy
>   p. chorioretinitis
>   p. curve
>   p. cystoid degeneration
>   p. field
>   p. fusion
>   p. glare
>   p. glioma
>   p. iridectomy (PI)
>   p. iridectomy operation
>   p. iris roll
>   p. nerve
>   p. neuropathy
>   p. posterior curve (PPC)
>   p. ray of light
>   p. retina
>   p. scotoma
>   p. tapetochoroidal
>   degeneration
>   p. uveitis
>   p. vision

peripheral pit
>   Herbert's p. p.

peripherophose

periphery
>   nasal p.
>   posterior pole and p.
>   (PP&P)

periphlebitis
>   p. retinae
>   retinal p.

periphoria
periretinal edema
periscleral space
periscleritis
perisclerotic
periscopic
>   p. concave lens
>   p. convex lens
>   p. lens
>   p. meniscus
>   p. spectacles

peristriate visual cortex
peritarsal network
peritectomy
peritomize
peritomy
perivascular sheathing
perivasculitis
periventricular lesion

PERK
>   prospective evaluation of radial
>   keratomy
>   PERK protocol

Perkins
>   P. applanation tonometer
>   P. brailler
>   P. tonometer

PERLA
>   pupils equal, reactive to light
>   and accommodation

Perlia's nucleus
Permaflex lens
Permalens lens
permanganate
>   potassium p.

permeability
>   oxygen p.

permeable
>   rigid gas-p. (RGP)

permeation
>   analgesia p.

pernicious
>   p. anemia
>   p. myopia

peroxide
>   hydrogen p.

peroxisomal disorder
perpendicular
perphenazine
Perritt
>   P. double-fixation forceps
>   P. forceps

PERRLA
>   pupils equal, round, reactive to
>   light and accommodation

persistent
>   p. anterior hyperplastic
>   primary vitreous
>   p. hyperplasia of primary
>   vitreous (PHPV)
>   p. hyperplastic primary
>   vitreous
>   p. hyperplastic vitreous
>   p. posterior hyperplastic
>   primary vitreous

Personnel
>   Joint Review Committee for
>   Ophthalmic Medical P.
>   (JRCOMP)

perspective
>   geometric p.
>   linear p.

Perspex
  P. CQ
  P. CQ-Shearing-Simcoe-
  Sinskey lens
  P. frame
perverted
  p. nystagmus
  p. ocular movement
P-ES
  Isopto P-ES
Peter's
  P. anomaly
  P. operation
Petit
  diplobacillus of P.
Petit's canal
petrificans
  keratitis p.
petrosal nerve
petrous
  p. bone
  p. ridge
Petrus single-mirror laser lens
Petzetakis-Takos syndrome
Petzval surface
Peutz-Jeghers syndrome
Peyman
  P. lens
  P. vitrectomy unit
  P. vitrector
  P. vitreophage unit
  P. wide field lens
Peyman-Green
  P.-G. vitrectomy lens
  P.-G. vitreous forceps
Peyman's
  P. full-thickness eye-wall
  resection
  P. iridocyclochoroidectomy
Peyman-Tennant-Green lens
Pfeiffer-Komberg method
P.F. Lee pediatric goniolens lens
PGC
  pontine gaze center
PH
  pinhole
phacitis
Phaco
  P. Cavitron
  irrigating/aspirating unit
  P. Emulsifier Cavitron Unit
phacoallergica
  endophthalmitis p.

phacoanaphylactic
  p. endophthalmitis
  p. uveitis
phacoanaphylaxis
phacoantigenic
phacoblade
  Myocure p.
phacocele
phacocyst
phacocystectomy
phacocystitis
phacodonesis
phacoemulsification,
  phakoemulsification
  Alcon p.
  p. cautery
  p. handpiece
phacoemulsifier
phacoemulsify
phacocrysis
phacoexcavation
phacoexcavator
phacofragmatome
phacofragmentation
phacogenetica
  endophthalmitis p.
phacogenic
  p. glaucoma
  p. uveitis
phacoglaucoma
phacohymenitis
phacoid
phacoiditis
phacoidoscope
phacolysin
phacolysis
phacolytic
  p. glaucoma
  p. uveitis
phacoma
phacomalacia
phacomatosis
phacometachoresis
phacometer
phacomorphic glaucoma
phacopalingenesis
phacoplanesis
phacosclerosis
phacoscope
phacoscopy
phacoscotasmus
phacotoxic uveitis
phacozymase

phagocytic dysfunction
phagocytized
phagocytosed cellular debris
phagocytosis
phagolysosomes
phagosome
Phakan
phakia
phakic
    p. cystoid macular edema
    p. eye
    p. macular edema
phakitis
phakodonesis
phakoemulsification (*var. of*
  phacoemulsification)
phakofragmatome
    Girard p.
phakogenic glaucoma
phakolytic glaucoma
phakoma
phakomatoses
phakomatosis
phakomatous choristoma tumor
phakomorphic glaucoma
phalangosis
phantom vision
Pharmacia
    P. Intermedics
    P. intraocular lens
    P. Visco J-loop lens
pharmacological
    p. blockade
    p. testing
pharmacologic manipulation
pharmacology
pharyngoconjunctival fever (PCF)
pharyngorhinitis
phase
    capillary p.
    venous p.
phemfilcon A
phenacaine
    p. hydrochloride
phenacetin
phenazopyridine
phenbenicillin
phencyclidine hydrochloride
phenelzine sulfate
Phenergan
phengophobia
pheniramine maleate and
  naphazoline HCl

phenmetrazine hydrochloride
phenobarbital
    p. sodium
phenol
phenolphthalein
phenomenon, pl. phenomena
    Alder-Reilly p.
    aqueous-influx p.
    Ascher's aqueous-influx p.
    Ascher's glass-rod p.
    Aubert's p.
    autokinetic visible light p.
    Bell's p.
    Bezold-Brücke p.
    Bielschowsky's p.
    blood-influx p.
    blue-field entoptic p.
    breakup p.
    Brücke-Bartley p.
    click p.
    crowding p.
    doll's head p.
    entopic p.
    escape p.
    extinction p.
    flicker p.
    Galassi's pupillary p.
    glass-rod negative p.
    glass-rod positive p.
    Gunn's jaw-winking p.
    hemifield slide p.
    Hertwig-Magendie p.
    interface phenomena
    jack-in-the-box p.
    jaw-winking p.
    Le Grand-Geblewics p.
    Marcus Gunn p.
    misdirection p.
    Mitzuo's p.
    orbicularis p.
    paradoxical pupillary p.
    phi p.
    Piltz-Westphal p.
    pseudo-Graefe's p.
    Pulfrich stereo p.
    Purkinje's p.
    Raynaud's p.
    Riddoch's p.
    setting-sun p.
    shot-silk p.
    Tournay's p.
    Tyndall's p.
    Uhthoff's p.

Westphal-Piltz p.
Westphal's p.
Phenoptic
phenothiazine
p. derivative
p. keratopathy
p. toxicity
phenotype
phenoxybenzamine hydrochloride
phentermine
phenylalanine
phenylbutazone
phenylephrine
p. hydrochloride
phenylethyl alcohol
phenylketonuria (PKU)
phenylmercuric
p. acetate
p. nitrate
phenylpropanolamine hydrochloride
Phenylzin
phenytoin
pheochromocytoma
Phillips fixation forceps
phi phenomenon
pHisoHex
phlebitis
phlebography
phlebolith
phlebophthalmotomy
phlebosclerosis
phlegmonous
p. dacryocystis
p. dacryocystitis
phlorhizin diabetes
phlycten
phlyctena, pl. **phlyctenae**
phlyctenar
phlyctenoid
phlyctenosis
phlyctenula, pl. **phlyctenulae**
phlyctenular
p. conjunctivitis
p. keratitis
p. keratoconjunctivitis
p. ophthalmia
p. pannus
phlyctenule
phlyctenulosis
allergic p.
conjunctival p.
corneal p.
tuberculous p.

PHM
posterior hyaloid membrane
PHNI
pinhole no improvement
phocomelia
Roberts-SC p.
phoresis
phoria
lateral p.
monofixational p.
vertical p.
phoriascope
phorometer
phorometry
phoro-optometer
phoropter
p. retractor
Ultramatic Rx Master p.
p. vision tester
phoroscope
phorotone
phosphatase
alkaline p.
Phosphate
Aralen P.
Decadron P.
phosphate
dexamethasone p.
dexamethasone sodium p.
p. diabetes
disodium hydrogen p.
naphazoline and
antazoline p.
potassium p
prednisolone sodium p.
sodium p.
phosphene
accommodation p.
phospholine
echothiophate p.
Phospholine Iodide
phosphonoformic acid
phosphoric acid
phosphorus
phosphothionate
S-3-(amino-2-
hydroxypropyl) p.
photalgia
photerythrous
photesthesia
photic
photoablation
photoablative

photobrown lenses
photocarbonization
photoceptor
photochemical
    p. process
    p. visual pigment
photochemistry
photochromic, photochromatic
    p. lens
    p. spectacles
photocoagulation
    argon laser p.
    laser p.
    macular p.
    panretinal p. (PRP)
    panretinal argon laser p.
    retinal scatter p.
    scatter p.
    xenon arc p.
photocoagulator
    American Optical p.
    Clinitex p.
    Ialo p.
    IOLAB I&A p.
    IOLAB
      irrigating/aspirating p.
    laser p.
    Mira p.
    Olivella-Garrigosa p.
    xenon p.
    xenon arc p.
    Zeiss p.
photocoreoplasty
photodisrupting laser
photodisruption
photodynamic therapy
photodynia
photodysphoria
photoelasticity
photoelectric
    p. oculography
    p. vibration
photofrin
photogene
photography
    cross-polarization p.
    fluorescence retinal p.
photogray lens
photokeratitis
photokeratoscope
    Allergan Humphrey p.
    Allergan Medical Optics p.
    computerized p.

    CooperVision p.
    CooperVision refractive p.
    CooperVision refractive
      surgery p.
photometer
    Bunsen grease spot-p.
    flame p.
    flicker p.
    Föerster p.
photometry
photomydriasis
    Clinitex p.
photon
photopapillometry
photophobia
photophobic
photophthalmia
photopia
photopic
    p. adaptation
    p. eye
    p. vision
photopigments
    cone p.
photopsia
photopsin
photopsy
photoptarmosis
photoptometer
    Föerster p.
photoptometry
photoreception
photoreceptive
photoreceptor cell
photorefractive
    p. keratectomy (PRK)
    p. keratoplasty (PRK)
photoretinitis
photoretinopathy
photos
    fundus p. (FP)
photoscopy
photosensitive lens
photosensitization
photosensor oculography
photostress
    macular p.
    p. test
photosun lens
phototherapeutic keratectomy
  (PTK)
phototherapy
Phototome System 2700

phototonus
phototoxicity
photovaporation laser
photovaporization
photovaporizing laser
PHPV
    persistent hyperplasia of primary
      vitreous
phthiriasis
phthisical eye
phthisis
    p. bulbi
    p. cornea
    essential p.
    essential p. bulbi
    ocular p.
phycomycosis
    cerebral p.
phylloquinone (K)
physical
    p. manipulation
    p. optics
Physick's operation
physiologic, physiological
    p. astigmatism
    p. blind spot
    p. cup
    p. excavation
    p. myopia
    p. nystagmus
    p. optics
    p. position of rest
    p. retina
    p. scotoma
physiology
physostigmine
    pilocarpine and p.
    p. and pilocarpine
    p. salicylate
    p. sulfate
phytanic acid storage disease
PI
    peripheral iridectomy
pia
pial
    p. arterial plexus
    p. sheath
PIC
    posterior intermediate curve
pick
    Burch p.
    Desmarres fixation p.
    fiberoptic p.

    fixation p.
    fixation/anchor p.
    Michel p.
    Olk vitreoretinal p.
    scleral p.
Pickford-Nicholson analmoscope
Pick's
    P. retinitis
    P. vision
pickup
    Shoch foreign body p.
    p. spatula suture
pico- (p)
picosecond
Pico's operation
picric acid
pictograph
picture chart
piebald eyelash
"pie on the floor" defect
Pierce
    P. coaxial
      irrigating/aspirating cannula
    P. I/A cannula
    P. I/A irrigating vectis
    P. I/A tripod implant
    P. I/A unit
    P. irrigating vectis
Pierre-Marie's ataxia
Pierre Robin syndrome
Pierse
    P. corneal Colibri-type
      forceps
    P. corneal forceps
    P. eye speculum
    P. fixation forceps
    P. forceps
Pierse-Hoskins forceps
Pierse-type Colibri forceps
"pie in the sky" defect
piezometer
piggyback
    p. contact lens
    p. probe
pigment
    p. cells
    clumped retinal p.
    p. clumping
    p. demarcation lines
    p. deposition
    p. derangement
    p. dispersion

pigment *(continued)*
  p. epithelial detachment (PED)
  p. epithelial detachment maculopathy
  p. epithelial dystrophy
  p. epithelial hypertrophy
  p. epitheliitis
  epitheliitis focal retinal p.
  p. epitheliopathy
  p. epithelium (PE)
  p. floater
  p. granules
  p. layer
  p. layer ectropion
  photochemical visual p.
  placoid p.
  p. precipitates
  p. seam
  visual p.
  xanthophyll p.

pigmentary
  p. deposits on lens
  p. dilution
  p. dispersion glaucoma
  p. dispersion syndrome
  p. dropout
  p. glaucoma
  p. halo
  p. migration
  p. perivenous chorioretinal degeneration
  p. rarefaction and clumping
  p. retinopathy

pigmentation
  clumped p.
  hematogenous p.
  Hudson-Stähli line of corneal p.
  orange punctate p.
  p. rarefaction

pigmented
  p. epithelium of iris
  p. keratic precipitates
  p. layer of ciliary body
  p. layer of eyeball
  p. layer of iris
  p. layer of retina
  p. lesions
  p. line of cornea
  p. paravenous chorioretinal atrophy

  p. stroma
  p. veils

pigmenti
  incontinentia p.

pigmento
  retinitis pigmentosa sine p.

pigmentosa
  retinitis p. (RP)
  sector retinitis p.

pigmentosum
  conjunctivitis xeroderma p.
  xeroderma p.

pigmentum nigrum

pigtail
  p. fixation
  p. probe

Pilagan

PilaSite

Pillat's dystrophy

pillow
  Richard p.

Pilo-20
  Ocusert P.

Pilo-40
  Ocusert P.

Pilocar

pilocarpine
  epinephrine and p.
  p. and epinephrine
  p. HCl
  p. nitrate
  p. and physostigmine
  physostigmine and p.
  p. test
  timolol and p.
  p. and timolol maleate

Pilocel

pilocyte

pilocytic astrocytoma

Pilofrin

Pilokair

pilomatrixoma tumor

Pilomiotin

Pilopine gel 4%

Pilopine HS

Piloptic

pilot application

Piltz's sign

Piltz-Westphal phenomenon

pimelopterygium

pin
  Pischel p.

Walker p.
Walker micro p.
pince-nez
pin-cushion distortion
pineal
    p. eye
    p. gland
pinealoma
ping-pong gaze
pinguecula, pinguicula
pingueculae
pingueculum
pinguicula (*var. of* pinguecula)
pinhole (PH)
    p. disk
    p. and dominance test
    p. goggle
    p. no improvement (PHNI)
    p. pupil
pink
    sharp and p. (S&P)
pinkeye
    p. conjunctivitis
    p. disk
Pinky ball
pinocytotic vesicle
pinpoint pupil
pinta
pipe light
piperacillin
piperazine
piperocaine hydrochloride
piqûre diabetes
Pischel
    P. electrode
    P. micropins
    P. pin
    P. scleral rule
pisciform cataract
pit
    congenital optic nerve p.
    Gaule's p.
    Herbert's p.
    Herbert's peripheral p.
    iris p.'s
    lens p.
    optic p.'s
    optic nerve p.
    orbital p.
    temporal p.'s
pitting
pituitarigenic
    p. oculopathy

pituitary
    p. ablation
    p. adenoma
    apoplexy of p.
    p. apoplexy
    p. body
    p. dwarfism
    p. gigantism
    p. gland
    p. tumor
Pityrosporum
    P. orbiculare
    P. ovale
pivot point
PK
    penetrating keratoplasty
PKP
    penetrating keratoplasty
PKU
    phenylketonuria
PL
    preferential looking
placebo
placement
    implant p.
Placido's disk
Placidyl
placode
    lens p.
    p. lens
placoid
    p. pigment
    p. pigmentation of
      epithelium
    p. pigment epitheliopathy
pladaroma, pladarosis
plagiocephaly
plain
    p. catgut suture
    p. collagen suture
    p. gut suture
plaited frill
plaiting
plana
    cornea p.
    pars p.
    trans pars p.
plane
    Broca's p.
    Broca's visual p.
    Daubenton's p.
    equivalent refracting p.
    eye/ear p.

plane *(continued)*
    Frankfort horizontal p.
    horizontal p.
    p. of incidence
    lens p.
    Listing's p.
    nodal p.
    orbital p.
    p. parallel plate
    principal p.
    p. of regard
    spectacle p.
    unity conjugacy p.'s
    vertical p.
    visual p.
plane-surface refraction
Plange spud
planitis
    cyclitis in pars p.
    pars p.
planned extracapsular cataract
    extraction
planoconcave lens
planoconvex
    p. lens
    p. nonridge lens
plano lens
Plano T lens
plant
planum
    p. orbitale
    os p.
    xanthoma p.
plaque
    cholesterol p.
    demyelinating p.
    eyelid p.
    gray p.
    Hollenhorst's p.
    hyaline p.
    p. keratopathy
    preretinal p.
    red scaly p.
    scaly p.
    subcapsular p.
Plaquenil
    P. Sulfate
plasma
    p. cell
    p. cell tumor
plasmacytoid infiltrate
plasmalemma
Plasmodium

plasmoid
    p. agglutination
    p. aqueous
    p. aqueous humor
    p. humor
plastic
    p. bifocal
    p. cyclitis
    p. disposable irrigating
       vectis
    p. eye shield
    p. frame
    p. iritis
    p. lens
    ocular p.
    p. prism
    p. repair of eyelid
    p. shield
    p. sphere implant
plasticity
plate
    cribriform p.
    embryonic p.
    foot p.
    Gelfilm p.
    Hardy-Rand-Littler p.
    Hardy-Rand-Littler
       screening p.
    Ishihara p.
    Ishihara
       pseudoisochromatic p.
    isochromatic p.
    Jaeger lid p.
    lid p.
    paper p.
    plane parallel p.
    pseudoisochromatic p.
    pseudoisochromatic
       color p.'s
    reticular p.
    scar p.
    Silastic p.
    Stahl caliper p.
    Storz lid p.
    tarsal p.
    Teflon p.
plateau
    p. iris
    p. iris syndrome
Plateau-Talbot law
platelet abnormality
platelet-fibrin embolus

Platina
- P. clip
- P. clip lens
- P. intraocular lens implant
- P. lens

platinum
- p. probe spatula
- p. salts
- p. spatula

platybasia
platycephaly
platycoria
platymorphia
platymorphic
platysmal reflex
pleiotropism
pleomorphic adenoma
pleomorphism
pleoptic
- Bangerter method of p.
- Cüppers method of p.
- p. exercise

pleoptophor
plesiopia
plethora
plethysmographic goggle
plethysmography
plexiform
- p. external layer
- p. inner layer
- p. internal layer
- p. layer
- p. neurofibroma
- p. neuroma
- p. outer layer

Plexiglas
- P. frame
- P. implant

plexus
- angular aqueous sinus p.
- annular p.
- brachial p.
- capillary p.
- ciliary ganglionic p.
- Hovius' p.
- intraepithelial p.
- intrascleral p.
- ophthalmic p.
- pericorneal p.
- pial arterial p.
- scleral p.
- stroma p.
- subepithelial p.

Pley
- P. extracapsular forceps
- P. forceps

Pliagel
plica, gen. and pl. **plicae**
- p. lacrimalis
- p. lunata
- p. palpebronasalis
- p. semilunaris
- p. semilunaris conjunctivae

plicata
- pars p.

plication
- retractor p.

Plitz's reflex
plombage operation
plug
- Berkeley Bioengineering brass scleral p.
- brass scleral p.
- Dohlman p.
- Eagle Vision-Freeman punctum p.
- Freeman punctum p.
- Herrick lacrimal p.
- punctal p.
- Teflon p.

plugging
- follicular p.

Plus
- Amvisc P.
- Econopred P.
- Lens P.
- Murine P.
- Tears P.
- Unisol P.
- Wet-N-Soak P.

plus
- cyclophoria p.
- p. cyclophoria
- cyclotropia p.
- p. disease
- p. lens
- p. spectacle lens

PMMA
- polymethyl methacrylate

PN
- periarteritis nodosa

pneumatic
- p. retinopexy
- p. tonometer

pneumatonograph (PTG)
- Alcon applanation p.

pneumatonographer
pneumatonometer
pneumococcal
  p. bacillus
  p. conjunctivitis
  p. ulcer
Pneumococcus
pneumococcus ulcer
Pneumocystis carinii
pneumoencephalography
pneumonia
pneumoniae
  Klebsiella p.
  Streptococcus p.
pneumonitis
  interstitial p.
  lymphocytic interstitial p.
pneumotomography
pneumotonometer
pneumotonometry
p.o.
  by mouth
POAG
  primary open-angle glaucoma
pocket operation
pod
POHS
  presumed ocular histoplasmosis
  syndrome
poikiloderma
  p. atrophicans and cataract
  p. congenitale
point
  anterior focal p.
  axial p.
  blur p.
  break p.
  cardinal p.
  central yellow p.
  congruent p.'s
  conjugate p.
  p.'s of convergence
  convergence p.
  correspondence p.'s
  corresponding p.
  corresponding retinal p.'s
  diathermy p.'s
  disparate p.
  disparate retinal p.'s
  p. of dispersion
  p. of divergence
  eye p.
  far p.

  p. of fixation
  fixation p.
  fixed p.
  focal p.
  focal image p.
  identical p.
  image p.
  incident p.
  lacrimal p.
  lustrous central yellow p.
  p. mutation
  near-p.
  near visual p. (NVP)
  neutral p.
  nodal p.
  null p.
  optical nodal p.
  pivot p.
  posterior focal p.
  principal p.
  p. of regard
  restoration p.
  secondary focal p.
  p. source
  stereo-identical p.
  supraorbital p.
  p. system test types
  virtual p.
  visual p.
  yellow p.
poisoning
  p. degenerative cataract
  food p.
  lead p.
polar cataract
polarimeter
polarimetry
polariscope
polariscopic
polariscopy
polarization
  bee p.
polarize
polarized light
polarizer
polarizing ophthalmoscope
Polaroid
  P. filter
  P. vectograph slide
pole
  anterior p.
  inferior p.

posterior p.
superior p.
polioencephalitis
superior p.
poliosis
polisher
capsule p.
Drews capsule p.
felt disc p.
Gills-Welsh capsule p.
Holladay posterior
capsule p.
Knolle p.
Knolle capsule p.
Kraff p.
Kraff capsule p.
Kratz p.
Look capsule p.
Terry silicone capsule p.
polisher/scratcher
Jensen p./s.
Kratz p./s.
Kratz-Jensen p./s.
polishing
posterior capsular p.
**Polle pod attachment for
ophthalmoscope**
Pollock
P. forceps
P. punch
Polocaine
poloxamer
polus
p. anterior bulbi oculi
p. anterior lentis
p. posterior bulbi oculi
p. posterior lentis
Polyak's operation
polyamide
polyarteritis nodosa
polycarbonate lens
polychondritis
atrophic p.
relapsing p.
polychromatic
p. luster
polyclonality
Polycon
P. I contact lens
P. II contact lens
polycoria
p. spuria
p. vera

Polycycline
polycythemia
p. rubra vera
p. vera
Polydek suture
polydipsia
polydystrophic dwarfism
polydystrophy
pseudo-Hurler p.
polyester suture
polyethylene
p. glycol (PEG)
p. implant
p. T-tube
p. tube
polygenic inheritance
polyglactin suture
polyglycolic acid suture
polygonal pigmented cells
polyhedral cells
polymacon
polymegathism
polymer
polymerization
polymethyl
p. methacrylate (PMMA)
p. methacrylate contact lens
p. methacrylate frame
polymorphic
p. macular degeneration of
Brayley
p. superficial keratitis
polymorphism
allelic p.
restriction fragment
length p. (RFLP)
polymorphonuclear
p. leukocyte
p. reaction
p. response
polymorphous dystrophy
polymyalgia
p. rheumatica
polymyositis
polymyxin
p. B
p. B sulfate
p. B sulfate sterile
p. B and Terramycin
p. E
polyneuritis
infectious p.
polyneuropathy

polyopia, polyopsia
    binocular p.
    p. monophthalmica
polyostotic fibrous dysplasia
polyoxethylene sorbitan fatty acid ester
polyoxyl 40 stearate
polyp
    choanal p.
    Hopmann's p.
    nasal p.
    presenile p.
Poly-Pred
polypropylene
Polyquad
polyquaternium-1
polyradiculopathy
polysinusectomy
polysinusitis
Polysporin
polystichia
polysulfone
polytome x-ray
polytomography
Polytrim
polyuria
polyvidone (PVP)
polyvinyl alcohol (PVA)
polyvinylpyrrolidone, povidone (PVP)
Pompe's disease
pons, pl. pontes
pontile
pontine
    p. gaze center (PGC)
    p. lesions
    p. paramedian reticular formation
Pontocaine
pontomesencephalic dysfunction
pooling
population
    finite p.
porcelain white end-point
porcupine lymphoma
porofocon
porphyria
porropsia
port
    Berkeley Bioengineering infusion terminal p.
    Gills-Welsh guillotine p.
    p. vitrectomy

portal
    aspiration p.
port-wine stain
porus opticus
position
    p. accommodation
    p. ametropia
    Bertel's p.
    cardinal p.
    convergence p.
    p. cyclophoria
    dissociated p.
    p. error
    p. eyepiece
    face-down p.
    fusion-free p.
    heterophoric p.
    midline p.
    primary p.
    p. of rest
    Rhese's p.
    p. scotoma
    secondary p.'s
    sulcus fixated p.
    tertiary p.'s
    vertical divergence p.
positional
    p. abnormalities of retina
    p. nystagmus
positive
    p. accommodation
    p. afterimage
    p. convergence
    cyclophoria p.
    cyclotropia p.
    p. eyepiece
    p. meniscus
    p. meniscus lens
    p. scotoma
    p. vertical divergence
Posner
    P. diagnostic gonioprism
    P. diagnostic lens
    P. gonioprism
    P. slit lamp
    P. surgical gonioprism
Posner-Schlossman syndrome
post
    p. chamber
    p. chiasmal
postbasic stare
postcanalicular system
postcataract bleb

posterior
p. apical radius (PAR)
camera bulbi p.
camera oculi p.
p. capsular polishing
p. capsular zonular barrier
p. capsular zonular disruption
p. capsulotomy
p. central curve (PCC)
p. cerebral artery
p. chamber (PC)
p. chamber intraocular lens (PCIOL)
p. chamber lens
p. chamber lens implant (PCLI)
p. chiasmatic commissure
p. choroiditis
p. ciliary artery
p. ciliary vein
p. commissure
p. conical cornea
p. conjunctival artery
p. conjunctival vein
p. corneal depression
p. discission
p. dislocation
p. embryotoxon
p. epithelium of cornea
p. explant
p. fixation suture
p. focal point
p. hyaloid membrane (PHM)
p. hydrophthalmia
p. incision
p. inferior cerebellar artery syndrome
p. intermediate curve (PIC)
p. keratoconus
p. lamina
lamina elastica p.
p. lamina raphe
p. limiting lamina
p. limiting ring
membrana capsularis lentis p.
p. optical zone (POZ)
p. peribulbar block
p. peripheral curve (PPC)
p. pigment epitheliopathy
p. pituitary ectopia
p. polar cataract
p. pole
p. pole of eye
p. pole of eyeball
p. pole of lens
p. pole and periphery (PP&P)
p. polymorphic dystrophy (PPMD)
p. polymorphous corneal dystrophy
p. polymorphous dystrophy
p. scleritis
p. sclerochoroiditis
p. sclerotomy
p. segment
p. staphyloma
p. subcapsular cataract (PSC)
p. symblepharon
p. synechia
p. thermal sclerostomy
p. tube shunt implant
p. uveal melanoma
p. uveitis
p. veins
p. visual pathway imaging
p. vitreal detachment (PVD)
p. vitrectomy

posteriores
limbal palpebrales p.

posteromedially

postganglionic

Post-Harrington erysiphake

postherpetic
p. headache
p. neuralgia

posticum
staphyloma p.

postinfective reactive arthritis

postinflammatory
p. atrophy
p. cataract

postkeratoplasty

postmarital amblyopia

postocular neuritis

postoperative
p. adjustment
p. amblyopia
p. blindness

postorbital

postplaced

postsurgical hyphema

posttraumatic
  p. headache
  p. iridocyclitis
postural exophthalmos
posture
  compensatory p.
  compensatory head p.
  head p.
  inverted p.
postvitrectomy fibrin
potassium (K)
  p. acetate
  p. citrate
  p. hydroxide (KOH)
  p. iodide
  p. permanganate
  p. phosphate
  p. sorbate
potential
  early receptor p. (ERP)
  evoked p.
  flash visual evoked p.
  oscillatory p.
  receptor p.
  S p.
  visual evoked p. (VEP)
  visual evoked cortical p. (VECP)
Potential Acuity Meter (PAM)
Potter-Bucky diaphragm
Potter's syndrome
pouch
  Rathke's p.
Poulard's
  P. entropion
  P. operation
povidone-iodine
Powder
  Ophthalmic Moldite P.
powder
  bleaching p.
Powell wand
power
  back vertex p.
  bending p.
  p. calculation
  contact lens vertex p.
  dioptric p.
  equivalent p.
  lacrimal p.
  lens p.
  magnifying p.
  optical p.

Prentice's position p.
  radiant p.
  resolving p.
  p. vergence
  vertex of p.
  vertex p.
  zero optical p.
Power's operation
POZ
  posterior optical zone
PP
  punctum proximum of convergence
p.p.
  punctum proximum
PPC
  peripheral posterior curve
  posterior peripheral curve
PPMD
  posterior polymorphic dystrophy
PP&P
  posterior pole and periphery
PPRF
  paramedian pontine reticular formation
PR
  presbyopia
Pr
  praseodymium
p.r.
  punctum remotum
practolol
Prader-Willi syndrome
Praeger iris hook
prairie conjunctivitis
Pram occluder
praseodymium (Pr)
Prausnitz-Kustner reaction
praziquantel
prazosin
preauricular
  p. adenopathy
  p. nodes
precancerous lesion
prechiasmal
  p. compression
  p. disorder
precipitate
  keratic p. (KP)
  keratitic p.
  mutton-fat keratic p.
  pigment p.'s

pigmented keratic p.'s
punctate keratic p.'s
Precision Cosmet
P. C. intraocular lens
implant
P. C. lens
Precision refractor
precorneal
p. film
p. tear film
Pred
P. Forte
P. Mild
Predair A
Predair Forte
Predamide
Predate
Pred-G
Pred-G S.O.P
predictive value
predisposing condition
Prednefrin Forte
Prednisolone
Isopto P.
prednisolone
p. acetate
atropine and p.
p. and atropine
p. sodium phosphate
prednisone
Predsulfair
Predulose
preferential looking (PL)
Preflex for Sensitive Eyes
Prefrin
P. Liquifilm
P. Z Liquifilm
Prefrin-A
pregnancy
toxemia of p.
preliminary iridectomy
premacular gliosis
premature infant
prematurity
p. cataract
cicatricial retinopathy of p.
p. myopia
retinopathy of p. (ROP)
p. retinopathy
premedication
premelanosome

Premiere
P. irrigation-aspiration unit
P. SmallPort Phaco System
Prentice's
P. position power
P. rule
preoperative
p. evaluation
p. fasting
preorbita
prepapillary vascular loops
preparation
fortified topical p.
preparatory iridectomy
preplaced suture
prepresbyopia
preproliferative diabetic retinopathy
preretinal
p. hemorrhage
p. membrane
p. neovascularization
p. plaque
presbycusis
presbyope
presbyopia (PR)
p. glasses
presbyopic
presbytia
presbytism
presenile
p. cataract
p. melanosis
p. polyp
preseptal
p. cellulitis
p. orbicularis muscle
p. space
Presert
preservation
visual p.
preservative
preservatives in solution
pressing
eye p.
molded p.
press-on
p.-o. Fresnel lens
p.-o. lenses
p.-o. prism
pressure
p. amaurosis
applanation p.
p. bandage

353

pressure *(continued)*
    digital p.
    p. dressing
    exophthalmos due to p.
    eye restored to
      normotensive p.
    intracranial p.
    intraocular p. (IOP)
    mercury p.
    Michaelson's counter p.
    osmotic p.
    p. patch dressing
    p. shield
    white without p.
presumed
    p. ocular histoplasmosis
    p. ocular histoplasmosis
      syndrome (POHS)
pretectal
    p. nucleus
    p. region
    p. syndrome
prevalence rate
preventricular leukomalacia
Prevost's sign
Preziosi's operation
prezonular space
Priestley-Smith retinoscope
prilocaine
primaquine
primary
    p. acquired melanosis
    p. acquired nasolacrimal
      duct obstruction (PANDO)
    p. action
    p. amyloidosis
    p. angle-closure glaucoma
    p. anophthalmia
    p. cataract
    p. color
    p. deviation
    p. dye test
    p. dysgenesis mesodermalis
    p. eye
    p. familial amyloidosis
    p. glaucoma
    p. infantile glaucoma
    p. infantile glaucoma
      blepharospasm
    p. lens
    p. lens implant
    p. line of sight
    p. mover

    p. myopia
    p. open-angle glaucoma
      (POAG)
    p. optic atrophy
    p. perivasculitis of the
      retina
    p. persistent hyperplastic
      vitreous
    p. pigmentary degeneration
      of retina
    p. position
    p. position of gaze
    p. visual cortex
    p. vitreous
Primbs suturing forceps
primidone
primordium, pl. **primordia**
    optic p.
Prince
    P. cautery
    P. clamp
    P. electrocautery
    P. forceps
    P. muscle clamp
    P. muscle forceps
Prince's rule
principal
    p. fiber
    p. foci
    p. focus
    p. line
    p. line of direction
    p. optic axis
    p. plane
    p. point
    p. visual direction
principle
    Fresnel's p.
    Imbert-Fick p.
    Sheiner's p.
printers' point system
prism
    p. adaptation test (PAT)
    Allen-Thorpe gonioscopic p.
    AO rotary p.
    apex of p.
    p. ballast
    ballast p.
    p. ballast contact lens
    p. ballasted contact lens
    p. ballast lens
    p. bar
    bar p.

base-down p.
base-in p. (*var. of* base in)
  (BI)
base-out p. (*var. of* base
  out) (BO)
base-up p. (*var. of* base up)
  (BU)
Becker gonioscopic p.
Berens p.
p. cover measurement
p. cover test
p. and cover test (P&C)
p. degree
diopter p.
p. diopter (PD)
p. diopters or pupillary
  distance
dispersion p.
Drews inclined p.
Fresnel p.
Fresnel press-on p.
Goldmann p.
Goldmann contact lens p.
Goldmann three-mirror p.
gonioscopic p.
hand-held rotary p.
Jacob-Swann gonioscopic p.
Keeler p.
Maddox p.
Nicol p.
oblique p.
plastic p.
press-on p.
reflecting p.
right-angle p.
Risley p.
Risley rotary p.
rotary p.
scanning p.
p. segment
p. shift test
p. spectacles
square p.
p. test
three-mirror p.
p. vergence test
Wolff-Eisner p.

prismatic
p. contact lens
p. dioptric value
p. effect
p. effect by lens
p. fundus

p. gonioscopic lens
p. gonioscopy lens
p. goniotomy lens
p. lens
p. spectacle lens
p. spectacles
prismoptometer
prismosphere
prisoptometer
Pritikin punch
PRK
  photorefractive keratectomy
  photorefractive keratoplasty
p.r.n.
  as needed
proband
probe
  Alcon vitrectomy p.
  Anel p.
  angled p.
  Bodian lacrimal pigtail p.
  Bodian mini lacrimal p.
  Bowman p.
  Bowman lacrimal p.
  Castroviejo lacrimal sac p.
  p. cataract
  Clinitex Charles
    endophotocoagulator p.
  cryopexy p.
  cryotherapy p.
  Ellis foreign body spud
    needle p.
  Ellis needle p.
  French lacrimal p.
  Frigitronics freeze-thaw
    cryopexy p.
  Harms trabeculotomy p.
  Hertzog pliable p.
  Ilg p.
  Iliff p.
  Iliff lacrimal p.
  Keeler-Amoils curved
    cataract p.
  Keeler-Amoils glaucoma p.
  Keeler-Amoils long-shank p.
  Keeler-Amoils long-shank
    retinal p.
  Keeler-Amoils Machemer
    retinal p.
  Keeler-Amoils micro curved
    cataract p.
  Keeler-Amoils ophthalmic
    curved cataract p.

probe *(continued)*
Keeler-Amoils ophthalmic long-shank p.
Keeler-Amoils ophthalmic Machemer retinal p.
Keeler-Amoils ophthalmic micro curved cataract p.
Keeler-Amoils ophthalmic retinal p.
Keeler-Amoils ophthalmic straight cataract p.
Keeler-Amoils ophthalmic vitreous p.
Keeler-Amoils retinal p.
Keeler-Amoils straight cataract p.
Keeler-Amoils vitreous p.
Knapp p.
Knapp iris p.
lacrimal p.
lacrimal intubation p.
Linde cryogenic p.
Manhattan Eye & Ear p.
Mannis p.
Microvit p.
nasolacrimal duct p.
p. needle
needle p.
Ocutome p.
O'Donoghue angled DCR p.
Parker-Heath piggyback p.
piggyback p.
pigtail p.
Quickert p.
Quickert-Dryden p.
Quickert lacrimal p.
Quickert lacrimal intubation p.
Rolf lacrimal p.
Rollet lacrimal p.
Simpson lacrimal p.
spatula p.
p. spatula
p. syringe
Theobald p.
trabeculotomy p.
Vygantas-Wilder retinal drainage p.
Werb right-angle p
Williams p.
Worst p.
Worst pigtail p.
Ziegler p.

probenecid
probing
p. lacrimonasal duct
p. lacrimonasal duct operation
procaine
p. hydrochloride
procarbazine
procedure
acuity card p.
advancement p.
Bick's p.
Cibis' liquid silicone p.
ciliary p.
Custodis' p.
Custodis' nondraining p.
cyclodestructive p.
Donders' p.
Faden's p.
Fasanella-Servat p.
filtering p.
Girard's p.
hamular p.
Harada-Ito p.
hex p.
Hill's p.
Hummelsheim's p.
Ito p.
Jensen's p.
Jensen's transposition p.
Jones' tube p.
Kestenbaum's p.
Knapp's p.
Krönlein's p.
Kuhnt-Szymanowski p.
lathing p.
lower lid sling p.
modified Wies p.
PAM p.
Quickert's p.
Ruiz' p.
Sato's p.
Savin's p.
Sayoc's p.
scleral buckling p.
sling p.
strip p.
tarsal strip p.
Toti's p.
tuck p.
tumbling p.
uncinate p.
up-and-down staircases p.

Wheeler's p.
Wies' p.
PRO CEM-4 microscope
procerus
    musculus p.
process
    ciliary p.'s
    fine iris p.'s
    iris p.
    lacrimal p.
    photochemical p.
    spin-cast p.
    zygomatico-orbital p.
processus
    p. ciliares
    p. frontosphenoidalis ossis
      zygomatici
    p. orbitalis ossis palatini
    p. zygomaticus maxillae
prochlorperazine
procyonis
    Baylisascaris p.
prodromal
    p. glaucoma
    p. myopia
Products
    Katena P.
Profenal
profile
    p. analyzer
    p. perimetry
**ProFree/GP weekly enzymatic
cleaner**
profunda
    keratitis punctata p.
    keratitis pustuliformis p.
progeria
progonoma
    melanotic p.
program
    diagnostic p.
progressive
    p. addition lens
    p. cataract
    p. choroidal atrophy
    p. cone degeneration
    p. cone dystrophy
    p. cone-rod dystrophy
    p. external ophthalmoplegia
    (PEO)
    p. foveal dystrophy
    p. hemifacial atrophy
    p. lens

    p. macular dystrophy
    p. multifocal lens
    p. multifocal
      leukoencephalopathy
    p. myopia
    p. myopic degeneration
    p. nuclear ophthalmoplegia
    p. ophthalmoplegia
    p. supranuclear palsy (PSP)
    p. systemic sclerosis
    p. tapetochoroidal dystrophy
    p. vaccinia
progressive-add bifocal
projecting staphyloma
projection
    erroneous p.
    false p.
    light p.
    p. perimeter
    perimeter p.
    visual p.
Project-O-Chart
    AO P.-O.-C.
    AO Reichert
      Instruments P.-O.-C.
    Ultramatic P.-O.-C.
projector
    acuity visual p.
    fiberoptic light p.
    Lancaster red-green p.
    Marco chart p.
    Topcon chart p.
    Ultramatic Project-O-
      Chart p. (UPOC)
**Pro-Koester wide-field SCM
microscope**
prolactinoma
prolactin-secreting adenoma
prolapse
    iris p.
    p. of iris
    mitral valve p.
    vitreous p.
prolene
Prolene suture
proliferating retinitis
proliferation
    anterior hyaloidal
      fibrovascular p.
    glial p.
    hyaloidal fibrovascular p.
    massive periretinal p.
    (MPP)

proliferative
    p. choroiditis
    p. diabetic retinopathy
      (PDR)
    p. lupus retinopathy
    p. retinitis
    p. retinopathy
    p. sickle-cell retinopathy
    p. vitreoretinopathy (PVR)
prolongation
    P2 p.
prolonged-wear contact lens
promethazine
prominence
    Ammon's scleral p.
prominent
    p. buckle
    p. indentation
    p. Schwalbe ring
Pro-Ophtha
    P.-O. drape
    P.-O. dressing
    P.-O. eye pad
    P.-O. sponge
    P.-O. stick
propamidine
    p. isethionate
proparacaine
    p. HCl
    p. hydrochloride
propellering
prophylactically
prophylactic antibiotic
prophylaxis
    Credé's p.
propicillin
Propine
propionate
    sodium p.
propionibacterium
Propionibacterium acnes
Propofol
propositus
propoxycaine
Propper-Heine ophthalmoscope
propranolol
propria
    substantia p.
proprioception
proprioceptive
    p. head-turning reflex
    p. oculocep halic reflex

proptometer
proptosis
    axial p.
    Moran's p.
    unilateral p.
proptotic
propylene glycol
prosopagnosia
prosopantritis
prospective
    p. evaluation of radial
      keratomy (PERK)
    p. study
prosthesis, pl. prostheses
    ocular p.
    orbital p.
    orbital floor p.
    shell p.
    socket p.
prosthetic lens
prosthetophacos
prosthokeratoplasty
Prostigmin test
protan color blindness
protanomal
protanomalopia
protanomalous
    protanope p.
protanomaly
protanope
    p. protanomalous
protanopia
protanopic
protanopsia
protective
    p. lens
    p. spectacles
protector
    Arroyo p.
    Arruga p.
    eye p.
    oculoplasty corneal p.
protein
    Bence-Jones p.
    C-reactive p.
    p. electrophoresis
    retinol binding p. (RBP)
    silver p.
proteinaceous
    p. aqueous exudation
    p. coating
    p. cyst

proteinosis
    lipid p.
    lipoid p.
Proteus
protocol
    PERK p.
protometer
proton beam
protozoan, protozoal
    p. disease
    p. uveitis
protriptyline hydrochloride
protruding eyes
protrusion
    conical p.
    corneal p.
provocative
    p. test
    p. testing
Prowazek-Greeff body
Prowazek-Halberstaedter body
Prowazek's inclusion body
proximal convergence
PRP
    panretinal photocoagulation
PRRE
    pupils round, regular, and equal
pruritus
    senescent p.
Prussian blue
psammoma bodies
PSC
    posterior subcapsular cataract
pseudoabducens palsy
pseudoacanthosis nigricans
pseudo Argyll-Robertson pupil
pseudoblepsia, pseudoblepsis
pseudobulbar palsy
pseudocancerous lesion
pseudochiasmal
pseudocoloboma
pseudodendritic keratitis
pseudoepitheliomatous hyperplasia
pseudoesotropia
pseudoexfoliation
    p. of lens capsule
    p. syndrome
pseudoexfoliative capsular glaucoma
pseudoexophoria
pseudoexophthalmos
pseudoexotropia
pseudofacility
pseudofluorescence

pseudo-Foster Kennedy's syndrome
pseudogerontoxon
pseudoglandular
pseudoglaucoma glaucoma
pseudoglioma
pseudo-Graefe's
    p.-G. phenomenon
    p.-G. sign
pseudoguttata
pseudoherpetic
pseudo-Hurler polydystrophy
pseudohypertelorism
pseudohypertropia
pseudohypoparathyroidism
pseudohypopyon
pseudoinflammatory
    p. macular dystrophy
    p. macular dystrophy of
    Sorsby
pseudointernuclear ophthalmoplegia
pseudoiritis
pseudoisochromatic
    p. color plates
    p. plate
pseudomelanoma
pseudomembrane
pseudomembranous
    p. conjunctivitis
    p. rhinitis
Pseudomonas
    P. aeruginosa
    P. pyocyanea
    P. stutzeri
pseudomycosis
pseudomyopia
pseudoneuritis
pseudonystagmus
pseudopannus
pseudopapilledema
pseudopapillitis
pseudopemphigoid
pseudophacos
pseudophake implant
pseudophakia
    p. adiposa
    p. fibrosa
pseudophakic
    p. detachment
    p. eye
pseudophakodonesis
pseudophakos
pseudopresumed ocular
    histoplasmosis syndrome

pseudoprolactinoma
pseudoproptosis
pseudopseudohypoparathyroidism
pseudopsia
pseudopterygia
pseudopterygium
pseudoptosis
pseudoretinitis pigmentosa
pseudoretinoblastoma
pseudorheumatoid nodules
pseudosarcomatous endothelial
  hyperplasia
pseudosclerosis
    spastic p.
pseudoscopic vision
pseudostrabismus
pseudotabes
    pupillotonic p.
pseudotemporal arteritis
pseudotrachoma
pseudotuberculous ophthalmia
pseudotumor
    p. cerebri
    lymphoid p.
    p. oculi
    orbital p.
pseudovernal conjunctivitis
pseudoxanthoma
    elastic p.
    p. elasticum (PXE)
psittaci
    Chlamydia p.
psoralens
psoriasis
psorophthalmia
PSP
    progressive supranuclear palsy
psychic blindness
psychogenic paralysis
psychosis
psychosomatic
pterion
pterygial tissue
pterygium, pl. pterygia
    active p.
    Arlt's p.
    belly of p.
    congenital p.
    epitarsus p.
    p. scissors
    p. unguis
pterygoid levator synkinesis

PTG
    pneumatonograph
Pthirus pubis
ptilosis
PTK
    phototherapeutic keratectomy
ptosed
ptosis, pl. ptoses
    p. adiposa
    age-related p.
    aponeurotic p.
    Berke's p.
    Blaskovics-Berke p.
    cerebral p.
    congenital p.
    congenital dystrophic p.
    p. crutch spectacles
    eyelid p.
    p. of eyelid
    false p.
    p. forceps
    Hiff's p.
    Horner's p.
    involutional p.
    involutional senile p.
    p. knife
    p. lipomatosis
    mechanical p.
    mechanical acquired p.
    morning p.
    myogenic p.
    myogenic acquired p.
    neurogenic p.
    neurogenic acquired p.
    p. scissors
    senescent p.
    p. sympathetica
    p. sympathica
    traumatic p.
    upside-down p.
    waking p.
ptotic
pubis
    Pthirus p.
pucker
    macular p.
puckering
    macular p.
puddler's cataract
puff of loose vitreous
Pulfrich stereo phenomenon
pulley
pulmonary function test

pulpit spectacles
Pulsair tonometer
pulsatile exophthalmos
pulsating exophthalmos
pulsation
    venous p.
pulse
    p. mode
    p. oximeter
    p. train
pulseless disease
pulsers
pulse-step
pulsion
pulverization
pulverulenta
    cataracta centralis p.
pump
    tear p.
pump-leak system
punch
    Berens p.
    Berens corneoscleral p.
    bone p.
    bone-biting p.
    Castrovicjo p.
    Castroviejo corneoscleral p.
    corneal p.
    corneoscleral p.
    Descemet p.
    Descemet membrane p.
    Gass corneoscleral p.
    Gass scleral p.
    Gass sclerotomy p.
    Hardy p.
    Holth p.
    Holth scleral p.
    Kelly-Descemet
      membrane p.
    Klein p.
    Pollock p.
    Pritikin p.
    Reiss punctal p.
    Rubin-Holth p.
    sclerectomy p.
    sclerotomy p.
    Storz corneoscleral p.
    Troutman p.
    Walser corneoscleral p.
    Walton p.
punched-out lesion
puncta

punctal
    p. cautery
    p. dilator
    p. lens
    p. occlusion
    p. openings
    p. plug
    p. stenosis
punctata
    p. albescens retinopathy
    Chondrodystrophia
      calcificans congenita p.
    hyalitis p.
punctate
    p. cataract
    p. epithelial erosion
    p. epithelial keratopathy
      (PEK)
    p. epithelial keratoplasty
    p. epithelial microcyst
    p. hemorrhage
    p. hyalitis
    p. hyalosis
    p. keratic precipitates
    p. keratitis
    p. keratopathy
    p. oculocutaneous albinism
    p. oculocutaneous
      albinoidism
    p. outer retinal
      toxoplasmosis
    p. retinitis
    p. staining
puncti
punctiform
punctographed
punctoplasty
punctum, pl. puncta
    p. aplasia
    p. caecum
    p. cecum
    dilation of p.
    p. dilator
    eversion of p.
    inferior p.
    lacrimal p.
    p. lacrimale
    lower p.
    p. luteum
    one-snip p.
    p. proximum (p.p.)
    p. proximum of
      accommodation

punctum *(continued)*
    p. proximum of
      convergence (PP)
    p. remotum (p.r.)
    p. stenosis
    superior p.
    three-snip p.
    upper p.
punctumeter
puncture
    anterior p.
    p. diabetes
    diathermy p.
    lumbar p.
    p. needle
    self-sealing scleral p.
    p. wound
    Ziegler's p.
puncture-tip needle
Puntenny forceps
pupil (p)
    Adie's p.
    Adie's tonic p.
    amaurotic p.
    Argyll-Robertson p.
    artificial p.
    Behr's p.
    p. block
    p. block glaucoma
    blown p.
    bounding p.
    Bumke's p.
    catatonic p.
    cat's eye p.
    cholinergic p.
    cogwheel p.
    constricted p.
    contraction of p.
    cornpicker's p.
    diabetic Argyll-Robertson p.
    dilated p.
    p. dilation
    p. dilator
    dilator muscle of p.
    entrance p.
    p.'s equal, reactive to light
      and accommodation
      (PERLA)
    p.'s equal, round, reactive
      to light and
      accommodation (PERRLA)
    exit p.
    fixed p.

    fixed dilated p.
    Gunn's p.
    hammock p.
    Holmes-Adie p.
    Horner's p.
    Hutchinson's p.
    iris and p. (I/P)
    irregular p.
    keyhole p.
    light response of p.
    Marcus Gunn p. (MG)
    p. miosis
    miotic p.
    myotonic p.
    neurotonic p.
    occluded p.
    paradoxical p.
    pear-shaped p.
    pinhole p.
    pinpoint p.
    pseudo Argyll-Robertson p.
    reverse Marcus Gunn p.
    rigid p.
    Robertson's p.
    p.'s round, regular, and
      equal (PRRE)
    Saenger's p.
    p. size
    skew p.
    sphincter muscle of p.
    p. spreader/retractor forceps
    spring p.
    stiff p.
    teardrop p.
    tonic p.
    updrawn p.
    white p.
pupilla, pl. **pupillae**
    caligo p.
    musculus dilator p.
    musculus sphincter p.
    sphincter p.
    synkinesis p.
pupillary
    p. aperture
    p. areflexia
    p. athetosis
    p. axis
    p. block
    p. block glaucoma
    p. capture
    p. contraction
    p. cyst

p. distance (PD)
p. entrapment
p. iris cyst
p. lens
p. light reflex
p. line
p. margin of iris
p. membrane
p. membrane remnant
p. miosis
p. paradoxic reflex
p. paralysis
p. reflex
p. sparing
p. sphincter akinesis
p. sphincter contractions
p. sphincter muscle
p. zone
pupilloconstrictor fibers
pupillograph
pupillography
pupillometer
reflex p.
pupillometry
pupillomotor
pupilloplegia
pupilloscope
pupilloscopy
pupillostatometer
pupillotonia
pupillotonic pseudotabes
pupils
pupil-to-root iridectomy
Puralube
pure
p. color
p. cyclitis
Purisol
Purkinje image tracker
Purkinje's
P. effect
P. fibers
P. figure
P. image
P. phenomenon
P. shadow
P. shift
Purkinje-Sanson
P.-S. image
P.-S. mirror image
purple
visual p.

purpura
Henoch-Scönlein p.
thrombocytopenia p.
purpurea
Digitalis p.
purpuriferous
purpuriparous
purpurogenous membrane
pursuit
cogwheel p.
p. mechanism
p. movement
saccadic p.
Purtscher's
P. angiopathic retinopathy
P. disease
P. retinopathy
purulent
p. conjunctivitis
p. cyclitis
p. iritis
p. keratitis
p. ophthalmia
p. retinitis
p. rhinitis
pusher
Aker lens p.
De LaVega lens p.
Martin Surefit lens p.
Visitec lens p.
push plus refraction technique
push/pull
Birks Mark II p./p.
Birks Mark II micro p./p.
Ilg p./p.
Kuglein p./p.
pustular blepharitis
Putenney's operation
Putterman
P. levator resection clamp
P. ptosis clamp
Putterman-Chaflin
P.-C. ocular
P.-C. ocular asymmetry
device
P.-C. ocular device
**Putterman-Mueller blepharoptosis
clamp**
PVA
polyvinyl alcohol
p value
P.V. Carpine
P.V. Carpine Liquifilm

PVD
  posterior vitreal detachment
PVP
  polyvidone
  polyvinylpyrrolidone
PVR
  proliferative vitreoretinopathy
PXE
  pseudoxanthoma elasticum
pyelonephritis
pyknotic
    p. keratitis
    p. nuclei
pyocele
pyocyanea
    Pseudomonas p.
pyocyaneal ulcer

pyocyaneus
    Bacillus p.
pyogenes
    Streptococcus p.
pyogenic granuloma
Pyopen
pyophthalmia
pyophthalmitis
pyramidal cataract
pyrazinamide
Pyrex
    P. eye sphere
    P. T-tube
    P. tube
Pyridium
pyridoxine
pyrimethamine

Q

Q
 Q fever
 Q switching
q arm
Q-banding
Q-switched
 Q.-s. laser
 Q.-s. neodymium YAG laser
 Q.-s. ruby laser
13q- syndrome
Quad cutting tip
quadrantanopsia, quadrantanopia
 homonymous q.
 superior q.
quadrant hemianopsia
quadrantic
 q. defect
 q. hemianopsia
 q. scotoma
Quaglino's operation
quality
 q. factor
 tear q.
quantitative
 q. echography
 q. perimetry
 q. static threshold
 q. threshold perimetry
quantity
 tear q.
quartz
quaternary
 q. ammonium chloride
 q. ammonium compound

Quevedo
 Q. fixation forceps
 Q. suturing forceps
Quickert
 Q. lacrimal intubation
  probe
 Q. lacrimal probe
 Q. probe
 Q. suture
 Q. three-suture technique
Quickert-Dryden
 Q.-D. probe
 Q.-D. tube
Quickert's procedure
quick left/right component
quiet
 q. chamber
 eye was q.
 q. iritis
quinacrine
 q. hydrochloride
quinamm
quinaquine
quinidine
quinine
 q. amblyopia
 q. sulfate
quinone
Quire mechanical finger forceps

Rabl's lamellae
raccoon eyes
racemose
    r. aneurysm
    r. angioma
    r. hemangioma
racemosum
    staphyloma corneae r.
racquet bodies
radial
    r. astigmatism
    r. cells of Mueller
    r. dilator muscle
    r. fiber
    r. iridotomy
    r. iridotomy scissors
    r. keratotomy (RK)
    r. keratotomy knife
    r. keratotomy marker
    r. vessel array
radially oriented
radian
radiance
radiant
    r. absorptance
    r. emittance
    r. energy
    r. flux
    r. intensity
    r. and luminous flux
    r. power
    r. reflectance
radiatio
    r. occipitothalamica
    r. optica
radiation
    beta r.
    r. burn
    r. cataract
    r. effect
    electromagnetic r.
    geniculocalcarine r.
    Goldmann's coherent r.
    heavy ion r.
    infrared r.
    r. injury
    ionizing r.
    r. keratitis
    occipitothalamic r.
    optic r.

    r. retinopathy
    solar r.
    r. therapy
    ultraviolet r.
    visual r.'s
radiation-induced
    r.-i. carcinoma
    r.-i. optic neuropathy
radical astigmatism
radicans
    Rhus r.
radices
radii
Radin-Rosenthal
    R.-R. eye implant
    R.-R. implant
radioactive
    r. iodine
    r. plaque brachytherapy
radiography
radioimmunoassay
radioisotope scan
radiology
    orbital r.
radioscope
    Lombert r.
radiotherapy
radius, pl. radii
    apical r.
    r. gauge
    r. of lens
    r. of lentis
    posterior apical r. (PAR)
radix, pl. radices
    r. lateralis tractus optici
    r. medialis tractus optici
    r. oculomotoria ganglii
    ciliaris
    r. sympathica ganglii ciliaris
Raeder's
    R. paratrigeminal syndrome
    R. syndrome
rag-wheel method
railroad nystagmus
rainbow
    r. symptom
    r. syndrome
    r. vision
Rainen clip-bending spatula
Rainin lens spatula

Raji cell assay
Raman's effect
Raman spectrum
ramollitio retinae
Ramsay Hunt syndrome
Ramsden eyepiece
ramus
    tentorii r.
Randolph
    R. cyclodialysis cannula
    R. irrigator
random dot stereogram
Randot's
    R. chart
    R. Dot stereo test
range
    r. of accommodation
    r. of convergence
ranitidine
rank
    log r.
RAPD
    relative afferent pupillary defect
raphe
    canthal r.
    horizontal r.
    lateral palpebral r.
    palpebral r.
    r. palpebralis lateralis
    r. palpebrarum
    r. plica semilunaris
    posterior lamina r.
    temporal r.
rapid
    r. eye movements (REM)
    r. plasma reagin (RPR)
rare earth magnet
rarefaction
    pigmentation r.
rasp
    Lundsgaard r.
    Lundsgaard-Burch corneal r.
rate
    erythrocyte sedimentation r.
    incidence r.
    prevalence r.
    sedimentation r.
    Westergren sedimentation r.
    zeta sedimentation r.
Rathke's
    R. pouch
    R. pouch tumor

ratio
    accommodation-
      convergence r.
    accommodative
      conver-
      gence/accommodation r.
      (AC/A)
    arteriovenous r.
    cup-to-disk r. (C/D)
    nuclear cytoplasmic r.
    optic cup-to-disk r.
    rim-to-disk r.
Raverdino's operation
ray
    convergent r.
    converging r.
    divergent r.
    emergent r.
    r. incident
    marginal r.'s
    medullary r.
    monochromatic r.'s
    parallel r.'s
    paraxial r.'s
Ray-Brunswick-Mack operation
Rayleigh's
    R. equation
    R. limit
    R. scattering
    R. test
ray of light
    emergent r. o. l.
    incident r. o. l.
Ray-McLean operation
Raymond-Cestan syndrome
Raynaud's phenomenon
Rayner-Choyce implant
Rayner lens
razor
    Bard-Parker r.
    r. blade
    r. bladebreaker
    r. blade knife
    r. needle
razor-tip needle
RBP
    retinol binding protein
RD
    retinal detachment
rDNA
    recombinant DNA
reaction
    adverse r.

anaphylactic r.
anterior chamber r.
Arthus' r.
basophilic r.
conjunctival r.
consensual r.
eosinophilic r.
hemiopic pupillary r.
hypersensitivity r.
immune r.
immunologic r.
indirect pupillary r.
Jarisch-Herxheimer r.
lid closure r.
Loewi's r.
Mazzotti's r.
mononuclear r.
near r.
ocular tilt r.
ophthalmic r.
orbicularis r.
pain r.
polymorphonuclear r.
Prausnitz-Kustner r.
toxic r.
vestibular pupillary r.
Weil-Felix r.
Wernicke's r.
reader
bar r.
reading
r. cards
r. chart
r. glasses
r. rectangle
readings
K r.
reagent strips
reagin
rapid plasma r. (RPR)
real
r. focus
r. image
reaper's
r. keratitis
r. ophthalmia
reattachment
r. of choroid
r. of choroid operation
hydraulic retinal r.
r. of retina
r. of retina operation
rebound nystagmus

receptive field
receptor
alpha r.
r. amblyopia
beta r.
r. potential
sensory r.
visual r.
recess
optic r.
recessed-angle glaucoma
recession
angle r.
bimedial r.
conjunctival r.
left inferior oblique r.
r. of muscle
r. of ocular muscle
operation
optic muscle r.
tendon r.
traumatic angle r.
recession-angle glaucoma
recession-resection (R&R)
recessive
r. dystrophic epidermolysis
bullosa
r. inheritance
r. keratosis palmoplantaris
recess-resect (R&R)
recessus
Arlt-Jaesche r.
r. opticus
rechutes
iritis blennorrhagique à r.
reciprocal innervation
reciprocity law
Recklinghausen's
R. disease
R. syndrome
reclination
recombinant DNA (rDNA)
reconstruction
r. of eyelid
socket r.
recrudescence
rectangle
reading r.
rectifier
delayed r.
inward r.
rectus
inferior r. (IR)

rectus *(continued)*
    lateral r. (LR)
    r. lateralis muscle
    medial r. (MR)
    r. medialis muscle
    r. muscle
    superior r. (SR)
recurrence
recurrent
    r. central retinitis
    r. choroiditis
    r. corneal erosion
    r. epithelial erosion
    r. erosion of cornea
    r. exophthalmos
    r. hypopyon
    r. pupillary sparing
recurrentis
    Borrelia r.
red
    r. blindness
    r. blush
    Congo r.
    r. desaturation
    r. eye
    r. filter
    r. free filter
    r. glare test
    r. glass test
    r. reflex
    r. rubber catheter
    r. scaly plaque
    r. vision
redeepening
red-eyed shunt syndrome
red-filter
    r.-f. test
    r.-f. therapy
red-green blindness
Reditron refractometer
Redmond-Smith operation
Red Reflex Lens Systems lens
reduced
    r. eye
    r. eye model
    r. vergence
reducer
    McCannell ocular
      pressure r.
    ocular pressure r.
reductase
    aldose r.
reduplicated cataract

reduplication cataract
Reed-Sternberg cell
Reeh scissors
reel aspiration cannula
re-epithelialization
Reese
    R. forceps
    R. muscle forceps
    R. ptosis knife
Reese-Cleasby operation
Reese-Jones-Cooper operation
Reese's
    R. operation
    R. ptosis operation
    R. syndrome
refined refraction
refixation
reflectance
    r. echo
    radiant r.
reflected
    r. colors
    r. echo
    r. light
reflecting
    r. prism
    r. retinoscope
    r. surface
reflection
    corneal r.
    shiny cellophane r.
    specular r.
reflective scattering
reflectivity
reflectometer
reflectometry
reflex
    r. accommodation
    accommodation r.
    r. amaurosis
    r. amblyopia
    Aschner's r.
    attention r.
    auditory r.
    auditory oculogyric r.
    Bekhterev's r.
    Bell's r.
    black r.
    blind r.
    blind spot r.
    blink r.
    cat's eye r.
    cerebral cortex r.

cerebropupillary r.
cervico-ocular r.
choked r.
ciliary r.
ciliospinal r.
cochleopupillary r.
conjunctival r.
consensual light r.
convergency r.
copper-wire r.
corneal r.
corneal light r.
corneomandibular r.
corneomental r.
corneopterygoid r.
corticopupillary r.
crossed r.
cutaneous pupillary r.
dazzle r.
direct r.
direct-light r.
doll's eye r.
emergency light r.
eye r.
eyeball compression r.
eyeball-heart r.
eye-closure r.
eyelid closure r.
fixation r.
foveal r.
foveolar r.
fundal r.
fundus r.
fusion r.
Gault's r.
Gifford-Galassi r.
Gifford's r.
Gunn's pupillary r.
gustatolacrimal r.
Haab's r.
head-turning r.
Hirschberg r.
iridoplegia r.
iris contraction r.
juvenile r.
lacrimal r.
lacrimation r.
lid r.
light r.
light optometer r.
Lockwood's light r.
McCarthy's r.
myopic r.

nasolacrimal r.
near r.
oculocardiac r.
oculocephalic r.
oculocephalogyric r.
oculodigital r.
oculogyric auricular r.
oculopharyngeal r.
oculopupillary r.
oculorespiratory r.
oculosensory r.
oculosensory cell r.
opticofacial r.
opticofacial winking r.
optokinetic r.
optomotor r.
orbicularis r.
orbicularis pupillary r.
palpebral oculogyric r.
paradoxical pupillary r.
platysmal r.
Plitz's r.
proprioceptive head-
  turning r.
proprioceptive oculocep
  halic r.
pupillary r.
pupillary light r.
pupillary paradoxic r.
r. pupillometer
red r.
reversed pupillary r.
Ruggeri's r.
r. secretion
senile r.
shot-silk r.
silver-wire r.
skin pupillary r.
stretch r.
supraorbital r.
synkinetic near r.
tapetal light r.
r. tear secretion
threat r.
trigeminal r.
trigeminus r.
r. trigeminus
utricular r.
vestibulo-ocular r.
visual orbicularis r.
water-silk r.
Weiss' r.
Westphal-Piltz r.

reflex *(continued)*
    Westphal's pupillary r.
    white r.
    white pupillary r.
    wink r.
    yellow r.
    yellow light r.
reflux
    blood r.
    r. vergence
reformation
    r. of chamber
    fornix r.
    inferior fornix r.
refract
refracted light
refractile
    r. body
    r. crystal
    r. deposit
refracting
    r. angle of prism
    r. media
refraction
    r. angle
    cycloplegic r.
    cylindric r.
    direct-light r.
    double r.
    dynamic r.
    fogging system of r.
    homatropine r.
    index of r. (n)
    index of r.
    manifest r.
    ocular r.
    plane-surface r.
    refined r.
    r. spectacles
    spherical r.
    static r.
    unrefined r.
refractionist
refractionometer
    Hartinger Coincidence r.
    vertex r.
    Zeiss vertex r.
refractive
    r. accommodative esotropia
    r. amblyopia
    r. ametropia
    r. anisometropia

    Barraquer-Krumeich
      Swinger r.
    r. contact lens
    r. error
    r. hyperopia
    r. keratoplasty
    r. keratotomy
    r. media
    r. myopia
    r. state
refractivity
refractometer
    Abbe r.
    Hoya HDR objective r.
    Hoya MRM objective r.
    meridional r.
    Reditron r.
    Rodenstock eye r.
    Topcon r.
    Topcon eye r.
    Topcon RM-A2300 auto r.
refractometry
    laser r.
    urine r.
refractor
    Agrikola r.
    Allergan Humphrey r.
    Amoils r.
    AR 1000 r.
    automated r.
    automatic r.
    Berens r.
    Brawley r.
    Bronson-Turz r.
    Campbell r.
    Canon r.
    Castallo r.
    Castroviejo r.
    Coburn r.
    CooperVision Diagnostic
      Imaging r.
    Desmarres r.
    Elschnig r.
    Ferris-Smith r.
    Ferris-Smith-Sewall r.
    Fink r.
    Goldstein r.
    Gradle r.
    Graether r.
    Green r.
    Groenholm r.
    Hartstein r.
    Hillis r.

Humphrey automatic r.
Kirby r.
Knapp r.
Kronfeld r.
Kuglein r.
Leland r.
Marco r.
McGannon r.
Meller r.
Mueller r.
Nidek AR-2000 Objective
  Automatic r.
objective r.
Precision r.
Reichert r.
Rizzuti r.
Rollet r.
Schepens r.
SR-IV Programmed
  Subjective r.
Stevenson r.
subjective r.
Topcon r.
Wilmer r.
refrangible
Refresh PM
refringence
refringent
Refsum's disease
Regan-Lancaster dial
Regan's chart
regard
area of conscious r.
object of r.
regeneration
aberrant r.
r. aberration
regeneration of nerve
aberrant r. o. n.
region
ciliary r.
ethmoidal r.
infraorbital r.
ocular r.
orbital r.
pretectal r.
retrochiasmatic r.
scutum r.
regional
r. block
r. enteritis
regress

regression
regular astigmatism
regurgitation test
rehabilitation
optical r.
Reichert
R. binocular indirect
  ophthalmoscope
R. camera
R. Ful-Vue binocular
  ophthalmoscope
R. Ful-Vue ophthalmoscope
R. Ful-Vue spot retinoscope
R. lensometer
R. noncontact tonometer
R. ophthalmodynamometer
R. radius gauge
R. refractor
R. retinoscope
R. slit lamp
R. spot retinoscope
R. tonometer
Reichert's membrane
Reichling corneal scissors
Reidel's thyroiditis
Reiger's syndrome
reimplantation
Reinecke-Carroll lacrimal tube
reinforcement
scleral r.
reinnervation
Reis-Bucklers
R.-B. corneal dystrophy
R.-B. disease
R.-B. dystrophy
R.-B. ring-shaped dystrophy
R.-B. superficial corneal
  dystrophy
Reisinger lens-extracting forceps
Reisman's sign
Reiss punctal punch
Reiter's
R. disease
R. disease conjunctivitis
R. syndrome
rejection
allograft corneal r.
r. line
Rekoss' disk
relapsing
r. fever
r. polychondritis

relationship
    agonist-antagonist r.
    object/image r.
relative
    r. accommodation
    r. afferent pupillary defect
    (RAPD)
    r. amblyopia
    r. convergence
    r. divergence
    first-degree r.
    r. hemianopsia
    r. hyperopia
    near-point r.
    r. scotoma
    second-degree r.
    r. size
    r. spectacle magnification
    r. strabismus
relaxant
    muscle r.
    nondepolarizing muscle r.
relaxing incision
release hallucination
relucency
REM
    rapid eye movements
remnant
    pupillary membrane r.
removal
    r. of foreign body
    r. of foreign body operation
    lens r.
remover
    Alger brush rust ring r.
    Bailey foreign body r.
    DMV II contact lens r.
    frog cortex r.
    Soft Mate protein r.
Remy separator
renal
    r. diabetes
    r. failure
    r. medullary cyst
    r. retinitis
    r. retinopathy
Rendu-Osler-Weber disease
Renewed
    Tears R.
Renografin
ReNu
    R. Effervescent enzymatic
    cleaner

    R. Multi-Purpose
    R. Thermal enzymatic
    cleaner
repair
    Arlt's epicanthus r.
    Arlt's eyelid r.
    Blair's epicanthus r.
    blepharochalasis r.
    blepharoptosis r.
    Jones' r.
    Kuhnt-Junius r.
    lacrimal gland r.
    levator aponeurosis r.
    medial canthal r.
    trichiasis r.
    Wheeler's halving r.
reparative giant cell granuloma
replaceable blade
replacer
    Green r.
    Green iris r.
    Smith-Fisher iris r.
reposited
repositioning
repositor
    iris r.
    Knapp iris r.
    Nettleship iris r.
resection
    levator r.
    Mohs' microsurgical r.
    muscle r.
    r. of muscle
    Peyman's full-thickness eye-
    wall r.
    scleral r.
    wedge r.
reserpine
reserve
    divergence r.'s
    fusional r.
residual
    r. accommodation
    r. astigmatism
    r. cortex
residue
    edema r.
resilience
    orbital r.
resistance
    impact r.
    outflow r.

resistor
 Guardian scalpel with
  depth r.
 Guardian scalpel with
  myoguard depth r.
Resochin
Resolution
 logarithmic Minimum Angle
  of R. (logMAR)
resolution acuity
Resolve/GP
resolving power
resonance
 nuclear magnetic r. (NMR)
respiratorium
 scleroma r.
respiratory
 r. hippus
 r. status
response
 acquired immune r.
 allergic r.
 consensual light r.
 consensual pupillary r.
 curve r.
 direct-light r.
 direct pupillary r.
 eosinophilic r.
 immune r.
 mononuclear r.
 near r.
 oculocalorie r.
 polymorphonuclear r.
 synkinetic near r.
 vestibulo-ocular r. (VOR)
 visual-evoked r. (VER)
 visual-vestibulo-ocular r.
rest
 Chan wrist r.
 physiologic position of r.
 position of r.
restoration
 Berens-Smith cul-de-sac r.
 r. point
**restriction fragment length
 polymorphism (RFLP)**
restrictive syndrome
result
 false-negative r.
 false-positive r.
retardation
 aniridia, genitourinary
  abnormalities, and

 mental r. (AGR triad,
  AGR triad)
rete mirabile
retention
 carbon dioxide r.
reticula
reticular
 r. cystoid degeneration
 r. dystrophy of cornea
 r. keratitis
 r. lymphoblast
 r. plate
reticulum
 r. cell
 r. cell lymphoma
 r. cell sarcoma
 endoplasmic r.
 extraconal fat r.
 fat r.
 rough endoplasmic r.
retina
 angiomatosis of r.
 arteriosclerosis of r.
 central r.
 central fovea of r.
 cerebral layer of r.
 cerebral stratum of r.
 cholesterol emboli of r.
 coarctate r.
 coloboma of r.
 concussion of the r.
 r. cyanosis
 detached r.
 disciform degeneration of r.
 disinserted r.
 disinsertion of r.
 dragged r.
 falciform fold of r.
 fat embolism of r.
 flecked r.
 ganglionic layer of r.
 ganglionic stratum of r.
 ganglion layer of r.
 giant cyst of r.
 glioma of r.
 inferior zone of r.
 inflammatory changes of r.
 inner r.
 lattice degeneration of r.
 leopard r.
 lipemic r.
 lower r.
 medial arteriole of r.

retina *(continued)*
    medial venulae of r.
    nasal r.
    nasal arteriole of r.
    nasal venule of r.
    neovascularization of r.
    nerve layer of r.
    neuroepithelial layer of r.
    outer r.
    peripheral r.
    physiologic r.
    pigmented layer of r.
    positional abnormalities
      of r.
    primary perivasculitis of
      the r.
    reattachment of r.
    sensory r.
    shot-silk r.
    stiff r.
    superior zone of r.
    tear of r.
    temporal r.
    temporal arteriole of r.
    temporal venule of r.
    temporal zone of r.
    tented up r.
    thrombosis in r.
    tigroid r.
    upper r.
    vessel abnormalities of r.
    watered-silk r.
    yellow spot of r.
retinae
    albedo r.
    angiomatosis r.
    arteriola medialis r.
    atrophia choroideae et r.
    coloboma r.
    commotio r.
    ischemic r.
    limbal luteus r.
    macula flava r.
    macula lutea r.
    ora serrata r.
    pars caeca r.
    pars ciliaris r.
    pars iridica r.
    pars nervosa r.
    pars optica r.
    pars pigmentosa r.
    periphlebitis r.
    ramollitio r.

rubeosis r.
stratum cerebrale r.
sublatio r.
vasa sanguinea r.
vasculitis r.
vena centralis r.
venula medialis r.
retinal
    r. abiotrophy
    r. adaptation
    r. angiomatosis
    r. anlage tumor
    r. aplasia
    r. apoplexy
    r. arterial occlusion
    r. arteriole
    r. arteriovenous
      malformation
    r. artery
    r. artery aneurysm
    r. artery occlusion
    r. asthenopia
    r. astrocytoma
    r. atresia
    r. blood
    r. blur spot
    r. break
    r. burn
    r. camera
    r. capillary bed
    r. circinate
    r. circulation
    cis-r.
    r. cone
    r. correspondence
    r. cyst
    r. degeneration
    r. detachment (RD)
    r. detachment hook
    r. detachment pencil
    r. detachment syringe
    r. dialysis
    r. disorder
    r. disparity
    r. dysplasia
    r. dystrophy
    r. edema
    r. element
    r. embolism
    r. epithelial pigment
      hyperplasia
    r. error
    r. excavation

r. exudate
r. fixed fold
r. flap
r. foveola
r. ganglion
r. Gelfilm implant
r. gliocyte
r. glioma
r. gliosarcoma
r. gliosis
r. hemorrhage
r. hole
r. ice ball
r. image
r. image size
r. imbrication
r. ischemia
r. isomerase
r. lattice degeneration
r. microembolism
r. migraine
r. necrosis
r. necrosis syndrome
r. neovascularization
r. neurons
r. periphlebitis
r. pigmentary dystrophy
r. pigment epithelial
  hypertrophy
r. pigment epitheliitis
r. pigment epitheliopathy
r. pigment epithelium (RPE)
r. quadrant
  neovascularization
r. rivalry
r. rod
r. scatter photocoagulation
r. spike
r. staphyloma
r. stress lines
r. surgery
r. tacks
r. tear
r. telangiectasia
r. telangiectasis
r. thrombosis
r. toxicity
r. tuft
r. vascular occlusion
r. vasculature
r. vasculitis
r. vein
r. vein occlusion

r. venous beading
r. venous occlusion
r. venule
r. vessel
r. visual cells
r. zone
retinal arteriole
  aneurysm of r. a.
  narrowing of r. a.
retinal points
  corresponding r. p.
retinal-slip velocity
retinal vein
  occlusion of r. v.
retinal vessel
  sheathing of r. v.
  tortuosity of r. v.
retinascope
retinectomy
retinene isomerase
retinitis
  actinic r.
  AIDS-related r.
  albuminuric r.
  apoplectic r.
  azotemic r.
  central angioplastic r.
  central angiospastic r.
  r. centralis serosa
  central serous r.
  r. circinata
  circinate r.
  Coats' r.
  cytomegalovirus r.
  diabetic r.
  r. disciformans
  exudative r., r. exudativa
  foveomacular r.
  gravid r.
  r. gravidarum
  gravidic r.
  r. haemorrhagica
  herpes simplex r.
  hypertensive r.
  Jacobson's r.
  Jensen's r.
  leukemic r.
  metastatic r.
  r. nephritica
  Pick's r.
  r. pigmentosa (RP)
  r. pigmentosa sine pigmento
  r. proliferans

retinitis *(continued)*
    proliferating r.
    proliferative r.
    r. punctata albescens
    punctate r.
    purulent r.
    recurrent central r.
    renal r.
    rubella r.
    r. sclopetaria
    secondary r.
    septic r.
    serous r.
    simple r.
    solar r.
    splenic r.
    r. stellata
    striate r.
    suppurative r.
    r. syphilitica, syphilitic r.
    uremic r.
    Wagener's r.
retinoblastoma
    bilateral sporadic r.
    r. cell
    familial r.
    r. locus
    trilateral r.
    unilateral sporadic r.
retinocerebellar angiomatosis
retinochiasmatic
retinochoroid
retinochoroidal
    r. coloboma
    r. infarction
    r. layer
retinochoroidectomy
retinochoroiditis
    birdshot r.
    r. juxtapapillaris
    toxoplasmic r.
retinochoroidopathy
    birdshot r.
    central serous r.
retinocortical
retinocytoma
retinodialysis
Rétinofocomètre
retinograph
retinography
retinoic acid embryopathy
retinoid

retinoillumination
retinol binding protein (RBP)
retinomalacia
retinomigraine
Retinopan 45 camera
retinopapillitis of premature infants
retinopathy
    angiopathic r.
    arteriosclerotic r.
    background r.
    background diabetic r.
    birdshot r.
    blood-and-thunder r.
    bull's eye r.
    cancer-associated r.
    canthaxanthine crystalline r.
    carbon monoxide r.
    carotid occlusive disease r.
    cellophane r.
    central angioplastic r.
    central angiospastic r.
    central disk-shaped r.
    central serous r. (CSR)
    chloroquine r.
    circinate r.
    compression r.
    crystalline r.
    diabetic r.
    drug abuse r.
    dysoric r.
    dysproteinemic r.
    eclamptic r.
    eclipse r.
    electric r.
    external exudative r.
    exudative r.
    foveomacular r.
    gold dust r.
    gravidic r.
    r. hemorrhage
    hemorrhagic r.
    hypertensive r.
    hypotensive r.
    inflammatory r.
    ischemic r.
    Keith-Wagener r.
    Leber's idiopathic stellate r.
    leukemic r.
    lipemic r.
    macular r.
    nonproliferative r.
    nonproliferative diabetic r.
      (NPDR)

particulate r.
pigmentary r.
r. of prematurity (ROP)
prematurity r.
preproliferative diabetic r.
proliferative r.
proliferative diabetic r.
  (PDR)
proliferative lupus r.
proliferative sickle-cell r.
punctata albescens r.
Purtscher's r.
Purtscher's angiopathic r.
radiation r.
renal r.
rubella r.
serous r.
sickle r.
sickle cell r.
solar r.
stellate r.
surface wrinkling r.
syphilitic r.
tamoxifen r.
tapetoretinal r.
toxemic r. of pregnancy
toxic r.
traumatic r.
Van Heuven's r.
vascular r.
venous stasis r. (VSR)
venous stenosis r.
X-linked juvenile r.
retinopexy
cyanoacrylate r.
pneumatic r.
retinopiesis
retinoschisis
acquired r.
congenital r.
familial foveal r.
juvenile r.
senescent r.
senile r.
X-linked r.
X-linked juvenile r.
retinoscope
Copeland r.
Copeland streak r.
Ful-Vue spot r.
Ful-Vue streak r.
Keeler r.
luminous r.

Priestley-Smith r.
reflecting r.
Reichert r.
Reichert Ful-Vue spot r.
Reichert spot r.
spot r.
streak r.
retinoscopy
Copeland's r.
cylinder r.
fogging r.
streak r.
retinosis
retinotomy
retinotopic
retinotoxic
retraction
endocrine lid r.
eyelid r.
lid r.
r. nystagmus
r. syndrome
thyroid lid r.
vitreous r.
retractor
Agrikola lacrimal r.
Agrikola lacrimal sac r.
Alexander-Ballen r.
Amenabar iris r.
Amoils r.
angled iris r.
Arruga r.
Ballen-Alexander orbital r.
Barraquer-Krumeich-
  Swinger r.
Bechert-Kratz cannulated
  nucleus r.
Berens r.
Berens lid r.
Blair r.
Brawley r.
Bronson-Turz r.
Campbell r.
Castallo r.
Castroviejo r.
Castroviejo lid r.
Coleman r.
conjunctiva r.
Conway lid r.
Coston-Trent iris r.
deep blunt rake r.
Desmarres r.
Desmarres lid r.

retractor *(continued)*
    Drews-Rosenbaum iris r.
    Duane r.
    Eliasoph lid r.
    Elschnig r.
    eyelid r.
    Fasanella r.
    Ferris-Smith r.
    Ferris-Smith-Sewall r.
    Fink r.
    Fink lacrimal r.
    Fisher lid r.
    Forker r.
    Givner lid r.
    Goldstein r.
    Goldstein lacrimal sac r.
    Good r.
    Gradle r.
    Graether r.
    Graether collar-button r.
    Graether collar-button micro
     iris r.
    Groenholm r.
    Gross r.
    Harrington r.
    Harrison r.
    Hartstein r.
    Hartstein irrigating iris r.
    Hill r.
    Hillis r.
    Jaeger r.
    Jaffe-Givner lid r.
    Jaffe lid r.
    Kaufman type II r.
    Keeler-Fison tissue r.
    Keeler-Rodger iris r.
    Keizer-Lancaster lid r.
    Kelman iris r.
    Kirby r.
    Kirby lid r.
    Knapp r.
    Knapp lacrimal sac r.
    Kronfeld r.
    Kuglein r.
    lacrimal sac r.
    lower lid r.
    MacVicar double-end
     strabismus r.
    McCool capsule r.
    McGannon r.
    Meller lacrimal sac r.
    Mueller lacrimal sac r.
    Nevyas r.

    Oklahoma iris wire r.
    Paul lacrimal sac r.
    Payne r.
    phoropter r.
    r. plication
    Rizzuti iris r.
    Rollet r.
    Rosenbaum-Drews r.
    Sanchez-Bulnes lacrimal
     sac r.
    Sato lid r.
    Schepens r.
    Schultz iris r.
    self-adhering lid r.
    self-retaining r.
    Senn r.
    Sewall r.
    Stevens lacrimal r.
    Stevenson lacrimal sac r.
    Teflon iris r.
    Thomas r.
    Ticho pliable iris r.
    Ultramatic Rx Master
     phoropter r.
    Vaiser-Cibis muscle r.
    Vasco-Posada orbital r.
    Visitec iris r.
    Welsh iris r.
    Wilder scleral r.
    Wilmer r.
retrieval device
retrobulbar
    r. abscess
    r. akinesia
    r. anesthesia
    r. block
    r. hemorrhage
    r. hemorrhage glaucoma
    r. injection
    r. lid block
    r. needle
    r. neuritis
    r. optic neuritis
    r. space
retrochiasmal pathway
retrochiasmatic region
retrocorneal membrane
retrodisplacement
retroflexion of iris
retrogeniculate lesion
retroilluminate
retroillumination
retroiridian

retrolaminar
retrolental fibroplasia (RLF)
retrolenticular
retromembranous
retro-ocular space
retro-orbital
retropupillary
retroscopic lens
retrospective study
retrotarsal fold
Reuss'
    R. color chart
    R. color tables
    R. table
Reverdin
    R. suture needle
reverse
    r. bobbing
    r. Marcus Gunn pupil
    r. optics
reverse-cutting needle
reversed
    r. astigmatism
    r. pupillary reflex
reverse-shape implant
reversible amblyopia
Rēv-Eyes
RFLP
    restriction fragment length
    polymorphism
RGP
    rigid gas-permeable
    rigid gas-permeable contact lens
rhabdomyoma
rhabdomyosarcoma
    orbital r.
rhegmatogenous
    r. detachment
    r. retinal detachment
Rhein fine foldable lens-insertion
    forceps
Rhese's position
rheumatic
    r. fever
    r. nodule
    r. valvular disease
rheumatica
    polymyalgia r.
rheumatoid
    r. arthritis
    r. factor
    r. related ulceration
    r. sclerouveitis

rheumatoid-associated nuclear
    antigen
rheumatoid-related disease
rhinitis
    acute catarrhal r.
    allergic r.
    atrophic r.
    r. caseosa
    chronic catarrhal r.
    croupous r.
    dyscrinic r.
    fibrinous r.
    gangrenous r.
    hypertrophic r.
    membranous r.
    pseudomembranous r.
    purulent r.
    scrofulous r.
    r. sicca
    syphilitic r.
    tuberculous r.
rhinocanthectomy
rhinodacryolith
rhinophyma
rhinoplasty
rhinoscleroma
rhinosporidiosis
rhinotomy
rhodogenesis
rhodophylactic
rhodophylaxis
rhodopsin
Rhus
    R. radicans
    R. toxicodendron
rhytidosis
rhytids
    eyelid r.
ribbon
    r. gauze dressing
    synaptic r.
ribbon-like keratitis
riboflavin
ribosome
Riccò's law
Richard pillow
Richet's operation
Richner-Hanhart syndrome
rickettsial
    r. blepharitis
    r. disease
Ridaura

Riddoch's
    R. phenomenon
    R. syndrome
ridge
    laser r.
    r. lens
    mesenchymal r.
    petrous r.
    supraorbital r.
    synaptic r.
riding bow temple
Ridley
    R. anterior chamber lens
      implant
    R. implant
    R. lens
    R. Mark II implant
    R. Mark II lens implant
Riedel needle
Rieger's
    R. anomaly
    R. syndrome
Rifadin rifampin
rifampin
    Rifadin r.
Rifkind's sign
rifle
    air r.
right
    r. deorsumvergence
    r. esotropia
    r. exotropia
    r. eye (OD)
    r. gaze
    r. gaze verticals
    r. hyperphoria
    r. hypertropia
    r. sursumvergence
right-angle prism
right-beating nystagmus
right-eyed
right/left corneoscleral scissors
rigid
    r. contact lens
    r. gas-permeable (RGP)
    r. gas-permeable contact
      lens (RGP)
    r. gas-permeable lens
    r. pupil
rigidity
    mydriatic r.
    ocular r.
    scleral r.

Riley-Day syndrome
Riley-Smith syndrome
rim
    inferior orbital r.
    neural r.
    neuroretinal r.
    orbital r.
    orbital inferior r.
    saucering of r.'s
rima
    r. cornealis
    r. palpebrarum
rimless frame
rim-to-disk ratio
ring
    abscess r.
    r. abscess
    anterior limiting r.
    Bonaccolto-Flieringa
      scleral r.
    Bonaccolto scleral r.
    Bores twist fixation r.
    Burr corneal r.
    Caspar r.
    cataract mask r.
    r. cataract mask eye shield
    r. cataract mask shield
    centering r.
    choroidal r.
    ciliary r.
    Coats' r.
    Coats' white r.
    collagenolytic trabecular r.
    collagenous trabecular r.
    common tendinous r.
    conjunctival r.
    corneal r.
    corneal transplant
      centering r.
    Dollinger's tendinous r.
    Donders' r.'s
    fixation r.
    fixation/anchor r.
    Fleischer's r.
    Fleischer's keratoconus r.
    Fleischer-Strumpell r.
    Flieringa r.
    Flieringa fixation r.
    Flieringa-Kayser copper r.
    Flieringa-Kayser fixation r.
    Flieringa-Legrand fixation r.
    Flieringa scleral r.
    r. forceps

r. form congenital cataract
Girard scleral-expander r.
glaucomatous r.
glial r.
greater r.
r. of iris
iris r.
iron Fleischer r.
Kayser-Fleischer r.
Kayser-Fleischer cornea r.
Klein-Tolentino r.
Landers irrigating
  vitrectomy r.
Landers vitrectomy r.
Landolt's r.
Landolt's broken r.
r. lens expressor
lenticular r.
lesser r.
Lowe's r.
Martinez corneal transplant
  centering r.
Maxwell's r.
McKinney fixation r.
McNeill-Goldmann r.
posterior limiting r.
prominent Schwalbe r.
rust r.
Saturn r.
Schwalbe's r.
Schwalbe's anterior
  border r.
scleral r.
scleral expander r.
scotoma r.
r. scotoma
r. of Soemmering
Soemmering's r.
symblepharon r.
tantalum r.
tantalum "O" r.
Thornton fixating r.
Tolentino r.
r. ulcer
r. ulcer of cornea
Vossius r.
Vossius lenticular r.
Wessely r.
white r.
Zinn's r.
Ringer's lactate solution
ring-like corneal dystrophy
Ring's D chromosome syndrome

ring-shaped
  r.-s. cataract
  r.-s. dystrophy
ringworm
Rinse
Riolan's
  R. muscle
Ripault's sign
ripe cataract
Risley
  R. prism
  R. rotary prism
ristocetin
Ritalin
**Ritch-Krupin-Denver eye valve
  insertion forceps**
Ritch trabeculoplasty laser lens
Ritter
Ritter's
  R. disease
  R. fiber
rivalry
  binocular r.
  r. of retina
  retinal r.
river blindness
rivus lacrimalis
Rizzuti
  R. expressor
  R. fixation forceps
  R. graft carrier spoon
  R. iris retractor
  R. lens expressor
  R. rectus forceps
  R. refractor
  R. scleral fixation forceps
Rizzuti-Bonaccolto instruments
Rizzuti-Fleischer instruments
**Rizzuti-Furness cornea-holding
  forceps**
Rizzuti-Kayser-Fleischer instruments
Rizzuti-Lowe instruments
Rizzuti-Maxwell instruments
**Rizzuti-McGuire corneal section
  scissors**
Rizzuti-Soemmering instruments
Rizzuti-Spizziri
  R.-S. cannula knife
  R.-S. knife
RK
  radial keratotomy
  RK marker

RLF
    retrolental fibroplasia
RLX
    R. coating
    R. lens
Roaf's syndrome
Robertson's
    R. pupil
    R. sign
Roberts-SC phocomelia
Robin chalazion clamp
Robinow's syndrome
Robin's syndrome
Robles' disease
Rochat's test
Rochon-Duvigneaud
    bouquet of R.-D.
    R.-D. bouquet of cones
Rocky Mountain spotted fever
rod
    r. achromatopsia
    bipolar r.
    r. cell
    r. and cone dystrophy
    r. fiber
    r. function
    graceful swirling r.'s
    gram-negative r.'s
    r. granule
    Maddox r.
    r. monochromasy
    r. monochromat
    r. monochromatism
    retinal r.
    scleral sponge r.
    r. spherule
    Viers r.
    vision r.
    r. vision
rod-cone
    r.-c. degeneration
    r.-c. dystrophy
Rodenstock
    R. eye refractometer
    R. lamp
    R. lens
    R. panfundoscope
    R. panfundus lens
    R. slit lamp
    R. System
rodent ulcer

Rodin
    R. implant
    R. orbital implant
rods and cones
roentgenogram
    orbital r.
Rolf
    R. dilator
    R. forceps
    R. lacrimal probe
    R. lance
roll
    iris r.
    peripheral iris r.
    scleral r.
rolled up epithelium with wavy border
roller forceps
Rollet
    R. irrigating/aspirating unit
    R. lacrimal probe
    R. refractor
    R. retractor
Rollet's syndrome
Romaña's sign
Romberg's
    R. sign
    R. syndrome
Romberg testing
Rommel
    R. cautery
    R. electrocautery
Rommel-Hildreth
    R.-H. cautery
    R.-H. electrocautery
rongeur
    Belz lacrimal sac r.
    biting r.
    bone r.
    Citelli r.
    Kerrison r.
    lacrimal sac r.
Ronne's nasal step
roof
    r. fracture
    r. of orbit
    orbital r.
room temperature vulcanizing (RTV)
RO Optho
root
    iris r.
    motor r.

oculomotor r.
sensory r.
ROP
retinopathy of prematurity
Roper alpha-chymotrypsin cannula
Roper-Hall
R.-H. localizer
R.-H. locator
ropy mucus
Rosa-Berens
R.-B. implant
R.-B. orbital implant
rosacea
acne r.
blepharoconjunctivitis r.
keratitis r.
r. keratitis
Roscoe-Bunsen law
rose
r. bengal
r. bengal red solution
r. bengal sodium I 125
r. bengal sodium I 131
r. bengal stain
r. bengal staining
roseata
iritis r.
Rosenbach's sign
Rosenbaum-Drews retractor
Rosenbaum pocket vision screener
Rosenblatt scissors
Rosenburg's operation
Rosengren's operation
Rosenmüller
valve of R.
Rosenmüller's
R. body
R. gland
R. node
R. valve
Rosenthal's fibers
Rosets
rosette
Flexner-Wintersteiner r.
Homer-Wright r.
Wintersteiner r.'s
Rosner tonometer
rostral interstitial nucleus
rotary
r. cutting tip
r. nystagmus
r. prism
rotating-type cutter

rotation
center of r.
r. center
eye r.
r. nystagmus
wheel r.
rotational
r. nystagmus
r. test
rotator
Bechert nucleus r.
Jaffe-Bechert nucleus r.
rotatory nystagmus
Roth-Bielschowsky
R.-B. deviation
R.-B. syndrome
Rothmund's syndrome
Rothmund-Thomson syndrome
Roth's
R. spots
R. spot syndrome
rotoextractor
Douvas r.
rotundum foramen
Rouget's muscle
rough endoplasmic reticulum
round
r. hemorrhage
r. top bifocal
roundworm
route
r. of administration
external r.
transconjunctival r.
Roveda
R. everter
R. lid everter
Roveda's operation
Rowbotham's operation
Rowinski's operation
Rowland keratome
Rowsey fixation cannula
RP
retinitis pigmentosa
RP hypertrophy
RPE
retinal pigment epithelium
RPR
rapid plasma reagin
R&R
recession-resection
recess-resect

RTV
room temperature vulcanizing
rubber dam
Rubbrecht's operation
rubella
r. cataract
r. retinitis
r. retinopathy
rubeola
r. conjunctivitis
rubeosis
r. iridis
iridis r.
r. iridis diabetica
r. retinae
Rubin-Holth punch
Rubinstein
R. cryoextractor
R. cryophake
R. cryoprobe
Rubinstein-Taybi syndrome
ruby
r. diamond knife
r. knife
r. laser
Rucker body
rudimentary eye
rudiment lens
Ruedemann
R. eye implant
R. implant
R. lacrimal dilator
R. tonometer
Ruedemann's operation
Ruedemann-Todd tendon tucker
ruffed canal
Ruggeri's reflex
Ruiz
R. fundus contact lens
R. fundus laser lens
R. fundus lens
R. plano fundus implant
R. plano fundus lens
implant
R. trapezoidal keratotomy
Ruiz-Nordan trapezoidal marker
Ruiz' procedure

rule
accommodation r.
Kestenbaum's r.
Knapp's r.
Kollner's r.
Krimsky-Prince
accommodation r.
Luedde's transparent r.
Pischel scleral r.
Prentice's r.
Prince's r.
ruler
biometric r.
Bio-Pen biometric r.
Hyde astigmatism r.
Scott No. 2 curved r.
Weck astigmatism r.
running nylon suture
rupture
choroidal r.
scleral r.
traumatic choroidal r.
ruptured globe
Rushton's ocular measurements
Russell bodies
Russell's
R. syndrome
Russian
R. forceps
R. four-pronged fixation
hook
rust
r. ring
r. ring of cornea
r. spots
Rutherford's syndrome
rutidosis
ruyschiana
membrana r.
r. membrane
Ruysch's
R. membrane
R. tunic
RV275
Tracoustic R.
Rycroft's operation
Rycroft tying forceps

S
Siemens
spherical lens
sulfur
Svedberg unit
S-3-(amino-2-hydroxypropyl)
phosphothionate
Sabin-Feldman dye test
Sabouraud's
S. agar
S. media
Sabreloc needle
saburral
s. amaurosis
s. amaurosis fugax
sac
conjunctival s.
diverticula of lacrimal s.
drainage of lacrimal s.
Föerster's lacrimal s.
s. formation
lacrimal s.
nasolacrimal s.
tear s.
saccade
hypometric s.
ocular s.
s. palsy
slow-to-no s.
saccadic
s. abnormality
s. eccentric target
s. eye movement
s. movement
s. movements of eye
s. pursuit
s. velocity
saccular aneurysm
sacculated
sacculus lacrimalis
saccus
s. conjunctivae
s. conjunctivalis
s. lacrimalis
Sachs' disease
Sachs tissue forceps
sacroiliac joint
saddle
s. bridge
Turkish s.

Saemisch's
S. operation
S. section
S. ulcer
Saenger's
S. pupil
S. sign
Safar's operation
safety
s. glasses
s. lens
s. spectacles
Safir Ophthalmetron
sagittal
s. axis
s. axis of eye
s. axis of Fick
s. depth
s. height
s. vault
sagittalization
Sainton's sign
Sakler erysiphake
salbutamol
salicylate
methyl s.
physostigmine s.
sodium s.
salicylic acid
saline
Blairex sterile s.
Hydrocare preserved s.
Lens Plus s.
Murine sterile s.
s. saturated wool dressing
Soft Mate s.
s. solution
sorbic acid Sorbi-Care s.
salivary gland
salmon
s. patch
s. patch hue
salmon-patch hemorrhage
salt and pepper
s. a. p. appearance
s. a. p. fundus
salts
calcium s.
gold s.
platinum s.

Salus'
    S. arch
    S. sign
Salzmann's
    S. corneal dystrophy
    S. degeneration
    S. dystrophy
    S. nodular corneal
      degeneration
    S. nodular corneal
      dystrophy
    S. nodular degeneration
Salz nucleus splitter
Samoan conjunctivitis
sampling error
Sampoelesi's line
Sanchez-Bulnes lacrimal sac
    retractor
Sanchez-Salorio syndrome
Sanders'
    S. disease
    S. disorder
    S. operation
Sanders-Castroviejo suturing
    forceps
Sandhoff's disease
Sandt forceps
Sanfilippo's
    S. disease
    S. disorder
    S. syndrome
sanguineous cataract
Sanson's image
S-antigen
Sanyal's conjunctivitis
saponification
Sappey's fiber
sapphire knife
sarcoid
    Boeck's s.
    s. granulomatous disease
sarcoidosis
    pediatric ocular s.
sarcoma, pl. **sarcomata**
    Ewing's s.
    granulocytic s.
    hemorrhagic s.
    Kaposi's s.
    melanotic s.
    multifocal hemorrhagic s.
    reticulum cell s.
sarcomatosum
    ectropion s.

    glioma s.
    s. senilis
    s. spasticum
    s. uveae
sarcomere
satellite
    s. cells
    s. lesion
Sato
    S. cataract needle
    S. corneal knife
    S. lid retractor
Sato's
    S. keratoconus
    S. operation
    S. procedure
Sattler's
    S. layer
    S. veil
saturated color
saturation
    color s.
Saturn
    S. II contact lenses
    S. ring
saturninus
    halo s.
saucering of rims
saucerization
saucer-shaped cataract
Sauer
    S. corneal debrider
    S. debrider
    S. forceps
    S. infant speculum
    S. speculum
    S. suture forceps
    S. suturing forceps
Sauflon
    S. lens
    S. PW lens
Sauvineau's ophthalmoplegia
Savin's
    S. operation
    S. procedure
saw
    Stryker s.
Sayoc's
    S. operation
    S. procedure
SBV
    single binocular vision

sc
  without correction
scaffold for new vessel growth
scalded skin syndrome
scale
  Esterman s.
  Snell-Sterling's visual
    efficiency s.
scalloped contours
scalloping
scalpel
  s. guard
  Guyton-Lundsgaard s.
  Myocure s.
  Myocure blade s.
  Oasis feather micro s.
scalp flap
scaly plaque
scan
  A-s.
  choroidal s.
  computed tomography s.
  Contact A- and B-s.
  cross-vector A-s.
  gallium s.
  isotope s.
  magnetic resonance
    imaging s.
  MRI s.
  radioisotope s.
  technetium s.
  Ultra-Image A-s.
scanning
  s. electron microscopy
  gallium s.
  s. prism
scaphocephaly
scaphoid
scar
  corneal s.
  facetted corneal s.
  gray-white corneal s.
  linear s.
  peripapillary s.
  s. plate
scarification
scarified
scarifier
  Desmarres s.
  s. knife
  Kuhnt corneal s.
Scarpa's staphyloma

scarring
  conjunctival s.
  corneal s.
  episcleral s.
  gossamer s.
scatter
  beam s.
  light s.
  s. pattern
  s. photocoagulation
  sclerotic s.
scattergram
scattering
  light s.
  Rayleigh's s.
  reflective s.
scatterplot
Schaaf
  S. forceps
  S. foreign body forceps
Schachar lens
Schacher's ganglion
Schachne-Desmarres
  S.-D. everter
  S.-D. lid everter
Schaedel cross-action towel clamp
Schaefer
  S. fixation forceps
  S. sponge holder
Schäfer's syndrome
Scharf lens
Schaumann's inclusion bodies
Scheie
  S. anterior chamber cannula
  S. blade
  S. cataract-aspirating
    cannula
  S. cataract-aspirating needle
  S. cautery
  S. electrocautery
  S. goniopuncture knife
  S. goniotomy knife
  S. knife
  S. needle
  S. ophthalmic cautery
  S. trephine
Scheie-Graefe fixation forceps
Scheie's
  S. akinesia
  S. classification
  S. operation
  S. syndrome

Scheie's *(continued)*
   S. technique
   S. thermal sclerostomy
Scheie-Westcott corneal section
   scissors
Scheiner's
   S. experiment
   S. theories
schematic eye
schenckii
   Sporothrix s.
Schepens
   S. binocular indirect
     ophthalmoscope
   S. depressor
   S. electrode
   S. forceps
   S. Gelfilm
   S. hollow hemisphere
     implant
   S. operation
   S. ophthalmoscope
   S. refractor
   S. retinal detachment unit
   S. retractor
   S. scleral depressor
   S. spoon
   S. technique
   S. thimble depressor
Schepens-Pomerantzeff
   ophthalmoscope
scheroma
Schiff
   periodic-acid S. (PAS)
Schilder's disease
Schillinger suture support
Schimek's operation
Schiötz
   S. tonofilms
   S. tonometer
Schirmer
   S. filter paper
   S. strips
Schirmer's
   S. operation
   S. syndrome
   S. tear quality test
   S. tear test
   S. test
schisis
schistosomiasis
   nodules in s.
Schlegel lens

Schlemm
   canal of S.
Schlemm's canal
Schlichting's dystrophy
Schmalz's operation
Schmid-Fraccaro syndrome
Schmidt's keratitis
Schmincke's tumor
Schnabel's
   S. cavern
   S. optic atrophy
Schnaitmann's bifocal
Schnyder's
   S. crystalline corneal
     dystrophy
   S. crystalline dystrophy
Schöbl's scleritis
Schocket
   S. anterior chamber tube
     shunt
   S. scleral depressor
Schöler's treatment
Schön's theory
school myopia
Schultz
   S. fiber baskets
   S. iris retractor
Schumann
   S. giant type eye magnet
   S. giant type magnet
Schwalbe
Schwalbe's
   S. anterior border ring
   S. line
   S. ring
   S. space
schwannoma
   malignant s.
Schwann's cells
Schwartz syndrome
Schweigger
   S. capsule forceps
   S. extracapsular forceps
   S. forceps
Schweigger's
   S. hand perimeter
   S. perimeter
SCID
   severe combined
     immunodeficiency
scieropia
scimitar scotoma

scintillans
    synchesis s.
scintillating
    s. granules
    s. scotoma
scintillation
scintillography
    lacrimal s.
scirrhencanthis
scirrhophthalmia
scissors
    Aebli corneal s.
    Aebli corneal section s.
    alligator s.
    anterior chamber
      synechia s.
    Atkinson corneal s.
    bandage s.
    Barraquer s.
    Barraquer-DeWecker s.
    Barraquer iris s.
    Barraquer vitreous strand s.
    Becker corneal section
      spatulated s.
    Berens s.
    Berens corneal transplant s.
    Berens iridocapsulotomy s.
    Berkeley Bioengineering
      mechanized s.
    Birks Mark II Instruments
      micro trabeculectomy s.
    Birks Mark II micro
      trabeculectomy s.
    Bonn iris s.
    canalicular s.
    capsulotomy s.
    Castroviejo s.
    Castroviejo anterior
      synechia s.
    Castroviejo corneal
      section s.
    Castroviejo corneal
      transplant s.
    Castroviejo
      iridocapsulotomy s.
    Castroviejo keratoplasty s.
    Castroviejo synechia s.
    Castroviejo-Vannas
      capsulotomy s.
    Cohan-Vannas iris s.
    Cohan-Westcott s.
    conjunctival s.
    corneal s.

    corneal section spatulated s.
    corneal spatulated s.
    corneoscleral s.
    corneoscleral right/left
      hand s.
    DeWecker s.
    DeWecker iris s.
    DeWecker-Pritikin s.
    dissecting s.
    enucleation s.
    eye s.
    eye suture s.
    Fine suture s.
    Frost s.
    Giardet corneal transplant s.
    Gill s.
    Gill-Hess s.
    Gills-Welsh s.
    Gills-Welsh-Vannas s.
    Gills-Welsh Vannas angled
      micro s.
    Girard corneoscleral s.
    Glasscock s.
    Grieshaber vertical
      cutting s.
    Grieshaber vitreous s
    Guist s.
    Guist enucleation s.
    Haenig irrigating s.
    Halsted strabismus s.
    Harrison s.
    Hoskins-Castroviejo
      corneal s.
    Hoskins-Westcott
      tenotomy s.
    House-Bellucci alligator s.
    Huey s.
    Hunt chalazion s.
    iridectomy s.
    iridocapsulotomy s.
    iridotomy s.
    iris s.
    Irvine s.
    Irvine probe-pointed s.
    Karakashian-Barraquer s.
    Katzin s.
    Keeler intravitreal s.
    keratectomy s.
    keratoplasty s.
    Kirby s.
    Knapp s.
    Knapp iris s.
    Kreiger-Spitznas vibrating s.

scissors *(continued)*
Lagrange s.
Lagrange sclerectomy s.
Lawton corneal s.
Lister s.
Littauer dissecting s.
Littler s.
Littler dissecting s.
Manson-Aebli corneal
 section s.
Mattis s.
Mattis corneal s.
Maunoir iris s.
Max Fine s.
Mayo s.
McClure iris s.
McGuire s.
McGuire corneal s.
McLean s.
McLean capsulotomy s.
McPherson s.
McPherson-Castroviejo s.
McPherson-Castroviejo
 corneal section s.
McPherson corneal
 section s.
McPherson-Vannas s.
McPherson-Vannas micro
 iris s.
McPherson-Westcott
 conjunctival s.
McPherson-Westcott stitch s.
McReynolds s.
McReynolds pterygium s.
mechanized s.
micro Westcott s.
mini-keratoplasty stitch s.
mini-keratoplasty stitch s.
Moore-Troutman corneal s.
s. movement
MPC automated
 intravitreal s.
Nadler superior radial s.
Noyes iridectomy s.
Noyes iris s.
Nugent-Gradle s.
O'Brien stitch s.
pterygium s.
ptosis s.
radial iridotomy s.
Reeh s.
Reichling corneal s.
right/left corneoscleral s.

Rizzuti-McGuire corneal
 section s.
Rosenblatt s.
Scheie-Westcott corneal
 section s.
Shield iridotomy s.
Smart s.
Spencer eye suture s.
Spring iris s.
Stevens eye s.
Stevens tenotomy s.
Storz-Westcott
 conjunctival s.
strabismus s.
superior radial tenotomy s.
Sutherland s.
Sutherland-Grieshaber s.
Thomas s.
Thorpe s.
Thorpe-Castroviejo s.
Thorpe-Westcott s.
Troutman s.
Troutman-Castroviejo
 corneal section s.
Troutman conjunctival s.
Troutman-Katzin corneal
 transplant s.
Troutman microsurgical s.
Troutman suture s.
Twisk micro s.
Vannas s.
Vannas capsulotomy s.
Verhoeff s.
vibrating s.
vitreous strand s.
Walker s.
Walker-Apple s.
Walker-Atkinson s.
Werb s.
Westcott s.
Westcott conjunctiva s.
Westcott stitch s.
Westcott tenotomy s.
Westcott utility s.
Wilmer s.
Wilmer conjunctival s.
Wincor enucleation s.
scissors-shadow
SCL
 soft contact lens
sclera, pl. **scleras, sclerae**
 blue s.
 buckling s.

ectasia of s.
foramen of s.
lamina cribrosa sclerae
lamina fusca sclerae
limbus of s.
massive granuloma of s.
melanosis sclerae
sinus venosus s.
sulcus s.
white s.

scleral
s. band
s. blade
s. buckle
s. buckling
s. buckling operation
s. buckling procedure
s. canal
s. cautery
s. channel
s. contact lens
s. crescent
s. cyst
s. degeneration
s. depressor
s. ectasia
s. exoplant
s. expander
s. expander ring
s. fistula
s. fistulectomy operation
s. flap
s. flap suture
s. framework
s. furrow
s. grip
s. hook
s. icterus
s. implant
s. lamina cribrosa
s. lip
s. marker
s. patch graft
s. pick
s. plexus
s. reinforcement
s. resection
s. resection knife
s. rigidity
s. ring
s. roll
s. rupture
s. search coil

s. search coil technique
s. shell
s. shell glaucoma
s. shortening clip
s. shortening operation
s. show
s. sponge rod
s. spur
s. staphyloma
s. substance
s. sulcus
s. supporter
s. trabecula
s. tunnel
s. twist
s. twist-grip forceps
s. venous sinus

scleralis
pars s.

scleralization

scleras

scleratitis

sclerectasia
partial s.
total s.

sclerectasis

sclerectoiridectomy

sclerectoiridodialysis

sclerectome

sclerectomy
Holth's s.
Iliff-House s.
s. punch
thermal s.

scleriasis

scleriritomy

scleritis
annular s.
anterior s.
brawny s.
deep s.
diffuse anterior s.
gelatinous s.
herpes simplex s.
malignant s.
s. necroticans
necrotizing s.
necrotizing nodular s.
nodular s.
posterior s.
Schöbl's s.
syphilitic s.

sclerocataracta

sclerochoroiditis
    anterior s.
    posterior s.
scleroconjunctival
scleroconjunctivitis
sclerocornea
sclerocorneal
    s. junction
    s. sulcus
sclerocytes
scleroderma
scleroiritis
sclerokeratectomy
sclerokeratitis
sclerokeratoiritis
sclerokeratosis
scleromalacia perforans
scleroma respiratorium
scleronyxis
sclero-optic
sclerophthalmia
scleroplasty operation
sclerosed
sclerosing
    s. keratitis
    s. orbital granuloma
    s. panencephalitis
    chorioretinitis
sclerosis, pl. scleroses
    arteriolar s.
    central areolar choroidal s.
    central choroidal s.
    choroidal s.
    choroidal primary s.
    diffuse choroidal s.
    multiple s.
    nuclear s. (NS)
    peripapillary s.
    progressive systemic s.
    systemic s.
    tuberous s.
sclerostomy
    s. needle
    posterior thermal s.
    Scheie's thermal s.
sclerotic
    s. coat
    s. scatter
    s. stroma
sclerotica
    tunica s.
scleroticectomy
scleroticochoroidal canal

scleroticochoroiditis
scleroticonyxis
scleroticopuncture
scleroticotomy
sclerotitis
sclerotome
    Alvis-Lancaster s.
    Atkinson s.
    Castroviejo s.
    Curdy s.
    Guyton-Lundsgaard s.
    Lundsgaard s.
    Lundsgaard-Burch s.
    Walker-Lee s.
sclerotomy
    anterior s.
    DeWecker's anterior s.
    foreign body s.
    Lindner's s.
    s. operation
    posterior s.
    s. punch
    s. removal of foreign body
    s. with drainage
    s. with exploration
sclerouveitis
    rheumatoid s.
Scobee
    S. muscle hook
    S. oblique muscle hook
S-cone
scoop
    Arlt s.
    Daviel s.
    enucleation s.
    Kirby intraocular lens s.
    Knapp s.
    Lewis s.
    Mules s.
    Wilder s.
scope
    Bjerrum s.
    tangent s.
    Welch-Allyn Pocket s.
scopolamine
    s. ear patch
    s. hyoscine
    s. patch
scoria
scoterythrous vision
scotodinia
scotograph
scotoma, pl. scotomata

absolute s.
altitudinal s.
annular s.
arc s.
arcuate s.
arcuate Bjerrum's s.
aural s.
bitemporal hemianopic s.
Bjerrum's s.
cecocentral s.
central s.
centrocecal s.
color s.
comet s.
congruous homonymous
  hemianopic s.
cuneate-shaped s.
double arcuate s.
eclipse s.
equatorial ring s.
flittering s.
focal s.
frame s.
glaucomatous nerve-fiber
  bundle s.
hemianopic s.
homonymous hemianopic s.
insular s.
ipsilateral centrocecal s.
junction s.
s. junction
junctional s.
motile s.
negative s.
paracentral s.
pericentral s.
peripapillary s.
peripheral s.
physiologic s.
position s.
positive s.
quadrantic s.
relative s.
ring s.
s. ring
scimitar s.
scintillating s.
Seidel's s.
sickle s.
superior arcuate s.
suppression s.
s. of Traquair

unilateral altitudinal s.
zonular s.
scotomagraph
scotomameter
scotomata
scotomatous
scotometer
  Bjerrum s.
scotometry
scotomization
scotopia
scotopic
  s. adaptation
  s. eye
  s. perimetry
  s. vision
scotopsin
scotoscope
scotoscopy
Scott
  S. lens-insertion forceps
  S. No. 2 curved ruler
scraper
  Knolle s.
  Knolle capsule s.
  Kratz s.
  Kratz capsule s.
scraping
  conjunctival s.'s
  epithelial s.
scratch
  s. resistant lens
  s. resistant spectacle lens
scratched contact lens
scratcher
  Jensen capsule s.
  Knolle capsule s.
  Kratz s.
  Kratz capsule s.
  Kratz-Jensen s.
screen
  Bernell tangent s.
  Bjerrum s.
  Grey-Hess s.
  Hess s.
  Hess diplopia s.
  Hess-Lee s.
  tangent s.
screener
  Rosenbaum pocket vision s.
screening
  genetic s.

scrofulous, scrofular
    s. conjunctivitis
    s. keratitis
    s. ophthalmia
    s. rhinitis
scrub
    lid s.
    Ocusoft s.
    s. typhus
scrubber
    Simcoe anterior chamber
      capsule s.
scurf
scurvy
scutum region
sea
    s. fan
    s. fan sign
    s. fronds
seam
    pigment s.
Searcy
    S. anchor/fixation
    S. chalazion trephine
    S. erysiphake
    S. oval cup erysiphake
sebaceous
    s. adenoma
    s. cell
    s. cell carcinoma
    s. cyst
    s. gland of conjunctiva
    s. g's of conjunctiva gland
sebaceum
    adenoma s.
seborrhea
seborrheic
    s. blepharitis
    s. keratosis
sebum palpebrale
seclusion
    s. of pupil
secobarbital sodium
Seconal
second
    s. cranial nerve
    s. sight
secondary
    s. action
    s. amyloidosis
    s. anophthalmia
    s. axis
    s. cataract

    s. deviation
    s. dye test
    s. exotropia
    s. eye
    s. focal point
    s. glaucoma
    s. keratitis
    s. lens
    s. lens implant
    s. malignant neoplasm
    s. membrane
    s. optic atrophy
    s. positions
    s. retinitis
    s. vitreous
second-degree relative
second-grade fusion
secretion
    basal s.
    basal tear s.
    oily s.
    reflex s.
    reflex tear s.
    tear s.
section
    nerve cross s.
    orbital s.
    Saemisch's s.
sector
    s. cuts
    s. defect
    s. iridectomy
    s. iridectomy operation
    s. pallor
    s. palsy
    s. retinitis pigmentosa
sectoranopia
sector-shaped defect
sedimentary cataract
sedimentation rate
seeding
    vitreous s.
Seeligmüller's sign
see-saw nystagmus
segment
    anterior s.
    anterior ocular s.
    bifocal s.
    compensated s.
    dissimilar s.
    extramedullary s.
    inner s.
    intramedullary s.

intratemporal s.
outer s.
posterior s.
prism s.
segmental
s. explant
s. implant
s. lens
Seidel's
S. scotoma
S. sign
S. test
seizure
selenium sulfide
self-adhering lid retractor
self-retaining
s.-r. infusion cannula
s.-r. irrigating cannula
s.-r. retractor
self-sealing scleral puncture
Selinger's operation
sella, pl. sellae
empty s.
J-shaped s.
tilt of s.
s. turcica
sellar calcification
semicircular canals
semifinished
s. blank
s. contact lens
s. glass
s. lens
semilunar
s. fold
s. folds of conjunctiva
semilunaris
plica s.
raphe plica s.
semiscleral contact lens
semishell implant
senescence
senescent
s. cataract
s. cortical degenerative
cataract
s. disciform macular
degeneration
s. ectropion
s. elastosis
s. enophthalmus
s. entropion
s. halo

s. keratosis
s. macular degeneration
s. macular exudative
choroiditis
s. macular hole
s. miosis
s. nuclear degenerative
cataract
s. pruritus
s. ptosis
s. retinoschisis
senile
s. atrophy
s. cataract
s. chorioretinitis
s. choroidal change
s. disciform degeneration
s. disciform macular
degeneration
s. ectropion
s. elastosis
s. entropion
s. exudative macular
degeneration
s. guttate choroidopathy
s. halo
s. keratosis
s. lenticular myopia
s. macular degeneration
(SMD)
s. macular exudative
choroiditis
s. miosis
s. nuclear sclerotic cataract
s. reflex
s. retinoschisis
s. sclerotic cataract
s. vitritis
senilis
cataract s.
choroiditis guttata s.
circus s.
ectropion s.
sarcomatosum s.
Senior-Loken syndrome
Senn retractor
senopia
sensation
corneal s.
decreased corneal s.
light s.
s. time

sense
> color s.
> form s.
> light s.
> stereognostic s.

Sensitive
> S. Eyes
> S. Eyes daily cleaner
> S. Eyes drops
> S. Eyes saline/cleaning
> solution

sensitivity
> contrast s.
> cornea s.
> increment threshold
> spectral s.
> light s.
> periocular drug s.
> spectral s.
> s. threshold

Sensorcaine
> S. with epinephrine

sensory
> s. amblyopia
> s. correspondence
> s. deprivation nystagmus
> s. esotropia
> s. exotropia
> s. fusion
> s. nerve
> s. receptor
> s. retina
> s. root
> s. root of ciliary ganglion
> s. system
> s. test
> s. visual pathway

sentinel
> Dalma's s.

separable
> s. acuity
> minimum s.

separate image test
separation
> s. difficulty
> s. of retina
> vitreous s.

separator
> Kirby cylindrical zonal s.
> Kirby flat zonal s.
> Remy s.

septate
septicemia

Septicon
septic retinitis
septo-optic
> s.-o. dysplasia
> s.-o. dysplasia syndrome

Septra
septum
> s. cavum pellucidum
> intermuscular s.
> orbital s.
> s. orbitale
> s. sequela
> tarsus orbital s.

sequela, pl. sequelae
> septum s.

Sequels
> Diamox S.

sequence
> linear sebaceous nevus s.

sequestered spaces
Sereine
serentil
series
> Kurova Shursite lens s.
> Zeiss slit-lamp s.

serofibrinous
serologic
> s. examination
> s. test

serosa
> choroiditis s.
> s. choroiditis
> retinitis centralis s.

serous
> s. chorioretinopathy
> s. cyclitis
> s. detachment
> s. detachment maculopathy
> s. iritis
> s. macular detachment
> s. membrane
> s. pigment epithelium
> s. retinitis
> s. retinopathy

Serpasil
serpent ulcer of cornea
serpiginous
> s. choroiditis
> s. choroidopathy
> s. corneal ulcer
> s. keratitis
> s. ulcer

serpiginous ulcer
    chronic s. u.
serpinginosum
    angioma s.
serrata
    ora s.
Serratia
    S. marcescens
serrefine
    s. clamp
    Dieffenbach s.
    Lemoine s.
serum
    s. protein electrophoresis
    s. sickness
Service
    Lighthouse Low Vision S.
sessile papilloma
set
    British Standards Institution
      optotype s.
    Catalano intubation s.
    Crawford lacrimal s.
    diagnostic fitting s.
    Jackson lacrimal
      intubation s.
    Jaffe lid retractor s.
    McIntyre infusion s.
    Mentanium vitreoretinal
      instrument s.
    Simcoe lens positioning s.
    Tolentino vitrectomy lens s.
seton operation
setting
    field diaphragm s.
setting-sun
    s.-s. phenomenon
    s.-s. sign
seventh
    s. cranial nerve
    s. nerve palsy
severe combined immunodeficiency
(SCID)
Severin
    S. implant
    S. lens
Sewall
    S. forceps
    S. retractor
sex-linked disease
Sézary's syndrome
SFP
    simultaneous foveal perception

shadow
    s. graph
    Purkinje's s.
    s. test
shadowing
    acoustical s.
    hollowing and s.
Shafer's sign
Shaffer's operation
Shaffer-Weiss classification
shaft vision
shagreen
    anterior capsule s.
    anterior mosaic crocodile s.
    crocodile s.
    s. pattern
shaking
    head s.
shallow
    s. chamber
    flat and s.
shallowing of chamber
sham-movement vertigo
shape
    verrucous s.
shaped cataract
sharp
    s. hook
    s. and pink (S&P)
Sharplan argon laser
Sharpoint
    S. knife
    S. microsurgical knife
    S. slit knife
    V-lance S.
    S. V-lance blade
Shearing
    S. intraocular lens
    S. lens
    S. planar posterior chamber
      intraocular lens
    S. posterior chamber
      intraocular lens implant
Shea's syndrome
sheath
    arachnoid s.
    bulbar s.
    dural s.
    eyeball s.
    fetal fibrovascular s.
    fibrovascular s.
    muscle s.
    nerve s.

sheath *(continued)*
    optic nerve s.
    pial s.
    s. syndrome
sheathing
    halo s.
    perivascular s.
    s. of retinal vessel
    venous s.
    vessel s.
    s. of vessel
Sheehan's syndrome
Sheehy-Urban sliding lens adaptor
sheet
    Barrier s.
    Eye-Pak II s.
    foil s.
    glassy s.'s
    ground glass s.
    Silastic s.
    Supramid s.
    Teflon s.
Sheets
    S. glide
    S. irrigating vectis
    S. lens
    S. lens glide
    S. lens-inserting forceps
    S. lens spatula
    S. micro iris hook
Sheets-McPherson tying forceps
Sheiner's principle
shelf-type implant
shell
    s. implant
    s. prosthesis
    scleral s.
shelving
Shepard
    S. forceps
    S. incision depth gauge
    S. incision irrigating
      cannula
    S. intraocular lens forceps
    S. intraocular utility forceps
    S. iris hook
    S. lens-inserting forceps
    S. micro iris hook
    S. optical center marker
    S. radial keratotomy
      irrigating cannula
    S. reversed iris hook
    S. tying forceps

Shepard-Reinstein forceps
Sheridan-Gardiner isolated letter-
  matching test
Sherman card
Sherrington's
    S. law
    S. law of reciprocal
      innervation
shield
    aluminum eye s.
    Barraquer s.
    Barraquer eye s.
    Buller s.
    Buller eye s.
    Cartella s.
    Cartella eye s.
    cataract mask s.
    collagen s.
    corneal light s.
    Expo Bubble s.
    Expo Bubble eye s.
    eye s.
    face s.
    Fox s.
    Fox aluminum s.
    Fox eye s.
    Grafco eye s.
    Green s.
    Green eye s.
    Guibor s.
    Hessburg corneal s.
    Hessburg eye s.
    Jardon eye s.
    Mueller s.
    Mueller eye s.
    Paton s.
    Paton eye s.
    plastic s.
    plastic eye s.
    pressure s.
    ring cataract mask s.
    ring cataract mask eye s.
    trigeminal s.
    Universal s.
    Universal eye s.
    Visitec corneal s.
    Weck s.
    Weck eye s.
Shield iridotomy scissors
Shields forceps
shield-shaped
shift
    Purkinje's s.

shingles
shiny cellophane reflection
shipyard
    s. conjunctivitis
    s. disease
    s. eye
    s. keratoconjunctivitis
Shoch
    S. foreign body pickup
    S. suture
shoelace stitch
short
    s. ciliary artery
    s. ciliary nerves
    s. C-loop lens
    s. posterior ciliary artery
    s. root of ciliary ganglion
    s. sight
Short Cut A-OK small-incision
   knife
shortening
short-scale contrast
shortsightedness
shot-silk
    s.-s. phenomenon
    s.-s. reflex
    s.-s. retina
show
    scleral s.
Shprintzen syndrome
shredded iris
Shugrue's operation
shunt
    dural s.
    Schocket anterior chamber
     tube s.
    s. vessels
    White glaucoma pump s.
shunting
    left-to-right s.
Shy-Drager syndrome
sialadenosis
sialidosis
sicca
    keratoconjunctivitis s. (KCS)
    rhinitis s.
    s. syndrome
siccus, pl. panni
    pannus s., pl. panni
Sichel
    S. blade
    S. knife
Sichel's disease

Sichi
    S. implant
    S. orbital implant
Sichi's operation
sickle
    s. cell anemia
    s. cell hemoglobin C
     disease
    s. cell hemoglobin D
     disease
    s. cell hemoglobinopathy
    s. cell retinopathy
    s. cell thalassemia
    s. cell thalassemia disease
    s. cell trait
    s. hemoglobinopathy
    s. retinopathy
    s. scotoma
sickness
    serum s.
    sleeping s.
side-biting spatula
side-cutting spatulated needle
side port cannula
sideratic cataract
siderophone
sideroscope
siderosis
    s. bulbi
    s. cataract
    s. conjunctivae
    s. lentis
    ocular s.
siderotic
sidewall infusion cannula
Sidler-Huguenin endothelioma
Siegrist-Hutchinson syndrome
Siegrist's
    S. spots
    S. streak
Siemens (S)
sight
    day s.
    far s.
    line of s.
    long s.
    near s.
    night s.
    old s.
    primary line of s.
    second s.
    short s.

sighted
    partially s.
sign
    Abadie's s.
    Abadie's s. of exophthalmic
        goiter
    Argyll-Robertson pupil s.
    Arroyo's s.
    Ballet's s.
    Bárány's s.
    Bard's s.
    Barré's s.'s
    Battle's s.
    Bekhterev's s.
    Berger's s.
    Bianchi's s.
    Bielschowsky's s.
    Bjerrum's s.
    black sunburst s.
    Boston's s.
    Braley's s.
    Brickner's s.
    Cantelli's s.
    Chvostek's s.
    Cogan's s.
    Collier's s.
    Cowen's s.
    Dalrymple's s.
    doll's eye s.
    s. of edema of lower eyelid
    Elliot's s.
    Enroth's s.
    Gianelli's s.
    Gifford's s.
    Goppert's s.
    Gower's s.
    Graefe's s.
    Griffith's s.
    Grocco's s.
    Gunn's s.
    Hoglund's s.
    Hutchinson's s.
    Jellinek's s.
    Jendrassik's s.
    Joffroy's s.
    Knie's s.
    Kocher's s.
    Larcher's s.
    Loewi's s.
    Lotze's local s.'s
    Macewen's s.
    Magendie-Hertwig s.
    Magendie's s.

Mann's s.
Marcus Gunn s.
Marcus Gunn pupillary s.
Maxwell-Lyons s.
May's s.
Means' s.
Metenier's s.
Möbius' s.
Möbius-von Graefe-
    Stellway s.
Munson's s.
Nikolsky's s.
ocular s.
orbicularis s.
Parrot's s.
peek s.
Piltz's s.
Prevost's s.
pseudo-Graefe's s.
Reisman's s.
Rifkind's s.
Ripault's s.
Robertson's s.
Romaña's s.
Romberg's s.
Rosenbach's s.
Saenger's s.
Sainton's s.
Salus' s.
sea fan s.
Seeligmüller's s.
Seidel's s.
setting-sun s.
Shafer's s.
Skeer's s.
Stellwag's s.
Stimson's s.
Suker's s.
swinging flashlight s.
Tellais' s.
Theimich's s.
Theimich's lip s.
Topolanski's s.
Tournay's s.
Trousseau's s.
Uhthoff's s.
von Graefe's s.
Weber-Rinne s.
Weber's s.
Wernicke's s.
Widowitz's s.
Wilder's s.
Woods' s.

Signet Optical lens
signet-ring
    s.-r. carcinoma
    s.-r. lymphoma
Silaclean
Sila Clean
silafilcon A
silafocon A
Silastic
    S. implant
    S. intubation
    S. plate
    S. scleral buckler implant
    S. sheet
    S. T-tube
silica gel
silicone
    s. acrylate
    s. acrylate contact lens
    s. acrylate contact lenses
    s. band
    s. button
    s. conformer
    s. contact lens
    s. elastomer lens
    s. explant
    s. eye sphere
    s. hemisphere
    s. implant
    s. introducer
    s. intubation
    s. lens
    s. lubricant
    s. mesh implant
    s. oil
    s. oil tamponade
    s. rod and sleeve forceps
    s. sponge explant
    s. sponge forceps
    s. strip
    s. tire
    s. tube
    s. tubing
siliculose, siliquose
    siliculose cataract
silk
    s. traction suture
    virgin s.
Silsoft contact lens
Silva-Costa operation
silver
    colloidal s.
    s. compound

    s. nitrate
    s. nitrate solution
    s. protein
Silver-Hildreth operation
silver nitrate, toughened
silver-wire
    s.-w. arteriole
    s.-w. reflex
    s.-w. vessels
Simcoe
    S. anterior chamber capsule
    scrubber
    S. aspirating needle
    S. corneal marker
    S. double cannula
    S. double-end lens loupe
    S. I&A system
    S. II PC aspirating needle
    S. II PC double cannula
    S. II PC lens
    S. II PC nucleus delivery
    loupe
    S. interchangeable tip
    S. irrigation-aspiration
    system
    S. lens
    S. lens implant forceps
    S. lens-inserting forceps
    S. lens positioning set
    S. loupe
    S. needle
    S. notched spatula
    S. nucleus delivery loupe
    S. nucleus erysiphake
    S. nucleus forceps
    S. nucleus lens loupe
    S. posterior chamber lens
    forceps
    S. reverse aperture cannula
    S. reverse irrigating-
    aspirating cannula
    S. speculum
    S. suture needle
    S. wire speculum
Simmonds' disease
Simmons
    occult temporal arteritis
    of S.
simple
    s. acute conjunctivitis
    s. astigmatism
    s. color
    s. conjunctivitis

simple *(continued)*
>   s. diplopia
>   s. episcleritis
>   s. glaucoma
>   s. heterochromia
>   s. hyperopic astigmatism
>   s. myopia
>   s. myopic astigmatism
>   s. optic atrophy
>   s. retinitis

simplex
>   s. glaucoma
>   herpes s.

Simpson lacrimal probe
Simulantest
simultanagnosia
simultaneous
>   s. contrast
>   s. foveal perception (SFP)
>   s. macular perception (SMP)
>   s. perception
>   s. prism cover test (SPC)

Singapore epidemic conjunctivitis
single
>   s. binocular vision (SBV)
>   s. cover test

single-cut contact lens
single-mirror goniolens
sinister
>   visio oculus s.

sinistrality
sinistrocular
sinistrocularity
sinistrogyration
sinistrotorsion
Sinskey
>   S. hook
>   S. intraocular lens
>   S. lens
>   S. lens hook
>   S. lens-manipulating hook
>   S. micro iris hook
>   S. micro lens hook
>   S. micro tying forceps

Sinskey-Wilson foreign body
  forceps
sinus
>   anterior chamber s.
>   Arlt-Jaesche s.
>   Arlt's s.
>   s. catarrh
>   cavernous s.
>   s. circularis iridis

>   ethmoid s.'s
>   ethmoidal s.
>   frontal s.
>   s. headache
>   s. of Maier
>   Maier's s.
>   s. mucocele
>   paranasal s.
>   scleral venous s.
>   sphenoid s.
>   s. venosus sclera
>   venous s.'s

sinusitis
>   frontal s.
>   maxillary s.
>   paranasal s.

sinusoidal
Sipple-Gorlin syndrome
Sipple's syndrome
SITE
>   SITE gillotine cutting tip
>   SITE irrigating/aspirating
>   needle
>   SITE macrobore needle
>   SITE macrobore plus needle
>   SITE needle
>   SITE Phaco I/A needle
>   SITE TXR diaphragmatic
>   microsurgical system
>   SITE TXR 2200
>   microsurgical unit
>   SITE TXR peristaltic
>   microsurgical system
>   SITE TXR
>   phacoemulsification system
>   SITE TXR
>   phacoemulsification system

site
>   inflammatory target s.

situs inversus
sixth
>   s. cranial nerve
>   s. cranial nerve palsy
>   s. nerve palsy

size
>   eye s.
>   lens s.
>   object s.
>   pupil s.
>   relative s.
>   retinal image s.
>   spot s.

Thornton guide for optical
zone s.
Sjögren-Larsson syndrome
Sjögren's
S. disease
S. reticular dystrophy
S. syndrome
Skeele curette
Skeer's sign
skein
Holmgren's s.
test s.'s
s. test
skeletal disorder
Skeleton fine forceps
skew
s. deviation
s. pupil
skiameter
skiametry
skiascope
skiascopy bar
skiascotometry
skin
s. autograft
s. diabetes
s. disorder
s. eruption
s. flap
s. graft
s. hook
s. marking pen
s. pupillary reflex
s. test
s. wheal
s. whorl
ski needle
skirt
vitreous s.
Sklar-Schiötz tonometer
skull
exophthalmos due to
tower s.
s. temple
slab-off
s.-o. grinding
s.-o. lens
slant
antimongoloid s.
mongoloid s.
s. muscle operation
s. operation
palpebral s.

**Slant haptic single-piece
intraocular lens**
SLE
slit-lamp examination
systemic lupus erythematosus
sleeping sickness
sleeve
anterior segment s.
Charles anterior segment s.
Charles infusion s.
Charles vitrector with s.
implant s.
s. implant
s. spreading forceps
Stevens-Charles s.
Watzke s.
slide
AO Vectographic Project-O-
Chart s.
epithelial s.
Polaroid vectograph s.
sliding flap
SlimFit
S. ovoid intraocular lens
S. small-incision ovoid lens
sling
Arion's s.
fascia lata s.
fascia lata frontalis s.
frontalis muscle s.
s. for implant
s. procedure
suture s.
tarsoligamentous s.
slit illumination
slit-lamp
s.-l. biomicroscopy
s.-l. examination (SLE)
s.-l. microscope
s.-l. ophthalmoscopy
SLK
superior limbic
keratoconjunctivitis
Sloan
S. letters
S. M system
S. reading card
sloping isopters
slot
slough
conjunctival s.
slow-to-no saccade
sludging of circulation

405

sluggish movements of eyes and eyelids
Sly syndrome
small aperture Steri-Drape
SmallPort Phaco System
smallpox
Smart
　　S. forceps
　　S. scissors
Smart-Leiske cross-action intraocular lens forceps
SMD
　　senile macular degeneration
smear
　　conjunctival s.
Smith
　　S. expressor
　　S. expressor hook
　　S. Indian technique
　　S. intraocular capsular amputator
　　S. knife
　　S. lid hook
　　S. modification of Van Lint lid block
　　S. orbital floor implant
　　S. speculum
Smith-Fisher
　　S.-F. iris replacer
　　S.-F. knife
　　S.-F. spatula
Smith-Green
　　S.-G. cataract knife
　　S.-G. knife
Smith-Indian operation
Smith-Kuhnt-Szymanowski operation
Smith-Leiske cross-action intraocular lens forceps
Smith-Lemli-Optiz syndrome
Smith-Riley syndrome
Smith's
　　S. eyelid operation
　　S. modification
　　S. operation
　　S. trabeculectomy
SMP
　　simultaneous macular perception
snail tracks
snare
　　Banner enucleation s.
　　Castroviejo s.
　　Castroviejo enucleation s.

enucleation wire s.
s. enucleator
Föerster enucleation s.
Foster enucleation s.
wire enucleation s.
Snellen
　　S. conventional reform implant
　　S. entropion forceps
　　S. fraction
　　S. implant
　　S. lens loupe
　　S. letters
　　S. line
　　S. reading cards
　　S. reform eye
　　S. soft contact lens
　　S. vectis
Snellen's
　　S. chart
　　S. operation
　　S. ptosis operation
　　S. test
　　S. test types
Snell's law
Snell-Sterling's visual efficiency scale
Sno Strips
snow
　　s. blindness
　　s. conjunctivitis
　　s. glasses
snowball opacity
snowbanks
snowflake cataract
snowstorm cataract
Snugfit eye patch
Snyder corneal spring forceps
SO
　　superior oblique
Soaclens
Soak
Soakare
Soaking
　　Wetting & S.
soaking solution
socket
　　anophthalmic s.
　　contracted s.
　　s. contracture
　　s. discharge
　　s. prosthesis
　　s. reconstruction

sodium
    s. acetate
    s. benzoate
    s. bicarbonate
    s. borate
    s. carbonate
    carboxymethylcellulose s.
    s. chloride
    s. chloride in solution
    s. citrate
    s. cromoglycate
    cromolyn s.
    dantrolene s.
    diclofenac s.
    s. ethylenediaminetet-
      raacetate
    s. ethylmercurithiosalicylate
    s. fluorescein
    fluorescein s.
    flurbiprofen s.
    foscarnet s.
    ganciclovir s.
    s. hexametaphosphate
    hyaluronate s.
    s. hyaluronate
    s. hyaluronate and
      chondroitin sulfate
    s. hydroxide
    s. hypochlorite
    s. lauryl sulfate
    naproxen s.
    pentobarbital s.
    phenobarbital s.
    s. phosphate
    s. propionate
    s. salicylate
    secobarbital s.
    s. sulfacetamide
    suramin s.
    thiopental s.
    valproate s.
    warfarin s.
Sodium Sulamyd
Soemmering's
    S. crystalline swelling
    S. foramen
    S. ring
    S. ring cataract
    S. spot
SOF
    superior orbital fissure

Soflens
    S. enzymatic contact lens
      cleaner
    S. lens
Sof/Pro-Clean
soft
    s. cataract
    s. contact lens (SCL)
    s. contact lens solution
    s. drusen
    s. exudate
    s. intraocular lens
    s. lens
    s. tissue swelling
Softcon
soft-finger tension
Soft Mate
    S. M. Comfort Drops for
      Sensitive Eyes
    S. M. Consept
    S. M. daily cleaning
      solution
    S. M. disinfection and
      storage solution
    S. M. Enzyme Alternative
    S. M. Enzyme Plus cleaner
    S. M. Hands Off daily
      cleaner
    S. M. protein remover
    S. M. saline
    S. M. Saline for Sensitive
      Eyes
solani
    Fusarium s.
solar
    s. blindness
    s. burn
    s. damage
    s. keratoma
    s. keratosis
    s. maculopathy
    s. radiation
    s. retinitis
    s. retinopathy
    s. urticaria
solid
    s. color
    s. silicone with Supramid
      mesh implant
    s. vision
solium
    Taenia s.
Solu-Cortef

Solu-Medrol
Solution
  One S.
Solution
solution
  Amvisc s.
  Amvisc Plus s.
  balanced saline s. (BSS)
  balanced salt s. (BSS)
  Barnes-Hind contact lens
    cleaning and soaking s.
  Barnes-Hind wetting s.
  boric acid s.
  Boston Advance
    conditioning s.
  Boston conditioning s.
  CooperVision balanced
    salt s.
  dexamethasone s.
  disinfecting s.
  eye irrigating s.
  Eye-Sed s.
  Eye-Sine s.
  Eye-Stream s.
  Eye Wash s.
  Feldman buffer s.
  fluorescein dye and stain s.
  Freeman s.
  graft preservation s.
  Healon s.
  hydrolysis of s.
  hypertonic s.
  hypotonic s.
  Indocin ophthalmic s.
  Iocare balanced salt s.
  irrigating s.
  isotonic s.
  K Sol preservation s.
  Miochol s.
  Occucoat s.
  ophthalmic s.
  oxidation of s.
  preservatives in s.
  Ringer's lactate s.
  rose bengal red s.
  saline s.
  Sensitive Eyes
    saline/cleaning s.
  silver nitrate s.
  soaking s.
  sodium chloride in s.
  soft contact lens s.
  Soft Mate daily cleaning s.
  Soft Mate disinfection and
    storage s.
  solvent s.
  Soquette contact lens
    soaking s.
  sterility of s.
  Trump's s.
  Visalens contact lens
    cleaning and soaking s.
  Viscoat s.
  wetting s.
  zinc sulfate s.
somatic cell
Sondermann's canal
sonolucent
  acoustical s.
Sonometric Ocuscan
Soothe Eye
S.O.P.
  Bleph-10 S.O.P.
  Blephamide S.O.P.
  Chloroptic S.O.P.
  FML S.O.P.
  Genoptic S.O.P.
  Lacri-Lube S.O.P.
Soper
  S. cone contact lens
  S. cone lens
Soquette
  S. contact lens soaking
    solution
sorbate
  potassium s.
sorbic acid Sorbi-Care saline
Sorbi-Care
sorbinil
sorbitan ester
sorbitol
Soriano's operation
Soria's operation
Sorsby
  pseudoinflammatory macular
    dystrophy of S.
Sorsby's
  S. macular degeneration
  S. maculopathy
  S. pseudoinflammatory
    dystrophy
  S. pseudoinflammatory
    macular degeneration
  S. pseudoinflammatory
    macular dystrophy
  S. syndrome

SOSS-10
soul blindness
soule
sound
    lacrimal s.
Sourdille's
    S. keratoplasty
    S. keratoplasty operation
    S. ptosis operation
Southern blot technique
Sovereign bifocal lens
sowda
S&P
    sharp and pink
space
    Berger's s.
    circumlental s.
    episcleral s.
    s. of Fontana
    Fontana's s.
    intercellular s.
    interfascial s.
    interlamellar s.
    s. of iridocorneal angle
    Kuhnt's s.'s
    s. myopia
    object s.
    s. occupying lesion
    perichoroidal s.
    periscleral s.
    preseptal s.
    prezonular s.
    retrobulbar s.
    retro-ocular s.
    Schwalbe's s.
    sequestered s.'s
    subpigment epithelial s.
    subretinal s.
    Tenon's s.
    zonular s.'s
Spaeth block
Spaeth's
    S. cystic bleb operation
    S. ptosis operation
span
Spanish silk suture
Spanlang-Tappeiner syndrome
spar
    Iceland s.
sparganosis
    nodules in s.
    ocular s.

sparing
    macular s.
    pupillary s.
    recurrent pupillary s.
Sparta micro forceps
spasm
    s. of accommodation
    accommodative s.
    ciliary s.
    convergence s.
    cyclic ocular motor s.
    facial s.
    hemifacial s.
    near-reflex s.
    nictitating s.
    s. nutans
    winking s.
spasmodic
    s. mydriasis
    s. strabismus
    s. torticollis
spasmus
    s. nutans
spastic
    s. ectropion
    s. entropion
    s. lagophthalmia
    s. miosis
    s. mydriasis
    s. pseudosclerosis
spasticity of conjugate gaze
spasticum
    ectropion s.
    entropion s.
    sarcomatosum s.
spatial
    s. acuity
    s. discrimination
    s. interaction
    s. localization
    s. summation
spatium, pl. spatia
    s. episclerale
    s. interfasciale
    s. intervaginale
    s. perichoroideale
spatula
    angled iris s.
    angulated iris s.
    Bangerter iris s.
    Barraquer s.
    Barraquer irrigator s.
    Berens s.

spatula *(continued)*
  Birks Mark II s.
  Birks Mark II micro s.
  Birks Mark ts push/pull s.
  capsule fragment s.
  Castroviejo s.
  Castroviejo cyclodialysis s.
  Castroviejo double-ended s.
  Castroviejo synechia s.
  Cleasby s.
  corneal fascia lata s.
  corneal graft s.
  Culler iris s.
  cyclodialysis s.
  double s.
  Drews-Sato suture pickup s.
  Elschnig s.
  Elschnig cyclodialysis s.
  Fisher-Smith s.
  French hook s.
  French lacrimal s.
  French pattern s.
  Gills-Welsh s.
  Green s.
  Green double s.
  Green lens s.
  Green replacer s.
  Hertzog lens s.
  Hirschman s.
  s. hook
  hook s.
  iris s.
  Jaffe s.
  Jaffe intraocular s.
  Jaffe lens s.
  Katena iris s.
  Kimura s.
  Kimura platinum s.
  Kirby angulated iris s.
  Kirby iris s.
  Knapp s.
  Knapp iris s.
  Knolle lens cortex s.
  Knolle lens nucleus s.
  Laird s.
  Lindner s.
  Manhattan Eye & Ear s.
  Maumenee vitreous sweep s.
  McIntyre s.
  McPherson s.
  McReynolds s.
  microvitreoretinal s.
  needle s.

  Obstbaum lens s.
  Obstbaum synechia s.
  Olk vitreoretinal s.
  Pallin lens s.
  Paton double s.
  Paton single s.
  Paton transplant s.
  platinum s.
  platinum probe s.
  probe s.
  s. probe
  Rainen clip-bending s.
  Rainin lens s.
  Sheets lens s.
  side-biting s.
  Simcoe notched s.
  Smith-Fisher s.
  spoon s.
  s. spoon
  suture pickup s.
  synechia s.
  Tan s.
  Tooke s.
  vitreous sweep s.
  Wheeler s.
  Wheeler iris s.
spatulated needle
spatule temple
SPC
  simultaneous prism cover test
spear
  s. cataract
  s. developmental cataract
  Merocel surgical s.
  Weck-cel surgical s.
Speas' operation
special
  s. sense vertigo
  s. spectacle lens
specificity
speckled corneal dystrophy
spectacle
  s. blur
  s. correction
  s. crown
  s. frame
  s. frame pad
  s. lens
  s. plane
spectacle-induced aniseikonia
spectacles
  aphakic s.
  Bartel s.

bifocal s.
bridge of s.
cataract s.
clerical s.
compound s.
decentered s.
divers' s.
divided s.
folding s.
Franklin s.
half-glass s.
Hallauer s.
hemianopic s.
industrial s.
Masselon s.
mica s.
orthoscopic s.
pantoscopic s.
periscopic s.
photochromic s.
prism s.
prismatic s.
protective s.
ptosis crutch s.
pulpit s.
refraction s.
safety s.
stenopeic s., stenopaic s.
telescopic s.
temples of s.
tinted s.
wire frame s.
spectacular image
spectinomycin
spectra
spectral
   s. sensitivity
Spectrocin
spectrocolorimeter
spectroscopy
spectrum, pl. **spectra, spectrums**
   chromatic s.
   color s.
   electromagnetic s.
   facio-auriculovertebral s.
   fortification s.
   ocular s.
   Raman s.
   visible s.
specula
specular
   s. glare
   s. image

   s. microscope
   s. microscopy
   s. reflection
Specular reflex slit lamp
speculum, pl. **specula**
   Alfonso s.
   Azar lid s.
   Barraquer s.
   Barraquer-Colibri s.
   Barraquer wire s.
   basket-style scleral
    supporter s.
   Becker-Park s.
   Bercovici wire lid s.
   Berens s.
   Bronson-Park s.
   Burch-Lester s.
   Castallo s.
   Castroviejo s.
   Clark s.
   Cook s.
   Culler s.
   Douvas-Barraquer s.
   eye s.
   eyelid s.
   Fanta s.
   fine-wire s.
   Floyd Barraquer wire s.
   Fox s.
   Gaffee s.
   Guist s.
   Guist-Bloch s.
   Guyton-Maumenee s.
   Guyton-Park s.
   Guyton-Park eye s.
   Guyton-Park lid s.
   Hirschman s.
   Iliff-Park s.
   Jaffe lid s.
   Kaiser s.
   Keeler-Pierse s.
   Keeler-Pierse eye s.
   Keizer-Lancaster s.
   Keizer-Lancaster eye s.
   Knapp s.
   Knapp-Culler s.
   Knapp eye s.
   Knolle lens s.
   Kratz-Barraquer wire eye s.
   Lancaster eye s.
   Lancaster lid s.
   Lancaster-O'Connor s.
   Lang s.

speculum *(continued)*
  Lange s.
  Lester-Burch s.
  lid s.
  Maumenee-Park s.
  Maumenee-Park eye s.
  McKee s.
  McKinney eye s.
  McPherson s.
  Mellinger s.
  Metcher s.
  Moria one-piece s.
  Mueller s.
  Murdock eye s.
  Murdock-Wiener eye s.
  Murdoon eye s.
  Omni-Park s.
  Park s.
  Park-Guyton s.
  Park-Guyton-Callahan s.
  Park-Guyton-Maumenee s.
  Park-Maumenee s.
  Paton single s.
  Paton transplant s.
  pediatric s.
  Pierse eye s.
  Sauer s.
  Sauer infant s.
  Simcoe s.
  Simcoe wire s.
  Smith s.
  stop s.
  Sutherland-Grieshaber s.
  Weeks s.
  Weiss s.
  Wiener s.
  Williams s.
  Williams pediatric eye s.
  wire lid s.
  Ziegler s.
Spencer
  S. chalazion forceps
  S. eye suture scissors
  S. silicone subimplant
Spencer-Watson
  S.-W. operation
  S.-W. Z-plasty
  S.-W. Z-plasty operation
Spero forceps
sph.
  sphere
  spherical
  spherical lens

sphacelation
sphenoccipital fissure
sphenocephaly
sphenoethmoidalis
  sutura s.
sphenoethmoiditis
sphenofrontalis
  sutura s.
sphenofrontal suture
sphenoid
  s. bone
  greater wing of the s.
  s. meningioma
  s. sinus
  s. wing meningioma
sphenoidal fissure
sphenoidalis
  ala minor ossis s.
  foramen s.
sphenomaxillary fissure
spheno-occipital
sphenoorbitalis
  sutura s.
spheno-orbital suture
sphenorbital
sphere (sph.)
  Carter s.
  Doherty s.
  s. implant
  s. introducer
  Morgagni's s.'s
  Mules s.
  Mules vitreous s.
  Pyrex eye s.
  silicone eye s.
spherical (sph.)
  s. aberration
  s. cornea
  s. equivalent
  s. equivalent lens
  s. implant
  s. lens (S, sph.)
  s. lens aberration
  s. refraction
Spherical Twirl
spherocylinder
spherocylindrical lens
spherocylindric lens
spherocytosis
  hereditary s.
spheroid degeneration
spherolith
spherometer

spherophakia
spherophakia-brachymorphia
  syndrome
spheroprism
spherule
    rod s.
sphincter
    s. erosion
    s. fiber
    s. iridis
    iris s.
    s. muscle
    s. muscle of pupil
    s. oculi
    s. oris
    s. pupilla
    s. tear
sphincterectomy
sphincterolysis
sphincterotomy
sphingolipidoses
sphingolipidosis
sphingomyelin
    s. lipidosis
spicule
    bone s.
spider
    s. angioma
    s. telangiectasia
    s. vasculature
Spielmeyer-Sjögren disease
Spielmeyer-Stock disease
Spielmeyer-Vogt disease
spike
    blue s.
    retinal s.
spinal
    s. cord
    s. miosis
    s. mydriasis
spina trochlearis
spin-cast
    s.-c. lens
    s.-c. process
spindle
    s. A melanoma
    Axenfeld-Krukenberg s.
    s. B melanoma
    cataract s.
    s. cataract
    s. cells
    Krukenberg's s.

    Krukenberg's corneal s.
    Krukenberg's pigment s.
spindle-shaped
    s.-s. area
    s.-s. cells
spinocerebellar degeneration
spiral
    s. field
    s. of Tillaux
    Tillaux's s.
spiralis
    Trichinella s.
spirochetal disease
spirochetemia
spirochetiform cataract
Spitz's nevus
Spizziri
    S. cannula knife
    S. knife
SPK
    superficial punctate keratitis
splaytooth forceps
splenic retinitis
splenium of corpus callosum
splinter hemorrhage
split fixation
splitter
    Salz nucleus s.
split-thickness autograft
splitting
    s. of lacrimal papilla
    s. lacrimal papilla operation
    macular s.
    Minsky's intramarginal s.
    stromal s.
spoke
    cortical s.'s
spoke-like sutural cataracts
spondylitis
    ankylosing s.
spondyloarthropathy
sponge
    Custodis s.
    s. explant
    Fuller silicone s.
    grooved silicone s.
    s. implant
    implant s.
    Krukenberg s.
    lens s.
    Lincoff s.
    Lincoff lens s.
    Masciuli silicone s.

sponge *(continued)*
    Merocel s.
    micro s.
    Microsponge Teardrop s.
    ophthalmic s.
    Packer tunnel silicone s.
    Pro-Ophtha s.
    Vaiser s.
    vitrectomy s.
    Weck s.
    Weck-cel s.
spongioblast
spongy
    s. appearance
    s. iritis
spontaneous
    s. congenital iris cyst
    s. ectopia lentis
    s. hyphema
spoon
    Bunge evisceration s.
    Castroviejo lens s.
    cataract s.
    Culler lens s.
    Cutler lens s.
    Daviel lens s.
    Elschnig s.
    enucleation s.
    evisceration s.
    Fisher s.
    graft carrier s.
    Hess s.
    Kalt s.
    Kirby intracapsular lens s.
    Knapp lens s.
    lens s.
    needle s.
    s. needle
    Rizzuti graft carrier s.
    Schepens s.
    s. spatula
    spatula s.
    Wells enucleation s.
Sporothrix schenckii
sporotrichosis
spot
    acoustic s.
    ash leaf s.
    baring of blind s.
    birdshot s.
    Bitot's s.
    blank s.
    blind s.

    blue s.
    blur s.
    Brushfield's s.
    café au lait s.'s
    cherry-red s.
    cluster of pigmented s.'s
    corneal s.
    cotton-wool s.
    cribriform s.
    depigmented s.
    dry s.
    Elschnig's s.
    eye s.
    flame s.'s
    Föerster-Fuchs black s.
    Föerster's s.
    Fuchs' s.
    Fuchs' black s.
    Gaule's s.
    histo s.'s
    Horner-Trantas s.
    Mariotte's s.
    Mariotte's blind s.
    Maxwell's s.
    mongolian s.
    physiologic blind s.
    retinal blur s.
    s. retinoscope
    Roth's s.'s
    rust s.'s
    Siegrist's s.'s
    s. size
    Soemmering's s.
    Tay's s.
    Tay's cherry-red s.
    white s.
    Wies' s.
    yellow s.
S potential
spotted fever
spotty corneal opacities
Spratt mastoid curette
spreader
    Athens suture s.
    conjunctiva s.
    Costenbader incision s.
    Gill incision s.
    incision s.
    Kwitko conjunctival s.
    Suarez s.
    Wilder band s.
spread function
spreading factor

spring
    s. catarrh
    s. conjunctivitis
    s. ophthalmia
    s. pupil
spring-inge temple
springing mydriasis
Spring iris scissors
springtime conjunctivitis
spud
    Alvis s.
    Alvis foreign body s.
    Bahn s.
    Corbett s.
    curved needle eye s.
    Davis s.
    Dix s.
    Dix foreign body s.
    Ellis s.
    Ellis foreign body s.
    eye s.
    Fisher s.
    flat eye s.
    foreign body s.
    Francis s.
    Goldstein golf club s.
    golf-club s.
    golf-club eye s.
    s. gouge
    gouge s.
    Hosford s.
    LaForce s.
    LaForce knife s.
    Levine s.
    s. needle
    needle s.
    O'Brien s.
    Plange s.
    Storz folding-handle eye s.
    Walter s.
    Walton s.
spur
    Fuchs' s.
    Grunert's s.
    Michel s.
    scleral s.
spuria
    polycoria s.
spurious cataract
Spurway's syndrome
Sputnik Russian razor blade
squamous
    s. blepharitis

    s. cell
    s. cell carcinoma
    s. cell carcinoma of eyelid
    s. seborrheic blepharitis
square prism
square-wave jerks
squashed-tomato appearance
Squid instrument/apparatus
squint
    accommodative s.
    angle s.
    s. angle
    comitant s.
    convergent s.
    deviation s.
    s. deviation
    divergent s.
    downward s.
    Duane's classification of s.
    external s.
    s. hook
    internal s.
    latent s.
    noncomitant s.
    upward s.
squinting eye
squirrel plague conjunctivitis
SR
    superior rectus
SR-IV Programmed Subjective refractor
SRK formula
SRM
    subretinal membrane
SRNV
    subretinal neovascularization
SSPE
    subacute sclerosing panencephalitis
stability
    tear film s.
Stableflex anterior chamber lens
stable vision
stage
    threshold s. III of retinopathy of prematurity (TS III ROP)
Stahl
    S. caliper block
    S. caliper plate
    S. calipers
    S. lens gauge
    S. nucleus expressor

Stähli's
  S. line
  S. pigment line
stain
  acid mucopolysaccharide s.
  acid-Schiff s.
  acridine orange s.
  alcian blue s.
  alkali Congo red s.
  calcofluor white s. (CFW)
  diastase s.
  eosin s.
  fluorescent s.
  Giemsa s.
  Gram's s.
  Hansel's s.
  hematoxylin s.
  lead citrate s.
  mucicarmine s.
  port-wine s.
  rose bengal s.
  Verhoeff's s.
staining
  s. agent
  arc s.
  arcuate s.
  basophilic s.
  blotchy positive s.
  coarse punctate s.
  conjunctival s.
  corneal s.
  fluorescein s.
  immunofluorescent s.
  punctate s.
  rose bengal s.
  stippling and s.
  three o'clock s.
staining pattern
  abnormal s. p.
stalk
  optic s.
Stallard-Liegard
  S.-L. operation
  S.-L. suture
Stallard's
  S. eyelid operation
  S. flap operation
stand
  Mayo s.
standard
  s. deviation
  s. notation
  s. thickness

stand-off
  edge s.-o.
Stangel modified Barraquer microsurgical needle holder
Staphcillin
staphylococcal
  s. allergic keratoconjunctivitis
  s. blepharitis
  s. blepharoconjunctivitis
  s. conjunctivitis
  s. keratoconjunctivitis
Staphylococcus
  S. aureus
  S. bacillus
  S. epidermidis
staphylococcus
staphyloma
  annular s.
  anterior s.
  anterior corneal s.
  ciliary s.
  s. corneae racemosum
  corneal s.
  equatorial s.
  intercalary s.
  posterior s.
  s. posticum
  projecting s.
  retinal s.
  Scarpa's s.
  scleral s.
  uveal s.
staphylomatous
staphylotomy
star
  epicapsular lens s.
  s. folds
  s. formation
  s. lens
  lens s.
  macular s.
  Winslow's s.
stare
  hyperthyroid s.
  postbasic s.
  thyroid s.
starfold
Stargardt's
  S. disease
  S. maculopathy
  S. syndrome
Star-Optic Eye Wash

Starr fixation forceps
star-shaped field
startle myoclonus
starvation
stasis, pl. **stases**
    axoplasmic s.
    papillary s.
    venous s.
Stat
    S. aspirator
    S. machine
    S. Scrub handwasher
      machine
state
    deturgescent s.
    dissociative s.
    refractive s.
static
    s. perimeters
    s. perimetry
    s. refraction
stationary
    s. cataract
    s. night blindness
statistics
statometer
Statrol
status
    respiratory s.
stave
Stay-Brite
Stay-Wet
Stay-Wet 3
steal syndrome
stearate
    polyoxyl 40 s.
Steclin
Steele-Richardson-Olszewski
    S.-R.-O. disease
    S.-R.-O. syndrome
steep contact lens
steepest meridian
Stefan's law
Steiger's curves
Steinhauser electromucotome
Stelazine
stella
    s. lentis hyaloidea
    s. lentis iridica
stellata
    retinitis s.

stellate
    s. cataract
    s. retinopathy
Stellwag's
    S. brawny edema
    S. sign
    S. symptom
stem
    brain s.
    s. cell
    s. palsy
stenochoria
stenocoriasis
stenopeic, stenopaic
    s. disk
    s. iridectomy
    s. spectacles
stenophotic
stenosal
stenosed
stenosis
    s. canaliculus
    carotid artery s.
    lacrimal punctal s.
    punctal s.
    punctum s.
stenotic
Stenstrom's ocular measurements
stent
    lacrimal s.
    lacrimal s.
step
    corneal graft s.
    s. graft operation
    nasal s.
    Ronne's nasal s.
Stephenson needle holder
Step-Knife diamond blade knife
step-ramp
stepwise fashion
Sterane
Sterapred
stereo
    s. acuity
    s. campimeter
stereoacuity
stereocampimeter
    Lloyd s.
stereognostic sense
stereogram
    random dot s.
stereo-identical point
stereo-ophthalmoscope

stereo-orthopter
stereophantoscope
stereophorometer
stereophoroscope
stereophotography
stereopsis
    Gross s.
    macular s.
    s. test
stereoscope
stereoscopic
    s. acuity
    s. diplopia
    s. parallax
    s. vision
stereoscopy
stereo test
Steri-Drape
    S.-D. drape
    3M small aperture S.-D.
    small aperture S.-D.
sterile
    s. adhesive bubble chamber
    s. adhesive bubble dressing
    s. corneal ulcer
    s. endophthalmitis
    s. melt
    polymyxin B sulfate s.
sterility of solution
sterilization
Steriseal disposable cannula
Steri-Strips
Stern-Castroviejo
    S.-C. forceps
    S.-C. locking forceps
    S.-C. suturing forceps
Sterofrin
    Isopto S.
steroid
    s. diabetes
    s. glaucoma
    s. therapy
steroid-induced
    s.-i. cataract
    s.-i. glaucoma
steroidogenic diabetes
Stevens
    S. eye scissors
    S. forceps
    S. hook
    S. iris forceps
    S. lacrimal retractor
    S. needle holder

    S. tenotomy hook
    S. tenotomy scissors
Stevens-Charles sleeve
Stevens-Johnson syndrome
Stevenson
    S. lacrimal sac retractor
    S. refractor
stick
    hockey s.
    needle s.
    Pro-Ophtha s.
Stickler's syndrome
sties
Stifel's figure
stiff
    s. folds
    s. pupil
    s. retina
    s. retinal fold
stigmatic
    s. image
    s. lens
stigmatometer
stigmatometric test card
stigmatoscope
stigmatoscopy
Stiles-Crawford effect
stiletto
    Berkeley Bioengineering s.
    Blair s.
    s. knife
stillicidium lacrimarum
Stilling
    canal of S.
Stilling's
    S. color tables
    S. color test
Stilling-Turk-Duane syndrome
Still's disease
Stimson's sign
stimulation
    bithermal caloric s.
    Ganzfeld s.
stimulator
    CAM s.
    Optokinetic s.
stimulatory antibody
stimulus, pl. stimuli
    s. deprivation
    flicker-fusion s.
    light s.
    optokinetic s.
    Vernier s.

sting
    bee s.
stippling
    s. and staining
stitch
    bow-tie s.
    cuticular s.
    s.-removal forceps
    s.-removing knife
    shoelace s.
    triple-throw square knot s.
    s. with twists
    zipper s.
St. Martin-Franceschetti cataract hook
Stocker-Holt dystrophy
Stocker-Holt-Schneider dystrophy
Stocker needle
Stocker's
    S. line
    S. operation
Stock's operation
Stock-Spielmeyer-Vogt syndrome
Stokes lens
stone
    tear s.
Stone implant
Stone-Jordan implant
stony-hard eye
stop
    Bowman needle s.
    Castroviejo corneal scissors
      with inside s.
    s. speculum
stopcock
    three-way s.
storage
    wet s.
Storz
    S. band
    S. calipers
    S. capsule forceps
    S. cataract knife
    S. cilia forceps
    S. corneal bur
    S. corneal forceps
    S. corneoscleral punch
    S. folding-handle eye spud
    S. keratome
    S. keratometer
    S. lid plate
    S. magnet
    S. microscope

    S. Microvit magnet
    S. Microvit vitrector
    S. tonometer
Storz-Atlas
    S.-A. hand eye magnet
    S.-A. hand magnet
    S.-A. magnet
Storz-Bell erysiphake
Storz-Bonn suturing forceps
Storz-Duredge steel cataract knife
Storz-Utrata forceps
Storz-Walker retinal detachment unit
Storz-Westcott conjunctival scissors
Stoxil
strabismal, strabismic
strabismometer
strabismus
    A-s.
    absolute s.
    accommodative s.
    alternate day s.
    alternating s.
    A-pattern s.
    Bielschowsky's s.
    bilateral s.
    binocular s.
    Braid's s.
    cicatricial s.
    comitant s.
    concomitant s.
    constant s.
    convergent s.
    cyclic s.
    s. deorsum vergens
    s. divergence
    divergent s.
    dynamic s.
    external s.
    s. fixus
    s. forceps
    s. hook
    incomitant s.
    incomitant vertical s.
    intermittent s.
    internal s.
    kinetic s.
    latent s.
    manifest s.
    mechanical s.
    mixed s.
    monocular s.
    monolateral s.

strabismus *(continued)*
>muscular s.
>noncomitant s.
>nonconcomitant s.
>nonparalytic s.
>paralytic s.
>periodic s.
>relative s.
>s. scissors
>spasmodic s.
>suppressed s.
>s. surgery
>s. sursum vergens
>unilateral s.
>uniocular s.
>variable s.
>vertical s.
>X-s.

strabometer
strabometry
strabotome
strabotomy
straightening
>arteriole s.

straight-eyed patient
straight-line bifocal
straight temple
Straith's
>S. eyelid operation
>S. operation

Strampelli
>S. implant
>S. lens
>S. lens implant

Strampelli-Valvo operation
strand
>glassine s.'s
>mucin s.'s
>mucous-like s.'s
>stromal s.'s
>vitreous s.'s

strap
>Velcro head s.

stratified
stratum
>s. cerebrale retinae

strawberry
>s. hemangioma
>s. nevus

streak
>angioid s.
>angioid retinal s.'s
>Knapp's s.

>lightning s.'s
>Moore's lightning s.
>s. retinoscope
>s. retinoscopy
>Siegrist's s.
>Verhoeff's s.

Streatfield-Fox operation
Streatfield-Snellen operation
Streatfield's operation
strephosymbolia
streptococcal
>s. bacillus
>s. blepharitis

Streptococcus
>*S. faecalis*
>*S. pneumoniae*
>*S. pyogenes*
>*S. viridans*

streptococcus, pl. streptococci
>β-hemolytic s.

streptokinase
streptomycin
streptotrichosis
stretch reflex
stria, gen. and pl. striae
>concentric s.
>corneal s.
>Haab's striae
>Knapp's striae
>striae retinae
>vertical s.

striascope
striatal nigral degeneration
striate
>s. cortex
>s. keratitis
>s. keratopathy
>s. melanokeratosis
>s. opacities
>s. retinitis
>s. visual cortex

striated glasses
striation
striatum
string of pearl
strip
>gliotic s.
>marginal tear s.
>s. procedure
>reagent s.'s
>silicone s.
>tear s.

stripe
    central reflex s.
stripper
    Crawford s.
    Crawford fascial s.
    fascia lata s.
    zonular s.
    zonule s.
stripping
    cortical s.
    s. membrane
Strips
    Sno S.
strips
    Schirmer s.
stroboscopic disk
stroma
    corneal s.
    iris s.
    s. of iris
    pigmented s.
    s. plexus
    sclerotic s.
    vitreous s.
    s. vitreum
stromal
    s. bed
    s. blood vessel
    s. corneal dystrophy
    s. disease
    s. dystrophy
    s. edema
    s. haze
    s. keratitis
    s. keratouveitis
    s. line
    s. matrix
    s. melt
    s. mucopolysaccharide
    s. necrosis
    s. neovascularization
    s. opacities
    s. splitting
    s. strands
    s. thickness
    s. ulcer
    s. vascularization
Stromberg's curves
Strow corneal forceps
Struble
    S. everter
    S. lid everter

structure
    angle s.
    Kolmer's crystalloid s.
strumous ophthalmia
strychnine
Stryker
    S. frame
    S. saw
Study
    Early Treatment Diabetic
        Retinopathy S. (ETDRS)
study
    case-control s.
    cohort s.
    double-blind s.
    family s.
    prospective s.
    retrospective s.
    vectographic s.
Sturge-Weber
    S.-W. disease
    S.-W. syndrome
Sturge-Weber-Dimitri syndrome
Sturm
    conoid of S.
    interval of S.
Sturm's
    S. conoid
    S. interval
stuttering velocities
stutzeri
        Pseudomonas s.
sty, stye, pl. **sties, styes**
    meibomian s.
    zeisian s.
Style S2 clear-loop lens
styrene contact lenses
Suarez spreader
Suarez-Villafranca operation
subacute sclerosing panencephalitis
    (SSPE)
subarachnoid
    s. bleed
    s. fluid
    s. hemorrhage
subcapsular
    s. cataract
    s. epithelium
    s. plaque
subchoroidal
subclinical diabetes
Subco needle

subconjunctival
  s. cyst
  s. edema
  s. emphysema
  s. hemorrhage
  s. injection
  s. needle
subconjunctivally
subconjunctivitis
subcortical alexia
subcutaneous fat atrophy
subduct
subduction
subdural hematoma
subendothelial
subepithelial
  s. keratitis
  s. nevus
  s. plexus
  s. punctate corneal infiltrate
subepithelialis
  keratitis punctata s.
subfoveal
subhyaloid hemorrhage
subimplant
  Spencer silicone s.
subinternal
subjective
  s. refraction test
  s. refractor
  s. vertigo
  s. vision
Subjective Autorefractor-7
subjectoscope
subjunctival hemorrhage
sublatio retinae
subluxated lens
subluxation
  s. of lens
subluxed lens
subnormal
  s. accommodation
  s. vision
suboptimal vision
suborbital
subperiosteal
  s. abscess
  s. implant
subpigment epithelial space
subretinal
  s. fluid
  s. fluid drainage
  s. hemorrhage

  s. membrane (SRM)
  s. neovascularization
    (SRNV)
  s. neovascular membrane
  s. space
subscleral
subsclerotic
subsector
substance
  corneal s.
  s. exophthalmos
  exophthalmos-producing s.
    (EPS)
  s. of lens
  s. P
  scleral s.
  toxic s.
substantia
  s. corticalis lentis
  s. lentis
  s. propria
  s. propria corneae
substrate
  anatomic s.
subtotal thyroidectomy
subvolution
Sucaryl
successive contrast
succinate
  ferrous s.
succinylcholine
succinylsulfathiazole
succulent vessel
Succus Cineraria Maritima
suction
  s. ophthalmodynamometer
  perilimbal s.
  s. trephine
  Vactro perilimbal s.
sudoriferous cyst
sugar cataract
sugar-induced cataract
sugar-loaf cornea
Suker's sign
Sulamyd
  Sodium S.
sulcus
  chiasmal s.
  ciliary s.
  corneoscleral s.
  s. fixated position
  s. fixation
  s. infraorbitalis maxillae

infrapalpebral s.
s. infrapalpebralis
intramarginal s.
lacrimal s.
optic s.
orbital s.
s. orbitales lobi frontalis
s. sclera
scleral s.
sclerocorneal s.
s. support
supraorbital s.
Sulf-10
Sulfacel 15
sulfacetamide
sodium s.
Sulfacort
sulfadiazine
sulfadimethoxine
sulfa drug
Sulfair 10
Sulfair Forte
sulfamethizole
sulfamethoxypyridazine
Sulfamide
sulfasalazine
Sulfasuxidine
Sulfate
Eserine S.
Plaquenil S.
sulfate
alkyl ether s.
atropine s.
chondroitin s.
dermatan s.
dimethyl s.
ferrous s.
heparan s.
hydroxychloroquine s.
keratan s.
neomycin s.
phenelzine s.
physostigmine s.
polymyxin B s.
quinine s.
sodium hyaluronate and
chondroitin s.
sodium lauryl s.
tranylcypromine s.
zinc s.
sulfide
selenium s.
sulfisoxazole

sulfite
sulfonamide
s. and decongestant
combination
s. and steroid combination
sulfonylurea
sulfur (S)
s. dioxide
s. gas
s. hexafluoride
sulfuric acid
sulindac
Sulphrin
Sulpred
Sulten-10
summation
spatial s.
Summerskill's operation
Sumycin
sunburst
black s.
s. dial
s. dial chart
s. effect
sunburst-type lesions
sunflower cataract
sunglasses
sunlight
sunrise syndrome
sunset syndrome
Superblade
Bishop-Harman S.
S. No. 75 blade
S. trapezoid
supercilia
superciliaris
arcus s.
superciliary
s. arch
s. muscle
supercilii
musculus corrugator s.
musculus depressor s.
supercilium
superduct
superduction
superficial
s. congestion
s. corneal line
s. keratectomy
s. keratitis
s. keratopathy
s. lamellar keratoplasty

superficial *(continued)*
  s. linear keratitis
  s. line of cornea
  s. punctate keratitis (SPK)
  s. punctate keratopathy
  s. reticular degeneration of Koby
superficialis
  keratitis ramificata s.
  xerosis s.
superimposition
superior
  s. arcade
  s. arcuate bundle
  s. arcuate scotoma
  arcus palpebralis s.
  arteriola macularis s.
  arteriola nasalis retinae s.
  arteriola temporalis retinae s.
  s. canaliculus
  s. cervical ganglion
  s. colliculus
  s. commissura of Meynert
  s. conjunctival fornix
  s. eyelid crease
  fissura orbitalis s.
  s. fornix
  glandula lacrimalis s.
  s. homonymous quadrantic defect
  s. lacrimal gland
  s. limbic keratoconjunctivitis (SLK)
  s. macular arteriole
  s. muscle
  musculus tarsalis s.
  s. myokymia
  s. nasal artery
  s. nasal vein
  s. oblique (SO)
  s. oblique extraocular muscles
  s. oblique muscle
  s. oblique myokymia
  s. oblique palsy
  s. oblique tendon
  s. oblique tendon sheath syndrome
  s. ophthalmic vein
  s. orbital fissure (SOF)
  s. orbital fissure syndrome
  s. palpebra

  s. palpebral furrow
  s. palpebral vein
  s. palsy
  s. pole
  s. polioencephalitis
  s. punctum
  s. quadrantanopsia
  s. radial tenotomy scissors
  s. rectus (SR)
  s. rectus extraocular muscles
  s. rectus forceps
  s. rectus muscle
  s. sector iridectomy
  s. tarsal muscle
  s. tarsus
  s. tarsus palpebrae
  s. temporal artery
  s. temporal vein
  temporal venulae retina s.
  s. tendon of Lockwood
  s. tendon sheath syndrome
  s. vascular arcade
  s. vena cava
  s. vena cava syndrome
  vena ophthalmica s.
  venula macularis s.
  venula nasalis retinae s.
  venula temporalis retinae s.
  s. zone of retina
superiores
  venae palpebrales s.
superioris
  levator palpebrae s.
  musculus levator palpebrae s.
superoccipital
superonasal
superonasally
Super Pinky ball
supersensitivity
  denervation s.
supertraction
  conus s.
  s. conus
superversion
supply
  vascular s.
support
  capsular s.
  iris s.
  Schillinger suture s.
  sulcus s.

supporter
  scleral s.
suppressed
  s. amblyopia
  s. strabismus
suppression
  s. amblyopia
  central s.
  facultative s.
  macular s.
  obligatory s.
  s. scotoma
suppressor T cell
suppuration
suppurativa
  hyalitis s.
suppurative
  s. choroiditis
  s. hyalitis
  s. keratitis
  s. retinitis
  s. ulcer
suprachoroid
  s. lamina
  s. layer
suprachoroidal hemorrhage
suprachoroidea
  lamina s.
supraciliary canal
supraduction
Supramid
  S. bridle collagen suture
  S. implant
  S. lens implant
  S. lens implant suture
  S. sheet
  S. suture
Supramid-Allen implant
supranuclear
  s. cataract
  s. control
  s. deviation
  s. disorder
  s. ocular palsy
  s. pathway
supraocular
supraoptic
  s. canal
  s. commissure
supraorbital
  s. akinesia
  s. arch
  s. arch of frontal bone

  s. artery
  s. canal
  s. foramen
  s. incisure
  s. margin of frontal bone
  s. margin of orbit
  s. nerve
  s. neuralgia
  s. notch
  s. point
  s. reflex
  s. ridge
  s. sulcus
  s. vein
supraorbitale
  foramen s.
supraorbitalis
  incisura s.
  nervus s.
suprascleral
suprasellar
  s. aneurysm
  s. meningioma
  s. tumor
**supratentorial arteriovenous
  malformation**
supratrochlear nerve
supravergence
supraversion
suprofen
suramin sodium
Surefit AC 85J lens
surface
  s. analgesia
  s. breakdown
  concave reflecting s.
  convex reflecting s.
  curved reflecting s.
  s. ectoderm
  ellipsoidal back s.
  s. implant
  s. irregularity
  Petzval s.
  reflecting s.
  toric s.
  s. wrinkling retinopathy
surfactant
  anionic s.
  ionic s.
  nonionic s.
Surgamid
surgery
  antiglaucoma s.

surgery *(continued)*
asymmetric s.
cataract s.
ciliodestructive s.
closed s.
closed-eye s.
corneal s.
cranio-orbital s.
decompressive s.
eye s.
eyelid s.
eye muscle s.
filtration s.
fistulizing s.
glaucoma s.
lacrimal s.
laser s.
laser-filtering s.
orbital s.
retinal s.
strabismus s.
symmetric s.
visco s.
vitreous s.
Surg-E-Trol
S.-E.-T. I/A/R System
S.-E.-T. System
irrigating/aspirating unit
surgical
s. calipers
s. gut suture
s. keratometry
s. marking pen
s. patch grafting
Surgicraft suture needle
Surgidev
S. intraocular lens
S. lens
S. PC BUV 20-24
intraocular lens
S. suture
Surgikos
S. disposable drape
S. drape
SurgiMed suture
SurgiScope
Marco S.
Surgisol
surplus field
sursumduction
alternating s.

sursumvergence
left s.
right s.
sursumversion
suspension
hydrocortisone s.
suspensory
s. ligament
s. ligament eye
Sus-Phrine
Sussman four-mirror gonioscope
sustentacular
s. fiber
s. tissue
Sutherland
S. lens
S. Rotatable Microsurgery
instruments
S. scissors
Sutherland-Grieshaber
S.-G. scissors
S.-G. speculum
sutura
s. ethmoidolacrimalis
s. ethmoidomaxillaris
s. frontolacrimalis
s. infraorbitalis
s. lacrimoconchalis
s. lacrimomaxillaris
s. palatoethmoidalis
s. palatomaxillaris
s. sphenoethmoidalis
s. sphenofrontalis
s. sphenoorbitalis
sutural
s. cataract
s. developmental cataract
suture
absorbable s.
adjustable s.
Alcon s.
anchor s.
anchoring s.
Arroyo encircling s.
Arruga encircling s.
Atraloc s.
16-bite nylon s.
black braided s.
black braided nylon s.
black braided silk s.
black silk sling s.
braided silk s.
braided Vicryl s.

bridge s.
bridle s.
buried s.
canaliculus rod and s.
cardinal s.
catgut s.
chromic s.
chromic catgut s.
chromic collagen s.
chromic gut s.
clove-hitch s.
coated Vicryl s.
compression s.
s. of cornea operation
Custodis s.
Dacron s.
Davis-Geck s.
Deknatel silk s.
Dermalon s.
Dexon s.
double-armed s.
Ethicon s.
Ethicon-Atraloc s.
Ethicon micropoint s.
Ethicon Sabreloc s.
s. of eyeball operation
Faden s.
fetal Y s.'s
figure-of-eight s.
fixation s.
Foster s.
frontolacrimal s.
frontosphenoid s.
Frost s.
Gaillard-Arlt s.
groove s.
guy s.
Guyton-Friedenwald s.
horizontal mattress s.
infraorbital s.
interrupted nylon s.
intracameral s.
iris s.
s. of iris operation
lacrimoconchal s.
lacrimoethmoidal s.
lacrimomaxillary s.
lacrimoturbinal s.
lancet s.
s. lancet
s. of lens
Look s.
Mannis s.

mattress s.
McCannel s.
McLean s.
Mersilene s.
micropoint s.
mild chromic s.
monofilament nylon s.
s. of muscle operation
nonabsorbable s.
Nurulon s.
nylon s.
nylon 66 s.
Ophthalon s.
palatomaxillary s.
s. pickup hook
pickup spatula s.
s. pickup spatula
plain catgut s.
plain collagen s.
plain gut s.
Polydek s.
polyester s.
polyglactin s.
polyglycolic acid s.
posterior fixation s.
preplaced s
Prolene s.
Quickert s.
running nylon s.
scleral flap s.
s. of sclera operation
Shoch s.
silk traction s.
s. sling
Spanish silk s.
sphenofrontal s.
spheno-orbital s.
Stallard-Liegard s.
Supramid s.
Supramid bridle collagen s.
Supramid lens implant s.
surgical gut s.
Surgidev s.
SurgiMed s.
Swiss silk s.
Tevdek s.
traction s.
twisted virgin silk s.
Verhoeff s.
Vicryl s.
virgin silk s.
white braided silk s.

suture *(continued)*
    Worst s.
    Y s.
suturing
    s. of eyelid
    s. forceps
    s. needle
Svedberg unit (S)
Swan
    S. discission knife
    S. incision
    S. knife
    S. lancet
    S. needle
Swan-Jacob gonioprism
Swan's
    S. syndrome
sweat gland
sweating
    gustatory s.
sweep
    Barraquer s.
    eye s.
    iris s.
sweeper
    Ticho zonule s.
Sweet
    S. locator
    S. original magnet
Sweet's method
swelling
    s. of disk
    Soemmering's crystalline s.
    soft tissue s.
Swets goniotomy knife cannula
swimming pool conjunctivitis
Swim'n Clear
swinging
    s. flashlight sign
    s. flashlight test
    s. light test
Swiss
    S. bladebreaker
    S. silk suture
switching
    Q s.
sycosiform
sycosis tarsi
Sydenham's chorea
syllabic blindness

Sylva
    S. anterior chamber
      irrigator
    S. irrigating/aspirating unit
Sylvian's aqueduct syndrome
symblepharon
    anterior s.
    posterior s.
    s. ring
    total s.
symblepharopterygium
symmetric surgery
sympathetic
    s. heterochromia
    s. inhibitor
    s. iridoplegia
    s. iritis
    s. nervous system
    s. ophthalmia
    s. pathway
    s. uveitis
sympathica
    ptosis s.
sympathizer
sympathizing eye
sympatholytic
sympathomimetic agent
symptom
    afferent visual s.
    Anton's s.
    Berger's s.
    Epstein's s.
    Haenel's s.
    halo s.
    Liebreich's s.
    Magendie's s.
    rainbow s.
    Stellwag's s.
    Wernicke's s.
symptomatic blepharospasm
synaphymenitis
synapse
synaptic
    s. connection
    s. ribbon
    s. ridge
synathroisis
syncanthus
synchesis
    s. corporis vitrei
    s. scintillans
synchysis
    s. scintillans

syndectomy
syndermatotic cataract
syndesmitis
syndrome
13q- s.
4p- s.
9p- s.
A s.
Aarskog s.
Aase s.
accommodative effort s.
acquired
  immunodeficiency s.
  (AIDS)
acute retinal necrosis s.
adherence s.
adhesive s.
Adie's s.
Ahlström's s.
Aicardi's s.
Albright's s.
Alezzandrini's s.
Alport's s.
Alström-Hallgren s.
Alström-Olsen s.
Alström's s.
Andersen's s.
Andosky's s.
Angelucci's s.
anterior chamber cleavage s.
anterior cleavage s.
Antley-Bixler s.
Anton-Babinski s.
Anton's s.
aortic arch s.
Apert's s.
arteriovenous strabismus s.
Ascher's s.
ataxia-telangiectasia s.
AV strabismus s.
Axenfeld's s.
Backhaus' s.
Balint's s.
Baller-Gerold s.
Bamatter's s.
Bardet-Biedl s.
bare lymphocyte s.
Barlow's s.
Baron-Bietti s.
Bartholin s.
basal cell nevus s.
Bassen-Kornzweig s.
Batten-Mayou s.

Batten's s.
battered-baby s.
battered-child s.
Béal's s.
Behçet's s.
Behr's s.
Benedikt's s.
Bernard-Horner s.
Bernard's s.
Bielschowsky-Jansky s.
Bielschowsky-Lutz-Cogan s.
Biemond's s.
Bietti's s.
big blind spot s.
blepharophimosis s.
blepharophimosis ptosis s.
blind spot s.
Bloch-Stauffer s.
Bloch-Sulzberger s.
Bonnet-Dechaume-Blanc s.
Bonnier's s.
brachial arch s.
brittle cornea s.
broad thumbs and broad
  toes s.
Brown-McLean s.
Brown's s.
Brown's tendon sheath s.
Brown's vertical
  retraction s.
Brushfield-Wyatt s.
capsular exfoliation s.
CAR s.
Carpenter's s.
cataract with Down s.
cat's cry s.
cat's eye s.
cavernous sinus s.
central scotoma s.
cerebrohepatorenal s.
cervico-oculo-acoustic s.
Cestan-Chenais s.
Cestan's s.
Chandler's s.
CHARGE s.
Charles-Bonnet s.
Charlin's s.
Chédiak-Higashi s.
cherry-red spot
  myoclonus s.
chiasma s.
chiasmal s.
chiasmatic s.

syndrome *(continued)*

    Churg-Strauss s.
    Claude-Bernard-Horner s.
    Claude's s.
    cleavage s.
    cleft s.
    Cockayne's s.
    co-contraction s.
    Coffin-Lowry s.
    Cogan-Reese s.
    Cogan's s.
    Cohen's s.
    Collins' s.
    congenital fibrous s.
    congenital rubella s.
    Conn s.
    Conradi's s.
    contact lens overwearing s.
    Cornelia de Lange s.
    cranial stenosis s.
    craniofacial s.
    CREST s.
    cri du chat s.
    Crouzon's s.
    Cushing's s.
    cutaneomucouveal s.
    DAF s.
    D chromosome ring s.
    Degos' s.
    DeGrouchy's s.
    DeJean's s.
    de Lange's s.
    DeMosier's s.
    diencephalic s.
    dispersion s.
    dorsal midbrain s.
    Down s.
    Doyne's s.
    Drews s.
    dry eye s.
    D trisomy s.
    Duane's s.
    Duane's retraction s.
    dural shunt s.
    dyscephalic s.
    E s.
    Eaton-Lambert s.
    Edwards' s.
    Ehlers-Danlos s.
    Ellingson's s.
    Elschnig's s.
    embryonic fixation s.
    empty sella s.

    exfoliation s.
    Fabry's s.
    Falls-Kertesz s.
    Fanconi's s.
    fetal alcohol s.
    fetal hydantoin s.
    fetal trimethadione s.
    fetal warfarin s.
    fibrosis s.
    Fiessinger-Leroy-Reiter s.
    Fisher's s.
    Fitz-Hugh-Curtis s.
    flaccid canaliculus s.
    flecked retina s.
    floppy eyelid s.
    Foix's s.
    Forsius-Eriksson s.
    Forssman's carotid s.
    Foster Kennedy's s.
    Foville's s.
    Foville-Wilson s.
    Franceschetti-Klein s.
    Franceschetti's s.
    François s.
    Fraser's s.
    Freeman-Sheldon s.
    Frenkel's anterior ocular
      traumatic s.
    Frey's s.
    Friedenwald's s.
    Friedreich's s.
    Fuchs' s.
    Fuchs-Kraupa s.
    Gardner's s.
    Gerstmann's s.
    Goldberg's s.
    Goldenhar's s.
    Goldmann-Favre s.
    Goltz s.
    Goltz-Gorlin s.
    Gradenigo's s.
    Graefe's s.
    Greig's s.
    Grönblad-Strandberg s.
    Gruber's s.
    Guillain-Barré s.
    Gunn's s.
    Hagberg-Santavuori s.
    Hallermann-Streiff s.
    Hallermann-Streiff-
      Francois s.
    Hallervorden-Spatz s.
    Hallgren's s.

Haltia-Santavuori type of
Batten's s.
Harada's s.
Hay-Wells s.
Heerfordt's s.
Heidenhaim's s.
hereditary benign
intraepithelial s.
hereditary benign
intraepithelial
dyskeratosis s.
heredodegenerative
neurologic s.
heredogenerative
neurologic s.
Hermansky-Pudlak s.
Hertwig-Magendie s.
HHH s.
Hippel-Lindau s.
histoplasmosis s.
Holmes-Adie s.
Holt-Oram s.
Homén's s.
Horner-Bernard s.
Horner's s.
Horton's s.
Hunter-Hurler s.
Hunter's s.
Hurler's s.
Hurler-Scheie s.
Hutchinson's s.
hyperophthalmopathic s.
hyperviscosity s.
hypoxic eyeball s.
ICE s.
internal capsule s.
iridocorneal endothelial s.
iridocorneal endothelial s.
(ICE)
iridocyclitis masquerade s.
iridoendothelial s.
iris-nevus s.
iris retraction s. of
Campbell
Irvine-Gass s.
ischemic chiasmal s.
ischemic ocular s.
Jacod's s.
Jahnke's s.
Jansky-Bielschowsky s.
jaw-winking s.
Jeune s.
Johnson's s.

Kasabach-Merritt s.
Kearns-Sayre s.
Kennedy's s.
Kiloh-Nevin s.
Kimmelstiel-Wilson s.
Klinefelter's s.
Klippel-Feil s.
Klippel-Trenaunay-Weber s.
Koeppe's s.
Koerber-Salus-Elschnig s.
Krause's s.
Kufs' s.
Kurz's s.
Langer-Giedion
trichorhinophalangeal s.
lateral medullary s.
Laurence-Biedl s.
Laurence-Moon s.
Laurence-Moon-Bardet-
Biedl s.
Laurence-Moon-Biedl s.
Lawford's s.
Leber's s.
Lenz's s.
LEOPARD s.
Letterer-Siwe s.
Lignac-Fanconi s.
Lofgren's s.
Louis-Bar s.
Lowe's s., Lowe-Terrey-
MacLachlan s.
Lowe's oculocerebrorenal s.
Lyle's s.
Magendie-Hertwig s.
malabsorption s.
malignant external otitis s.
Marchesani's s.
Marcus Gunn s.
Marcus Gunn jaw-
winking s.
Marfan's s.
Marinesco-Sjögren s.
Maroteaux-Lamy s.
Marshall s.
masquerade s.
Meckel-Gruber s.
Meigs' s.
Melkersson-Rosenthal s.
Melkersson's s.
Menière's s.
Menkes' s.
microtropic s.
Mieten's s.

syndrome *(continued)*
    Mikulicz's s.
    milk-alkali s.
    Millard-Gubler s.
    Miller-Fisher s.
    Miller's s.
    Milles' s.
    Möbius' s.
    Monakow's s.
    monofixation s.
    monosomy G s.
    morning glory s.
    Morquio-Brailsford s.
    Morquio's s.
    multiple evanescent white
      dot s. (MEWDS)
    multiple lentigines s.
    myasthenia s.
    myasthenia-like s.
    Naegeli's s.
    Nager's s.
    nail-patella s.
    nephrotic s.
    neurodegenerative s.
    neuroleptic malignant s.
    neurologic s.
    Nezelof s.
    Nieden's s.
    Noonan's s.
    Norman-Wood s.
    Nothnagel's s.
    nystagmus blockage s.
    ocular histoplasmosis s.
    ocular ischemic s.
    ocularmucous membrane s.
    oculobuccogenital s.
    oculocerebral s.
    oculocerebrorenal s.
    oculocutaneous s.
    oculoglandular s.
    oculopharyngeal s.
    oculorenal s.
    OMM s.
    one and one-half s.
    optic tract s.
    orbital s.
    orbital apex s.
    Osler-Rendu-Weber s.
    Ota's nevus s.
    overwear s. (OWS)
    Pallister-Hall s.
    Pancoast s.
    Pancoast superior sulcus s.

    parasellar s.
    Parinaud-plus s.
    Parinaud's s.
    Parinaud's oculoglandular s.
    Parry-Romberg s.
    Patau's s.
    periaqueductal s.
    Petzetakis-Takos s.
    Peutz-Jeghers s.
    Pierre Robin s.
    pigmentary dispersion s.
    plateau iris s.
    Posner-Schlossman s.
    posterior inferior cerebellar
      artery s.
    Potter's s.
    Prader-Willi s.
    presumed ocular
      histoplasmosis s. (POHS)
    pretectal s.
    pseudoexfoliation s.
    pseudo-Foster Kennedy's s.
    pseudopresumed ocular
      histoplasmosis s.
    Raeder's s.
    Raeder's paratrigeminal s.
    rainbow s.
    Ramsay Hunt s.
    Raymond-Cestan s.
    Recklinghausen's s.
    red-eyed shunt s.
    Reese's s.
    Reiger's s.
    Reiter's s.
    restrictive s.
    retinal necrosis s.
    retraction s.
    Richner-Hanhart s.
    Riddoch's s.
    Rieger's s.
    Riley-Day s.
    Riley-Smith s.
    Ring's D chromosome s.
    Roaf's s.
    Robinow's s.
    Robin's s.
    Rollet's s.
    Romberg's s.
    Roth-Bielschowsky s.
    Rothmund's s., Rothmund-
      Thomson s.
    Roth's spot s.
    Rubinstein-Taybi s.

Russell's s.
Rutherford's s.
Sanchez-Salorio s.
Sanfilippo's s.
scalded skin s.
Schäfer's s.
Scheie's s.
Schirmer's s.
Schmid-Fraccaro s.
Schwartz s.
Senior-Loken s.
septo-optic dysplasia s.
Sézary's s.
Shea's s.
sheath s.
Sheehan's s.
Shprintzen s.
Shy-Drager s.
sicca s.
Siegrist-Hutchinson s.
Sipple-Gorlin s.
Sipple's s.
Sjögren-Larsson s.
Sjögren's s.
Sly s.
Smith-Lemli-Optiz s.
Smith-Rilcy s.
Sorsby's s.
Spanlang-Tappeiner s.
spherophakia-
  brachymorphia s.
Spurway's s.
Stargardt's s.
steal s.
Steele-Richardson-
  Olszewski s.
Stevens-Johnson s.
Stickler's s.
Stilling-Turk-Duane s.
Stock-Spielmeyer-Vogt s.
Sturge-Weber s.
Sturge-Weber-Dimitri s.
sunrise s.
sunset s.
superior oblique tendon
  sheath s.
superior orbital fissure s.
superior tendon sheath s.
superior vena cava s.
Swan's s.
Sylvian's aqueduct s.
tectal midbrain s.
tegmental s.

temporal crescent s.
tendon sheath s.
Terry's s.
Terson's s.
Thomson's s.
tight lens s. (TLS)
Tolosa-Hunt s.
tonic pupil s.
Touraine's s.
Treacher Collins' s.
Turner's s.
UGH s.
Uhthoff's s.
Ullrich's s.
Usher's s.
uveal effusion s.
uveitis-vitiligo-alopecia-
  poliosis s.
uveocutaneous s.
uveoencephalitic s.
uveo-encephalitic s.
uveomeningeal s.
uveomeningitis s.
Uyemura's s.
V s.
van der Hoeve's s.
varicella s.
velocardiofacial s.
vertical retraction s.
visceral larva migrans s.
visual deprivation s.
vitreoretinal
  choroidopathy s.
vitreoretinal traction s.
vitreous wick s.
Vogt-Koyanagi s.
Vogt-Koyanagi-Harada s.
Vogt's s.
Vogt-Spielmeyer s.
von Graefe's s.
Von Hippel-Lindau s.
von Recklinghausen's s.
Waardenburg-Klein s.
Waardenburg-like s.
Waardenburg's s.
Wagner's s.
Wallenberg's s.
Wallenberg's lateral
  medullary s.
Warburg s.
Weber-Dubler s.
Weber's s.
Weill-Marchesani s.

syndrome *(continued)*
    Werner's s.
    Wernicke's s.
    Weyers-Thier s.
    white dot s.
    Wildervanck's s.
    Williams s.
    Wilson's s.
    windshield wiper s.
    wipe-out s.
    Wiskott-Aldrich s.
    Wolf's s.
    Wyburn-Mason s.
    XXXXX s.
    XXXXY s.
    XXXY s.
    Zellweger's s.
synechia, pl. synechiae
    annular s.
    anterior s.
    Castroviejo's anterior s.
    circular s.
    iris s.
    peripheral anterior s. (PAS)
    posterior s.
    s. spatula
    total s.
    total anterior s.
    total posterior s.
synechialysis
synechiotomy
    Paufique's s.
synechotome
synechotomy
synephris
syneresis of vitreous
synergism
synergist
    contralateral s.
synizesis
    s. pupillae
synkinesis
    external pterygoid levator s.
    facial s.
    oculomotor s.
    pterygoid levator s.
    s. pupilla
    trigemino-oculomotor s.
synkinetic
    s. movement
    s. near reflex
    s. near response
synophrys

synophthalmia, synophthalmos, synophthalmus
synophthalmos *(var. of* synophthalmia)
synoptophore
synoptoscope
syntenic genes
synthetic penicillin
syphilis
    congenital s.
    ocular s.
syphilitic
    s. cataract
    s. chorioretinitis
    s. choroiditis
    s. dacryocystis
    s. dacryocystitis
    s. episcleritis
    s. iritis
    s. keratitis
    s. ocular disease
    s. optic perineuritis
    s. retinitis
    s. retinopathy
    s. rhinitis
    s. scleritis
syringe
    Anel s.
    Fink-Weinstein two-way s.
    Fragmatome flute s.
    Fuchs retinal detachment s.
    Fuchs two-way s.
    Goldstein s.
    Goldstein anterior
     chamber s.
    Goldstein lacrimal s.
    lacrimal s.
    Parker-Heath anterior
     chamber s.
    probe s.
    retinal detachment s.
    two-way s.
    Yale Luer-Lok s.
syringoma
    eyelid s.
    s. tumor
System
    Alcon Closure S. (ACS)
    Autoswitch S.
    BKS Refractive S.
    Blairex S.
    Combiline S.
    Digital B S.

Dioptimum S.
Humphrey Instruments
Vision Analyzer
Overrefraction S.
Kowa Fluorescein S.
Lens Plus Oxysept S.
Malis Bipolar
Coagulating/Cutting S.
Massachusetts XII
Vitrectomy S. (MVS)
Micropigmentation S.
Microvit Probe S.
MiraSept S.
M-TEC 2000 Surgical S.
Ocutome II
Fragmentation S.
Opti-Pure S.
Premiere SmallPort
Phaco S.
Rodenstock S.
SmallPort Phaco S.
Surg-E-Trol I/A/R S.
Ultrascan Digital B S.
Vision
Analyzer/Overrefraction S.
Visulab S.
Zeiss Fiber Optic
Illumination S.

system

afocal optical s.
American Optical contrast
sensitivity s.
autonomic nervous s.
Bio-Optics telescope s.
British N s.
Cavitron
irrigation/aspiration s.
Cavitron-Kelman
irrigation/aspiration s.
central nervous s. (CNS)
closed-loop s.
Coburn
irrigation/aspiration s.
complement s.
delivery s.
dioptric s.
Dyer nomogram s. of lens
ordering
extrapyramidal s.
gaussian optical s.
Grieshaber power injector s.
Grolman photographic s.

Hessburg subpalpebral
lavage s.
hyaloid s.
immune s.
irrigation-aspiration s.
IVEX s.
Jaeger s.
Jaeger grading s.
Koeller illumination s.
lacrimal s.
McGuire I/A s.
McIntyre coaxial irrigating-
aspirating s.
McIntyre I/A s.
McIntyre
irrigation/aspiration s.
micropigmentation s.
Mot-R-Pak vitrectomy s.
nomogram s.
oculomotor s.
OCVM s.
Odyssey
phacoemulsification s.
optical s.
osseous s.
parasympathetic nerve s.
postcanalicular s.
printers' point s.
pump-leak s.
sensory s.
Simcoe irrigation-
aspiration s.
SITE TXR diaphragmatic
microsurgical s.
SITE TXR peristaltic
microsurgical s.
SITE TXR
phacoemulsification s.
SITE TXR
phacoemulsification s.
Sloan M s.
sympathetic nervous s.
T s.
tear drainage s.
tear duct s.
United Sonics J shock
phaco fragmentor s.
vertebrobasilar s.
vestibular s.
visual sensory s.
vortex s.
Wheeler cyclodialysis s.
zoom s.

systemic
   s. bacterial endophthalmitis
   s. disease
   s. drug
   s. glucocorticoid
   s. lupus erythematosus
   (SLE)

   s. sclerosis
   s. toxicity
Szymanowski-Kuhnt operation
Szymanowski's operation

TA
  temporal arteritis
tabes dorsalis
tabetic
  t. optic atrophy
table
  Reuss' t.
  Reuss' color t.'s
  Stilling's color t.'s
tachistesthesia
tachistoscope
tacks
  retinal t.
taco test
tactile tension
Taenia solium
tag
  vitreoretinal t.
Taillefer's valve
Takahashi
  T. forceps
  T. iris retractor forceps
Takata laser
Takayasu
  idiopathic arteritis of T.
Takayasu's disease
talantropia
Talbot
  T. law
  T. unit
talbutal
talc
tamoxifen
  t. retinopathy
tamponade
  gas t.
  intraocular silicone oil t.
  silicone oil t.
tamponage
tangency
tangent
  t. scope
  t. screen
  t. screen testing
tangential
Tangier's disease
Tanne corneal cutting block
Tansley's operation
Tan spatula

tantalum
  t. clip
  t. mesh
  t. mesh implant
  t. "O" ring
  t. ring
TAP
  tension by applanation
tap
  anterior chamber t.
  choroidal t.
  vitreous t.
tape
  Blenderm t.
  brow t.
  optokinetic t.
  Transpore eye t.
taper-cut needle
taper-point needle
tapetal light reflex
tapetochoroidal
  t. degeneration
  t. dystrophy
tapetoretinal
  t. degeneration
  t. retinopathy
tapetoretinopathy
tapetum
  t. choroideae
  t. lucidum
  t. nigrum
  t. oculi
tapioca
  t. iris melanoma
  t. melanoma
tapir
  bouche de t.
target
  accommodative t.
  fixation t.
  saccadic eccentric t.
tarsadenitis
tarsal
  t. artery
  t. asthenopia
  t. canal
  t. cartilage
  t. cyst
  t. ectropion
  t. gland

tarsal *(continued)*
    t. laceration
    t. membrane
    t. muscle
    t. plate
    t. portion of eyelid
    t. strip procedure
tarsales
    glandulae t.
tarsalis
tarsectomy
    Blaskovics' t.
    Kuhnt's t.
tarsi
    sycosis t.
    tinea t.
tarsitis
    tuberculous t.
tarsocheiloplasty
tarsoconjunctival
    t. flap
    t. gland
tarsoligamentous sling
tarsomalacia
tarsoorbital
tarsophyma
tarsoplasia
tarsoplasty
tarsorrhaphy
tarsotomy
    transverse t.
tarsus
    inferior t.
    t. orbital septum
    t. osseus
    superior t.
tartaric acid
tartrate
    ergotamine t.
    levallorphan t.
Tasia's operation
taste test
tattoo
    t. of cornea operation
tattooed
tattooing needle
tax double needle
Tay's
    T. cherry-red spot
    T. choroiditis
    T. disease
    T. spot
Tay-Sachs disease

T-cell helper/inducer
T-cell lymphoma
Teale-Knapp operation
tear
    artificial t.'s
    t. break-up time
    breakup time of t.
    conjunctival t.
    crocodile t.'s
    t. drainage system
    t. duct
    t. duct patency
    t. duct system
    t. film
    t. film break-up time
    t. film stability
    fishmouth t.
    t. gas
    giant t.
    horseshoe t.
    iatrogenic retinal t.
    t. lake
    t. layer
    t. of meniscus
    mucin of t.
    operculated t.
    t. pump
    t. quality
    t. quantity
    t. of retina
    retinal t.
    t. sac
    t. secretion
    sphincter t.
    t. stone
    t. strip
teardrop pupil
Tear-Efrin
Tearfair
Teargard
Teargen
tear-induced retinal detachment
tearing
Tearisol
Tears
    Artificial T.
    Comfort T.
    I-Liqui T.
    Isopto T.
    Just T.
    Liquifilm T.
    Milroy Artificial T.
    Natural T.

T. Naturale
T. Naturale Free
T. Naturale II
T. Plus
T. Renewed
Ultra T.
technetium scan
technique
agglutination t.
Armaly-Drance t.
Atkinson's t.
bare scleral t.
blind-spot projection t.
Boyden's chamber t.
Brockhurst's t.
Brown-Beard t.
capsule forceps t.
Crawford's t.
erysiphake t.
feeder-frond t.
flicher-fusion frequency t.
Fraunfelder's "no touch" t.
frontalis sling t.
Goldmann's kinetic t.
Goldmann's static t.
high-tension suturing t.
Hughes' modification of
  Burch t.
immunohistochemical t.
Knoll's refraction t.
letterbox t.
masquerade t.
McLean's t.
McReynolds' t.
O'Brien's t.
O'Brien's akinesia t.
Okamura's t.
open-sky t.
Papanicolaou t.
push plus refraction t.
Quickert three-suture t.
Scheie's t.
Schepens t.
scleral search coil t.
Smith Indian t.
Southern blot t.
tumbling t.
Van Lint's t.
Van Lint's modified t.
Van Milligen's eyelid
  repair t.
technology
imaging t.

tectal midbrain syndrome
tectonic
t. epikeratoplasty
t. keratoplasty
Teflon
T. implant
T. iris retractor
T. plate
T. plug
T. sheet
tegmental syndrome
Tegretol
teichopsia
tela, pl. **telae**
t. cellulosa
t. conjunctiva
t. elastica
telangiectasia
essential t.
hereditary t.
hereditary hemorrhagic t.
retinal t.
spider t.
telangiectasis
retinal t.
telangiectatic glioma
telebinocular
telecanthus
teleopsia
telephoto effect
Telescope
Hopkins Rod Lens T.
telescope
Galilean t.
monocular t.
telescopic
t. lens
t. spectacles
television
closed-circuit t.
Telfa
T. dressing
T. pad
T. plastic film dressing
Tellais' sign
Teller acuity cards
TEM
triethylenemelamine
TE MOO mode beam laser
template
temple
cable t.
curl t.

temple *(continued)*
   hockey-end t.
   t. length
   library t.
   loafer t.
   paddle t.
   riding bow t.
   skull t.
   spatule t.
   spring-inge t.
   straight t.
temples of spectacles
temporal
   t. arcade
   t. arteriole of retina
   t. arteritis (TA)
   t. artery
   t. artery biopsy
   t. artery pallor
   t. bone
   t. bulbar conjunctiva
   t. crescent
   t. crescent syndrome
   t. hemianopsia
   t. island of visual field
   t. lobe
   t. lobe field defect
   t. loop
   t. pits
   t. raphe
   t. retina
   t. venulae retina superior
   t. venule of retina
   t. wedge
   t. zone of retina
temporalis
   commissura palpebrarum t.
   t. muscle
temporary
   t. diabetes
   t. intracanalicular collagen
     implant
temporo-occipital artery
temporoparietal lobe
TEN
   toxic epidermal necrolysis
tenaculum
tendinous insertion
tendo
   t. oculi
   t. palpebrarum
tendon
   t. advancement

   Brown's t.
   canthal t.
   lateral canthal t.
   Lockwood's t.
   medial canthal t.
   t. recession
   t. sheath syndrome
   superior oblique t.
   tenotomy of ocular t.
   t. tucker
   Zinn's t.
tendotome
tendotomy
tenectomy
Tennant
   T. Anchorflex AC lens
   T. anchor lens-insertion
    hook
   T. hook
   T. implant
   T. lens
   T. lens forceps
   T. lens-inserting forceps
   T. lens-manipulating hook
   T. titanium suturing forceps
Tennant-Colibri corneal forceps
Tennant-Troutman superior rectus
  forceps
Tenner
   T. lacrimal cannula
   T. titanium suturing forceps
tenonectomy
tenonitis
   brawny t.
tenonometer
Tenon's
   T. capsule
   T. fascia bulbi
   T. fascia lata
   T. membrane
   T. space
tenontotomy
Tenormin
tenosynovitis
tenotome
tenotomist
tenotomize
tenotomy
   Arroyo's t.
   Arruga's t.
   curb t.
   free t.
   graduated t.

t. hook
intrasheath t.
t. of ocular tendon
t. operation
Z t.
Z marginal t.
tensile strength of vessels
Tensilon
T. implant
T. test
tension (TN)
applanation t. (AT)
t. by applanation (TAP)
t. of eye
finger t. (FAN)
hard-finger t.
intraocular t.
normal-finger t.
ocular t. (Tn)
soft-finger t.
tactile t.
t. test
zonular t.
tension, normal (TN)
tension oculus dextra (tension of right eye) (TOD)
tension oculus sinister (tension of left eye) (TOS)
tensor insertion
tented up retina
tenting
tentorial nerve
tentorii ramus
tenuis, pl. panni
pannus t.
Tenzel
T. elevator
T. forceps
T. rotational cheek flap
tepoxalin
teratogen
teratogenicity
teratoma
teratoneuroma
Terg-A-Zyme
terminaux
boutons t.
terminus
incision t.
Terra-Cortril
Terramycin
polymyxin B and T.

Terrien's
T. degeneration
T. marginal degeneration
T. ulcer
Terry
T. keratometer
T. silicone capsule polisher
Terry's syndrome
Terson
T. capsule forceps
T. extracapsular forceps
Terson's
T. operation
T. syndrome
tertiary
t. positions
t. vitreous
tertius palpebra
tessellated fundus
tessellation
Tessier's
T. classification
T. clefting
T. operation
Test
Bailey-Lovie Near T.
Binocular Visual Acuity T. (BVAT)
Brightness Acuity T. (BAT)
Pepper Visual Skills for Reading T.
test
afterimage t.
alternate cover t. (ACT)
alternate cover-uncover t.
alternating light t.
Amsler's t.
Amsler's grid t.
anaglyph t.
a-wave t.
Bagolini's t.
Bagolini's striated glasses t.
Bárány's caloric t.
Barraquer-Krumeich t.
4Δ base-out t.
Behçet's skin puncture t.
Berens' pinhole and dominance t.
Berens' three-character t.
Bielschowsky-Parks head-tilt three-step t.
Bielschowsky's t.
Bielschowsky's head-tilt t.

test *(continued)*

Bielschowsky's three-step, head-tilt t.
biochrome t.
biopter t.
blindness t.
breakup time t.
Bruchner's t.
caloric t.
t. card
cardinal field t.
Catford visual acuity t.
chi-squared test
cocaine t.
Coccidioides skin t.
color t.
color vision t.
complement fixation t.
confrontation visual field t.
contour stereo t.
corneal staining t.
cover t. (CT)
cover-uncover t.
creatinine clearance t.
cross cover t.
Cuignet's t.
D-15 t.
dark-room t.
dissimilar image t.
dissimilar target t.
DIVA t.
Dix-Hallpike t.
double Maddox rod t.
duction t.
duochrome t.
Dupuy-Dutemps dacryocystorhinostomy dye t.
dye t.
dye disappearance t. (DDT)
edrophonium t.
edrophonium chloride t.
Ehrmann's t.
electrophysiological t.
Farnsworth-Munsell color t.
Farnsworth-Munsell 100-hue color t.
Farnsworth-Munsell 100-hue color vision t.
Farnsworth's t.
fistula t.
flashlight t.
fluorescein t.

fluorescein angiogram t.
fluorescein dilution t.
fluorescein dye disappearance t.
fluorescein instillation t.
fluorescent antibody t.
fluorescent treponemal antibody t.
fly t.
FM-100 t.
forced-duction t.
forced generation t.
forward traction t.
four-dot t.
Fridenberg's stigometric card t.
FTA-absorption t.
glare t.
hair bulb incubation t.
hand-motion visual acuity t.
hand-movement visual acuity t.
Hardy-Rand-Ritter t.
Harrington-Flocks t.
HATTS t.
head-tilt t.
hemagglutination t.
hemagglutination treponemal t.
hemagglutination treponemal t. for syphilis (HATTS)
Hering-Bielschowsky after-image t.
Hering's t.
Hess screen t.
Hirschberg's t.
histoplasmin skin t.
Holmgren's color t.
Holmgren's wool skein t.
HOTV t.
indirect fluorescent antibody t.
interference visual acuity t.
intravenous thyrotropin-releasing hormone t.
Ishihara's t.
Ishihara's color t.
isoniazid therapeutic t.
Jaeger's t.
Jaeger's visual t.
Jenning's t.
Jones' t.

Jones' dye t.
Keystone t.
Keystone View steopsis t.
Kirby-Bauer disk
  sensitivity t.
Kirsch's t.
Krimsky's t.
Krimsky's prism t.
Kveim t.
lacrimal irrigation t.
Lancaster-Regan t.
Lancaster's red-green t.
Lancaster's screen t.
Landolt's broken-ring t.
lantern t.
letter t.
t. letter
light projection t.
light-stress t.
limulus lysate t.
linear visual acuity t.
lupus erythematosus cell t.
Maddox's rod t.
Maddox's wing t.
major amblyoscope t.
Marlow's t.
Mauthner's t.
Mecholyl t.
methylene blue dye t.
MHA-TP t.
microhemagglutination t.
monocular confrontation
  visual field t.
mydriatic t.
mydriatic provocative t.
Nagel's t.
near vision t.
neostigmine t.
neutral density filter t.
nudge t.
nystagmus t.
t. object
objective t.
Octopus t.
Octopus 201 perimeter t.
ocular motility t.
ophthalmic t.
ornithine tolerance t.
parallax t.
Paredrine t.
Parks-Bielschowsky three-step
  head-tilt t.
passive forced duction t.

perimeter corneal reflex t.
photostress t.
pilocarpine t.
pinhole and dominance t.
primary dye t.
prism t.
prism adaptation t. (PAT)
prism cover t.
prism shift t.
prism vergence t.
Prostigmin t.
provocative t.
pulmonary function t.
Randot's Dot E stereo t.
Rayleigh's t.
red-filter t.
red glare t.
red glass t.
regurgitation t.
Rochat's t.
rotational t.
Sabin-Feldman dye t.
Schirmer's t.
Schirmer's tear t.
Schirmer's tear quality t.
secondary dye t.
Seidel's t.
sensory t.
separate image t.
serologic t.
shadow t.
Sheridan-Gardiner isolated
  letter-matching t.
simultaneous prism cover t.
  (SPC)
single cover t.
skein t.
t. skeins
skin t.
Snellen's t.
stereo t.
stereopsis t.
Stilling's color t.
subjective refraction t.
swinging flashlight t.
swinging light t.
t. symbols
t t.
taco t.
taste t.
Tensilon t.
tension t.
three-character t.

test *(continued)*
three-step t.
thyrotropin-releasing
hormone t.
Titmus t.
Titmus stereo t.
Titmus stereoacuity t.
Titmus vision t.
TNO t.
TNO stereo t.
traction t.
transillumination t.
Treponema pallidum
immobilization t.
TRH t.
triiodothyronine
suppression t.
tuberculin skin t.
tumbling E t.
t. type
tyrosinase t.
VDRL t.
Venereal Disease Research
Laboratory t.
vertical prism t.
Vistech 6500 contrast t.
Visuscope motor t.
Visuscope sensory t.
water-drinking t.
water provocative t.
W4D t.
Welland's t.
Werner's t.
Westcott's t.
Wilbrand's prism t.
Wirt's stereo t.
Wirt's stereopsis t.
Wirt's vision t.
Wolff-Eisner t.
Worth's four-dot t. (W4D
test)
χ^2 t.
tester
Miller-Nadler glare t.
phoropter vision t.
Topcon vision t.
testing
caloric t.
dark-room t.
electrophysiological t.
forced-duction t.

four base-out prism t.
hematologic t.
hypothesis t.
near acuity t.
near vision t.
pharmacological t.
provocative t.
Romberg t.
tangent screen t.
visual field t.
test types
Jaeger's t. t.
point system t. t.
Snellen's t. t.
tetani
Clostridium t.
tetany
t. cataract
zonular t.
tetartanope
tetartanopia
tetartanopic
tetartanopsia
tetraacetate
tetracaine
t. hydrochloride
tetrachloride
carbon t.
tetrachromic
Tetracon
tetracycline
Tetracyn
tetrad
Konoto's t.
tetraethylammonium chloride
tetrafilcon A
tetrahydrocannabinol
tetrahydrozoline
tetranopsia
tetrastichiasis
Tevdek suture
text blindness
TG-140 needle
thalamolenticular
thalamus
optic t.
thalassemia
sickle cell t.
thalidomide
thaw-freeze
Thayer-Martin agar

Theimich's
    T. lip sign
    T. sign
Thelazia
    T. callipaeda
thelaziasis
Theobald probe
Theodore's keratoconjunctivitis
theory
    Alhazen's t.'s
    color t.
    duplicity t. of vision
    Helmholtz t. of
      accommodation
    Helmholtz t. of color vision
    Hering's t. of color vision
    Hering's t. of color vision
    Ladd-Franklin t.
    migration t.
    molecular dissociation t.
    opponent colors t.
    Scheiner's t.'s
    Schön's t.
    trichromatic color t.
    Unna's abtropfung t.
    von Frisch's t.
    Wollaston's t.
    Young-Helmholtz t. of color
      vision
therapeutic
    t. contact lens
    t. iridectomy
Therapy
    Dry Eye T.
therapy
    cobalt t.
    corticosteroid t.
    laser t.
    maximum tolerated
      medical t. (MTMT)
    miotic t.
    mydriatic-cycloplegic t.
    occlusion t.
    photodynamic t.
    radiation t.
    red-filter t.
    steroid t.
thermal
    t. adhesions
    t. burn
    t. cataract
    t. disinfection

    t. keratoplasty (TKP)
    t. sclerectomy
thermocautery
thermokeratoplasty
thermosclerectomy
thermosclerostomy
thermosclerotomy
thermosector
thiabendazole
thiamine
thick lens
thickness
    central t.
    contact lens t.
    t. of contact lens
    standard t.
    stromal t.
Thill Aniseikonia Worksheet
thimerosal
thin lens
thinning
    corneal t.
thioglycolate
thiomalate
    gold sodium t.
thiopental
    t. sodium
thioridazine
    t. hydrochloride
Thiotepa
thiothixene
third
    t. cranial nerve
    t. nerve palsy
third-grade fusion
Thomas
    T. brush
    T. calipers
    T. cannula
    T. cryoextractor
    T. cryoprobe
    T. cryoptor
    T. cryoretractor
    T. fixation forceps
    T. forceps
    T. irrigating-aspirating
      cannula
    T. Kapsule instruments
    T. Kapsule instruments
    T. retractor
    T. scissors
Thomas' operation
Thomson's syndrome

Thorazine
Thornton
   T. fixating ring
   T. fixation forceps
   T. guide for optical zone
     size
   T. optical center marker
Thorpe
   T. calipers
   T. conjunctival forceps
   T. corneal forceps
   T. forceps
   T. foreign body forceps
   T. four-mirror goniolaser
   T. four-mirror goniolaser
     lens
   T. four-mirror goniolens
   T. four-mirror vitreous
     fundus laser lens
   T. scissors
   T. slit lamp
   T. surgical gonioscope
Thorpe-Castroviejo
   T.-C. calipers
   T.-C. corneal forceps
   T.-C. fixation forceps
   T.-C. goniolens
   T.-C. scissors
   T.-C. vitreous foreign body
     forceps
Thorpe-Westcott scissors
Thrasher lens implant forceps
thread
   mucous t.
threat reflex
three-character test
three-mirror
   t.-m. contact lens
three-mirror
   t.-m. lens
   t.-m. prism
three o'clock staining
three-point touch
three-snip
   t.-s. operation
   t.-s. punctum
   t.-s. punctum operation
three-step test
three times a day (t.i.d.)
three-toothed forceps
three-way stopcock
threshold
   achromatic t.

brightness difference t.
displacement t.
final t.
light differential t.
minimum light t.
quantitative static t.
sensitivity t.
t. stage III of retinopathy
  of prematurity (TS III
  ROP)
tolerance t.
visual t., t. of visual
  sensation
thromboangiitis obliterans
thrombocytopenia
   t. purpura
thromboendarterectomy
thrombophlebitis
thrombosed artery
thrombosis
   cavernous sinus t.
   t. in retina
   retinal t.
thrombus
   fibrin t.
thrush
   lid t.
thumb occluder
Thurmond nucleus-irrigating
cannula
Thygeson's
   T. chronic follicular
     conjunctivitis
   T. disease
   T. keratitis
   T. superficial punctate
     keratitis
   T. superficial punctate
     keratopathy
thymic hypoplasia
thymidine
thymoma
thymoxamine
Thymoxid
thyroid
   t. disease
   t. disorder
   t. exophthalmos
   t. eye disease
   t. lid retraction
   t. ophthalmopathy
   t. orbitopathy
   t. stare

thyroidectomy
    subtotal t.
thyroiditis
    Hashimoto's t.
    Reidel's t.
thyroid-releasing hormone (TRH)
thyrotoxic exophthalmos
thyrotoxicosis
    t. ophthalmoplegia
thyrotropic exophthalmos
thyrotropin-releasing
    t.-r. hormone (TRH)
    t.-r. hormone test
thyroxine, thyroxin
TIA
    transient ischemic attack
tic
    t. douloureux
    local t.
    motor t.
ticarcillin
Ticho
    T. pliable iris retractor
    T. zonule sweeper
t.i.d.
    three times a day
tie-over
    t.-o. dressing
    t.-o. Sellotape dressing
tight
    t. contact lens
    t. lens syndrome (TLS)
tigre
tigroid
    t. background
    t. fundus
    t. retina
Tilderquist needle holder
Tillaux
    extraocular muscles of T.
Tillaux's spiral
Tillett's operation
Tillyer
    T. bifocal lens
    T. lens
tilorone
tilt
    pantoscopic t.
    t. of sella
    visual t.
tilted disk

tilting
    t. lens
    t. lens atresia
time
    breakup t. (BUT)
    fading t.
    sensation t.
    tear break-up t.
    tear film break-up t.
timolol
    t. and pilocarpine
Timoptic
    T. in Ocudose
    T. Ocudose
Timoptic Ocudose
Timpilo
tinea
    t. capitis
    t. tarsi
tinnitus
    gaze evoked t.
tinted
    t. contact lens
    t. lens
    t. spectacles
tinting
    t. of lens
    t. of spectacle lens
tip
    Binkhorst t.
    diathermy t.
    endolaser probe t.
    Girard irrigating t.
    guillotine cutting t.
    Keeler lancet t.
    Keeler micro t.
    Keeler micro round t.
    Keeler micro spear t.
    Keeler puncture t.
    Keeler razor t.
    Keeler triple facet t.
    Quad cutting t.
    rotary cutting t.
    Simcoe interchangeable t.
    Welsh flat-olive t.
tire
    276 t.
    implant t.
    t. implant
    silicone t.
    Watzke t.
tisiris

tissue
    t. adhesive
    adipose t.
    conjunctiva-associated
      lymphoid t.
    connective t.
    cutaneous t.
    donor t.
    ectopic t.
    episcleral t.
    nuclear t.
    orbital adipose t.
    pericanalicular connective t.
    pterygial t.
    sustentacular t.
Titan
titanium
    t. needle
    t. suturing forceps
Titmus
    T. stereoacuity test
    T. stereo test
    T. test
    T. vision test
titrated
titration
titubation
    head t.
TKP
    thermal keratoplasty
T lens
TLS
    tight lens syndrome
T lymphocyte
TM
    trabecular meshwork
TN
    tension
    tension, normal
Tn
    ocular tension
TNO
    T. stereo test
    T. stereo test
    T. test
tobacco/alcohol amblyopia
tobacco amblyopia
TobraDex
tobramycin
Tobrex
α-tocopherol
Toctron EA-290

TOD
    tension oculus dextra (tension of
    right eye)
Todd
    T. cautery
    T. electrocautery
    T. gouge
Todd's paralysis
tolazamide
tolbutamide
Tolentino
    T. cutter
    T. prism lens
    T. ring
    T. vitrectomy lens
    T. vitrectomy lens set
    T. vitreous cutter
tolerance threshold
Tolman micrometer
Tolosa-Hunt syndrome
Tomas
    T. iris hook
    T. suture hook
tomato-ketchup fundus
tomogram
tomography
    axial t.
    complex motion t.
    computed t. (CT)
    orbital t.
tonic
    t. accommodation
    t. convergence
    t. lids
    t. pupil
    t. pupil syndrome
    t. vergence
tonicity
tonofibrils
    t. tendinous xanthoma
    t. tuberous xanthoma
tonofilament
tonofilms
    crescent t.
    Schiötz t.
tonogram
tonograph
tonography
tonomat
Tonomat applanation tonometer
tonometer
    air-puff t.
    air-puff contact t.

air-puff noncontact t.
Alcon t.
Allen-Schiötz t.
AO applanation t.
AO Reichert Instruments
 applanation t.
applamatic t.
applanation t.
Aus Jena-Schiötz t.
Berens t.
Bigliano t.
biprism applanation t.
Carl Zeiss t.
Challenger t.
Challenger digital
 applanation t.
Coburn t.
Digilab t.
Draeger t.
Durham t.
electronic t.
Goldmann t.
Goldmann applanation t.
Harrington t.
impression t.
indentation t.
Intermedics intraocular t.
Keeler t.
Keeler Pulsair t.
Krakau t.
Lombert t.
MacKay-Marg t.
MacKay-Marg electronic t.
Maklakoff t.
McLean t.
Mueller electronic t.
noncontact t.
Pach-Pen t.
Perkins t.
Perkins applanation t.
pneumatic t.
Pulsair t.
Reichert t.
Reichert noncontact t.
Rosner t.
Ruedemann t.
Schiötz t.
Sklar-Schiötz t.
Storz t.
Tonomat applanation t.
Tono-Pen t.
tonometry
applanation t.

digital t.
indentation t.
Tono-Pen
Oculab T.-P.
T.-P. tonometer
tonsil
cerebellar t.
Tooke
T. corneal knife
T. cornea-splitting knife
T. knife
T. spatula
Tooke-Johnson corneal knife
Topcon
T. aspheric lens
T. camera
T. chart projector
T. digital lensometer
T. eye refractometer
T. lens
T. lensometer
T. LM P5 digital
 lensometer
T. microscope
T. perimeter
T. refractometer
T. refractor
T. RM-A2300 auto
 refractometer
T. slit lamp
T. vision tester
topical
t. anesthesia
t. anesthetic
t. drug
t. glucocorticoid
topicamide
hydroxyamphetamine HBr
 and t.
Topic-M
Topisporin
topogometer
topographic
t. agnosia
t. echography
topography
corneal t.
Topolanski's sign
Toradol
toric
t. ablation
t. contact lens
t. lens

toric *(continued)*
    t. spectacle lens
    t. surface
toricity
Toric-Optima series lens
toroidal contact lens
torpor
    t. retinae
torque
torsiometer
torsion
torsional
    t. deviation
    t. diplopia
    t. movement
    t. nystagmus
torticollis
    ocular t.
    spasmodic t.
tortuosity
    t. of retinal vessel
    vascularized t.
    venous t.
tortuous
torulosis
TOS
    tension oculus sinister (tension of left eye)
Total
total
    t. anterior synechia
    t. astigmatism
    t. blindness
    t. cataract
    t. hydrophthalmia
    t. hyperopia (Ht)
    t. hyphema
    t. keratoplasty
    t. ophthalmoplegia
    t. posterior synechia
    t. sclerectasia
    t. symblepharon
    t. synechia
totale
    ankyloblepharon t.
Toti-Mosher operation
Toti's
    T. operation
    T. procedure
toto
    eye removed in t.

touch
    three-point t.
    vitreous t.
Touraine's syndrome
Tournay's
    T. phenomenon
    T. sign
Touton's
    T. cell
    T. giant cells
Townley-Paton operation
toxemia of pregnancy
toxemic retinopathy of pregnancy
toxic
    t. amaurosis
    t. amblyopia
    t. cataract
    t. conjunctivitis
    t. diabetes
    t. epidermal necrolysis (TEN)
    t. follicular conjunctivitis
    t. maculopathy
    t. optic neuropathy
    t. reaction
    t. retinopathy
    t. substance
toxicity
    t. of alcohol
    cell-mediated t.
    digitalis t.
    ocular t.
    oxygen t.
    phenothiazine t.
    retinal t.
    systemic t.
    vitamin D t.
toxicodendron
    Rhus t.
toxicogenic conjunctivitis
toxicology
toxin
    botulinum t.
Toxocara
    T. canis
toxocariasis
    t. endophthalmitis
    ocular t.
Toxoplasma
    T. gondii
toxoplasmic
    t. choroiditis

t. retinochoroiditis
t. uveitis
toxoplasmosis
t. chorioretinitis
congenital t.
fulminant ocular t.
ocular t.
punctate outer retinal t.
Toynbee's corpuscle
TPI
Treponema pallidum
immobilization
trabecula, gen. and pl. trabeculae
anterior chamber t.
scleral t.
trabecular
t. fiber
t. membrane
t. meshwork (TM)
t. network
t. outflow
trabeculectomy
Cairn's t.
t. operation
Smith's t.
trabeculitis
t. glaucoma
trabeculodysgenesis
trabeculopexy
argon laser t. (ALT)
trabeculoplasty
argon laser t. (ALTP)
laser t.
trabeculopuncture
trabeculotome
Allen-Burian t.
Harms t.
McPherson t.
trabeculotomy
t. probe
trabeculum
corneoscleral t.
trachoma
Arlt-Jaesche t.
Arlt's t.
t. body
brawny t.
follicular t., granular t.
gland t.
t. gland
t. inclusion conjunctivitis
trachomata

trachomatis
Chlamydia t.
trachomatosus
pannus t.
trachomatous
t. conjunctivitis
t. dacryocystis
t. dacryocystitis
t. keratitis
t. pannus
tracker
Purkinje image t.
tracks
bear t.
snail t.
Tracor Northern
Tracoustic RV275
tract
geniculocalcarine t.
leiomyoma of uveal t.
optic t.
uveal t.
traction
t. band
t. detachment
diabetic t.
Moss' t.
t. suture
t. test
vitreous t.
tractional
t. retinal degeneration
t. retinal detachment
train
pulse t.
training
vision t.
Trainor-Nida operation
Trainor's operation
trait
autosomal dominant t.
sickle cell t.
trajectory
Tramacort
trampoline
tranexamic acid
tranquilization
tranquilizer
transantral decompression
transcleral
transconjunctival route
Transducer
Ocuscan 400 T.

transducer
transfer
    t. factor
    t. function
transferase
    lecithin:cholesterol acyl t.
    (LCAT)
transferred ophthalmia
transfixion
    t. of iris
    t. of iris operation
transient
    t. ametropia
    t. blindness
    t. congestion
    t. early exophthalmos
    t. ischemia
    t. ischemic attack (TIA)
    t. layer of Chievitz
    t. myopia
    t. obscurations of vision
    t. obscuration of vision
    t. vertebrobasilar ischemia
    t. visual obscuration
transillumination test
transilluminator
    Finnoff t.
transitional zone
transition zone
translimbal
translocation
translucent
transmissibility
    oxygen t.
transmission
    light t.
transmitted light
transocular
transorbital leukotomy
transparent ulcer of the cornea
trans pars plana
transplant
    corneal t.
    lamellar corneal t.
    McReynolds' pterygium t.
    ocular muscle t.
    penetrating corneal t.
transplantation
    t. antigen
    corneal t., t. of cornea
    t. of muscle operation
    organ t.
Transpore eye tape

transport
    axonal t.
    axoplasmic t.
transposition
    muscle t.
transpupillary cyclophotocoagulation
transsynaptic
transudate
transverse
    t. axis of Fick
    t. suture of Krause
    t. tarsotomy
transvitreal
Trantas'
    T. dot
    T. operation
tranylcypromine sulfate
trapdoor scleral buckle operation
trapezoid
    Superblade t.
trapezoidal
    t. incision
    t. keratotomy
trap incision
Traquair
    junctional scotoma of T.
    scotoma of T.
Traquair's island
trauma
    birth t.
    blunt t.
    corneal t.
    ocular t.
    orbital t.
    orbitocranial t.
traumatic
    t. amblyopia
    t. angle recession
    t. aniridia
    t. atrophy
    t. cataract
    t. choroidal rupture
    t. choroiditis
    t. corneal abrasion
    t. corneal cyst
    t. degenerative cataract
    t. glaucoma
    t. gliosis
    t. hyphema
    t. mydriasis
    t. ptosis
    t. pupillary miosis

t. retinopathy
t. scleral cyst
tray
    I-tech cannula t.
Treacher Collins' syndrome
treatment
    Imre's t.
    Schöler's t.
tree
    vascular t.
trematode infection
trematodiasis
tremor
    head t.'s
tremulous
    t. cataract
    t. iris
trepanation
    corneal t., t. of cornea
trephination
    open-sky t.
trephine
    Arroyo t.
    Arruga t.
    Arruga lacrimal t.
    automated t.
    automatic t.
    Bard-Parker t.
    Barraquer t.
    Barron t.
    Barron epikeratophakia t.
    t. blade
    Bonaccolto t.
    bone t.
    bone-biting t.
    Boston t.
    Brown-Pusey corneal t.
    Cardona corneal
      prosthesis t.
    Castroviejo t.
    Castroviejo corneal
      transplant t.
    Castroviejo improved t.
    chalazion t.
    corneal t.
    corneal prosthesis t.
    Davis t.
    Dimitry chalazion t.
    disposable t.
    Elliot t.
    Elliot corneal t.
    Elschnig t.
    Gradle corneal t.

Green t.
Grieshaber t.
Grieshaber corneal t.
Grieshaber-type corneal t.
Guyton corneal transplant t.
Hanna t.
Hessburg-Barron t.
Hessburg-Barron suction t.
Hessburg-Barron vacuum t.
Iliff t.
Iliff lacrimal t.
Katena t.
Katzin t.
King corneal t.
lacrimal t.
Lichtenberg corneal t.
lid t.
Londermann corneal t.
Lopez-Enriquez scleral t.
Martinez disposable
  corneal t.
Moria t.
Mueller t.
Mueller electric corneal t.
Paton t.
Paton corneal t.
Paufique t.
Schcic t.
Searcy chalazion t.
suction t.
Troutman t.
Troutman tenotomy t.
Walker t.
Treponema
    T. pallidum
    T. pallidum immobilization
      (TPI)
    T. pallidum immobilization
      test
treponemal antibody
tretinoin trifluorothymidine
TRH
    thyroid-releasing hormone
    thyrotropin-releasing hormone
      TRH test
triad
    AGR t.
      aniridia, genitourinary
        abnormalities, and
        mental retardation
    Charcot's t.
    Hutchinson's t.

triad *(continued)*
  near t.
  t. of retinal cone
trial
  t. case
  t. case and lens
  clinical t.
  t. clip
  t. frame
  t. lens
triamcinolone
triangle
  Arlt's t.
  color t.
  fitting t.
  frontal t.
  Wernicke's t.
triangular capsulotomy
trichiasis
  t. repair
trichilemmomas
Trichinella spiralis
trichinosis
trichloracetic acid
trichlorethylene
trichoepithelioma
trichofolliculoma tumor
trichoma
trichomatosis
trichomatous
trichophytosis
trichosis carunculae
trichroic
trichroism
trichromasy
trichromat
trichromatic, trichromic
  t. color theory
trichromatism
  anomalous t.
trichromatopsia
  anomalous t.
tricurve contact lenses
triethylenemelamine (TEM)
trifacial neuralgia
trifluoperazine
  t. hydrochloride
trifluorothymidine
  tretinoin t.
trifluperidol hydrochloride
triflupromazine
trifluridine

trifocal
  executive t.
  t. glasses
  t. lens
trigeminal
  t. nerve (N.V)
  t. neuralgia
  t. neuropathic keratopathy
  t. reflex
  t. shield
trigemino-oculomotor synkinesis
trigeminus
  nervus t.
  reflex t.
  t. reflex
trigger mechanism
trigone
  Mueller's t.
trihexosyl ceramide
triiodothyronine suppression test
Trilafon
trilamellar
trilateral retinoblastoma
trimethadione
trimethaphan camsylate
trimethidium methosulfate
trimethoprim
trimethoprim-sulfamethoxazole
triopathy
Tri-Ophtho
triparanol
triphosphatase
  adenosine t. (ATPase)
triphosphate
  adenosine t. (ATP)
Tripier's
  T. operation
  T. operation throw square
    knot
  T. operation triple
  T. operation vision
Triple
  T. Antibiotic
  T. Antibiotic with HC
triple
  t. symptom complex
  Tripier's operation t.
  t. vision
triple-facet-tip needle
Triple-Gen
triple-throw square knot stitch
triploidy
triplokoria

triplopia
tripod
triptokoria
triradiate line
trisodium phosphonoformate hexahydrate
Trisol
trisomy
    t. 13
    t. 18
    t. 21
    t. D
    D_1 t.
    E t.
    t. 9 mosaic
    t. 4p
    t. 9p
    t. 20p
tristichia
trisulfopyrimidine
tritan
tritanomal
tritanomalous
tritanomaly
tritanope
tritanopia
tritanopic
Tri-Thalmic
Tri-Thalmic HC
Triton
trocar
    Veirs t.
trochlea
    t. musculi obliqui superioris bulbi
    t. musculi obliqui superioris oculi
    t. of superior oblique muscle
trochlear
    t. fossa
    t. fovea
    t. hamulus
    t. muscle
    t. nerve (N.IV)
    t. tubercle
trochlearis
    fossa t.
    fovea t.
    nervus t.
    spina t.
Trokel lens
Trokel-Peyman laser lens

troland
tromethamine
Troncoso
    T. gonioscope
    T. gonioscopic implant
    T. gonioscopic lens implant
trophic
    t. change
    t. keratitis
    t. retinal degeneration
tropia
    alternating t.
    constant monocular t.
    t. deviation
    intermittent t.
    vertical t.
Tropicacyl
tropicamide
    t. and hydroxyamphetamine HBr
tropic deviation
tropometer
troposcope
trough level
Trousseau's sign
Troutman
    T. bladebreaker
    T. cannula
    T. conjunctival scissors
    T. corneal dissector
    T. corneal knife
    T. forceps
    T. implant
    T. lamellar dissector
    T. lens loupe
    T. microsurgical scissors
    T. needle holder
    T. punch
    T. rectus forceps
    T. scissors
    T. suture scissors
    T. tenotomy trephine
    T. trephine
    T. tying forceps
Troutman-Barraquer
    T.-B. corneal fixation forceps
    T.-B. corneal utility forceps
Troutman-Castroviejo
    T.-C. corneal fixation forceps
    T.-C. corneal section scissors

**Troutman-Katzin corneal transplant
scissors**
Troutman-Llobera fixation forceps
Troutman's operation
Troutman-Tooke corneal knife
TRU
    turbidity-reducing units
Truc's
    T. flap
    T. operation
true
    t. exfoliation
    t. hemianopsia
    t. image
    t. visual acuity (TVA)
Trump's solution
truncated contact lens
trunks
    vascular t.
TruVision lens
trypanosomiasis
tryptophan
T-sign
TS III ROP
    threshold stage III of retinopathy
    of prematurity
T system
t **test**
T-tube
    cul-de-sac irrigation T.-t.
    Houser cul-de-sac
     irrigator T.-t.
    lacrimal duct T.-t.
    polyethylene T.-t.
    Pyrex T.-t.
    Silastic T.-t.
    vinyl T.-t.
tubarine
tube
    angled suction t.
    anterior chamber t.
    Bowman t.
    cathode ray t. (CRT)
    corneal t.
    Crawford t.
    encircling t.
    encircling polyethylene t.
    endotracheal t.
    fil d'Arion silicone t.
    fusion t.
    Guibor t.
    Guibor duct t.
    Guibor Silastic t.

    Houser cul-de-sac
     irrigator t.
    Jones t.
    Jones Pyrex t.
    Jones tear duct t.
    laser t.
    L.T. Jones tear duct t.
    Luer t.
    Moulton lacrimal duct t.
    neural t.
    polyethylene t.
    Pyrex t.
    Quickert-Dryden t.
    Reinecke-Carroll lacrimal t.
    silicone t.
    vinyl t.
tuber
    frontal t.
tubercle
    t. bacillus
    caseating t.
    lacrimal t.
    lateral orbit t.
    lateral orbital t.
    lateral palpebral t.
    trochlear t.
    Whitnall's t.
tuberculin skin test
tuberculoid leprosy
tuberculoma
tuberculosis
    Mycobacterium t.
tuberculosis
    t. conjunctivitis
tuberculous
    t. dacryocystis
    t. dacryocystitis
    t. iritis
    t. keratitis
    t. phlyctenulosis
    t. rhinitis
    t. tarsitis
    t. uveitis
tuberous sclerosis
tubing
    silicone t.
Tübinger perimeter
tubular
    t. vision
    t. visual fields
tuck
    iris t.

left superior oblique t.
    t. procedure
tucked lid of Collier
tucker
    Bishop-Peter tendon t.
    Bishop tendon t.
    Burch-Greenwood t.
    Burch-Greenwood tendon t.
    Burch tendon t.
    Fink tendon t.
    Green muscle t.
    Green strabismus t.
    Ruedemann-Todd tendon t.
    tendon t.
tucking
Tudor-Thomas
    T.-T. graft
    T.-T. operation
tuft
    neovascular t.
    retinal t.
    vitreoretinal t.
    zonular-traction retinal t.
tularemia
    oculoglandular t.
tularemic conjunctivitis
tularensis
    Francisela t.
Tulevech cannula
tulle gras dressing
tumbling
    t. E test
    t. procedure
    t. technique
    t. technique operation
in tumbling fashion
tumefaction
tumor
    anemone cell t.
    benign t.
    brain t.
    Brooke's t.
    cerebellar astrocytoma t.
    cerebellopontine angle t.
    choristoma t.
    Coerens t.
    congenital limbal corneal
      dermoid t.
    conjunctival lymphoid t.
    craniofacial fibro-osseous t.
    cystic hydrocystoma t.
    dermoid t.

embryonal t. of ciliary
    body
ependymoma t.
epithelial t.
eyelid t.
t. of eyelid
fibro-osseous t.
fossa t.
hair follicle t.
t. of interior of eye
interior eye t.
intrasellar t.
Koenen's t.
lacrimal gland t.
lacrimal gland epithelial t.
lymphoid t.
lymphoproliferative t.
malignant t.
malignant epithelial t.
medulloblastoma t.
mesenchymal t.
metastasis of t.
t. metastasis
metastatic t.
mixed t.
mucinous adenocarcinoma t.
neurogenic t.
nonepithelial t.
ocular t.
ocular adnexal t.
t. of optic nerve
optic nerve t.
orbital t.
Pancoast t.
papilliform t.
phakomatous choristoma t.
pilomatrixoma t.
pituitary t.
plasma cell t.
Rathke's pouch t.
retinal anlage t.
Schmincke's t.
suprasellar t.
syringoma t.
trichofolliculoma t.
vascular t.
Warthin's t.
waxy t.
Wilms' t.
tunable dye laser
tungsten-halogen lamp
tunic
    Brücke's t.

tunic *(continued)*
fibrous t.
fibrovascular t.
Ruysch's t.
vascular t.
tunica
t. adnata oculi
t. albuginea oculi
t. conjunctiva
t. conjunctiva bulbi oculi
t. conjunctiva palpebra
t. fibrosa bulbi
t. fibrosa oculi
t. interna bulbi
t. nervea
t. nervosa oculi
t. sclerotica
t. senoria bulbi
t. uvea
t. vascularis oculi
t. vasculosa bulbi
t. vasculosa lentis
t. vasculosa oculi
tunicary
tunnel
scleral t.
t. vision
tunneled implant
turbidity
turbidity-reducing units (TRU)
turbo-tip of phacoemulsification unit
turcica
sella t.
Turkish saddle
Turk's line
Turner's syndrome
turning
head t.
tutamina oculi
TVA
true visual acuity
Tween
tweezers
jeweler t.
twelfth nerve palsy
twenty/twenty argon-fluoride excimer laser
Twenty/Twenty drops
twilight
t. blindness
t. vision
twin cone

Twirl
Spherical T.
twirling method
Twisk micro scissors
twist
t. fixation hook
scleral t.
stitch with t.'s
twisted virgin silk suture
two-angled polypropylene loop
two-light discrimination
two-plane lens
two-way
t.-w. cataract-aspirating cannula
t.-w. syringe
t.-w. towel clip
Tycos manometer
tying forceps
tying/stitch removal forceps
tyloma
t. conjunctivae
tylosis, pl. tyloses
t. ciliaris
tylotic
tyloxapol
Tyndall's
T. effect
T. phenomenon
type
t. I diabetes
t. II diabetes
t. l herpes simplex virus
test t.
typhlology
typhlosis
typhoid vaccine
typhus
epidemic t.
scrub t.
typical
t. achromatopsia
t. coloboma
typing
HLA t.
typoscope
Tyrell
T. iris hook
T. tympanic membrane hook
tyrosinase
t. test

tyrosinase-negative type
  oculocutaneous albinism
tyrosinase-positive type
  oculocutaneous albinism

tyrosinemia
tyrosinosis
Tyzine

ubiquitous
UGH
    uveitis glaucoma hyphema
    UGH syndrome
Uhthoff's
    U. phenomenon
    U. sign
    U. syndrome
Ulanday double cannula
ulcer
    acne rosacea corneal u.
    annular u.
    aphthous u.
    bacterial u.
    bacterial corneal u.
    catarrhal corneal u.
    central u.
    central corneal u.
    chronic serpiginous u.
    conjunctival u.
    corneal u.
    dendriform u.
    dendritic u.
    dendritic corneal u.
    dendritic herpes simplex
      corneal u.
    fascicular u.
    fungal corneal u.
    geographic herpes simplex
      corneal u.
    herpes simplex corneal u.
    herpetic u.
    hypopyon u.
    Jacob's u.
    marginal u.
    marginal catarrhal u.
    marginal corneal u.
    marginal ring u. of cornea
    metaherpetic u.
    Mooren's u.
    Mooren's corneal u.
    oval-shaped vernal u.
    pneumococcal u.
    pneumococcus u.
    pyocyaneal u.
    ring u.
    ring u. of cornea
    rodent u.
    Saemisch's u.
    serpent u. of cornea
    serpiginous u.
    serpiginous corneal u.
    sterile corneal u.
    stromal u.
    suppurative u.
    Terrien's u.
    transparent u. of the cornea
    Von Hippel's internal
      corneal u.
    xerophthalmic u.
ulcera
ulcerate
ulceration
    catarrhal marginal u.
    u. of cornea
    herpes epithelial tropic u.
    rheumatoid related u.
ulcerative
    u. keratitis
ulcerogenic
ulcerogranuloma
ulceromembranous
ulcerous
ulcus, pl. ulcera
    u. serpens corneae
ulectomy
ulerythema ophryogenes
Ulloa's operation
Ullrich's syndrome
Ultex
    U. bifocal
    U. implant
    U. lens
    U. lens implant
Ultima
    Dioptron U.
Ultracaine
ultrafiltration
Ultra-Image A-scan
Ultramatic
    U. Project-O-Chart
    U. Project-O-Chart projector
      (UPOC)
    U. Rx Master phoropter
    U. Rx Master phoropter
      retractor
Ultrapred
ultrascan
    Digital B System u.
Ultrascan Digital B System

Ultrasonic
    U. lancet needle
ultrasonic
    u. cataract removal lancet
    u. cataract-removal lancet
      needle
    u. micrometer
ultrasonogram
    A-scan u.
    B-scan u.
    Doppler u.
    gray-scale u.
ultrasonographic
ultrasonography
    A- & B-scan u.
    A-scan u.
    B-scan u.
    CooperVision u.
    Doppler u.
ultrasound
    Axisonic II u.
    CooperVision u.
    Ocuscan A-scan
      biometric u.
Ultra Tears
UltraThin surgical blade
ultraviolet
    u. burn
    u. filter
    u. keratoconjunctivitis
    u. light
    u. radiation
    u. ray ophthalmia
Ultravue lens
ultrazyme
Ultrazyme enzymatic cleaner
umbilicated cataract
umbra
umbrella iris
uncinate
    u. procedure
    u. process of lacrimal bone
unconventional outflow
uncrossed diplopia
uncut
    u. lens
    u. spectacle lens
underaction
    congenital superior
      oblique u.
undercorrection
underlying conus
underwater diathermy unit

undine
Undine dropper
undissociated alkaloid
undulate
undulatory nystagmus
unequal retinal image
unguis
    os u.
    pterygium u.
unharmonious ARC
unifocal optic nerve lesion
unilateral
    u. altitudinal scotoma
    u. arcus
    u. conjunctivitis
    u. hearing loss
    u. hemianopsia
    u. microtremor
    u. proptosis
    u. ptosis of eyelid
    u. sporadic retinoblastoma
    u. strabismus
uniocular
    u. hemianopsia
    u. strabismus
uniplanar
Uniplanar style PC II lens
Unisol
    U. Plus
Unisol 4
Unit
    Cilco Ultrasound U.
    Cooper I&A U.
    Intermedics Phaco I/A U.
    Krymed Cryopexy U.
    OMS Empac
      Irrigation/Aspiration U.
    Phaco Emulsifier
      Cavitron U.
unit
    Alcon cryosurgical u.
    Alcon irrigating/aspirating u.
    Alcon phacoemulsification u.
    Aloe reading u.
    Amoils cryosurgical u.
    Ångström u.
    AO Ful-Vue diagnostic u.
    AO Reichert Instruments
      Ful-Vue diagnostic u.
    Bishop-Harman
      irrigating/aspirating u.
    Bovie u.
    Bovie electrocautery u.

Got a Good Word for STEDMAN'S?

Help us keep STEDMAN'S products fresh and up-to-date with new words and new ideas!

Do we need to add or revise any items? Is there a better way to organize the content?

Be specific! How can we make this STEDMAN'S product the best medical word reference possible for you? Fill in the lines below with your thoughts and recommendations. Attach a separate sheet of paper if you need to—*you* are our most important contributor and we want to know what's on *your* mind. Thanks!

(PLEASE TYPE OR PRINT CAREFULLY)

Terms you believe are incorrect:

Appears as: Suggested revision:

_____   _____

_____   _____

_____   _____

New terms you would like us to add:

_____

_____

Other comments:

_____

_____

_____

All done? Great, just mail this card in today. No postage necessary, and thanks again!

Name / Title: _____

Facility / Company: _____

Address: _____

City / State / Zip: _____

Day Telephone No. (   ) _____

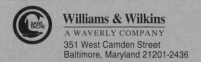

Williams & Wilkins
A WAVERLY COMPANY
351 West Camden Street
Baltimore, Maryland 21201-2436

To order or to receive a catalog call toll free 1-800-527-5597.

#079522-OPHTHALMOLOGY

Bovie electrosurgical u.
Bovie retinal detachment u.
Bracken
  irrigating/aspirating u.
Cavitron u.
Cavitron
  irrigating/aspirating u.
Cavitron-Kelman
  irrigating/aspirating u.
Charles
  irrigating/aspirating u.
Coburn
  irrigation/aspiration u.
u. of convergence
Cooper
  irrigating/aspirating u.
CooperVision
  irrigating/aspirating u.
CooperVision
  irrigation/aspiration u.
cryosurgical u.
DeVilbiss
  irrigating/aspirating u.
diathermy u.
Dougherty
  irrigating/aspirating u.
Drews
  irrigating/aspirating u.
Drews-Rosenbaum
  irrigating/aspirating u.
Empac-Cavitron
  irrigation/aspiration u.
Fink irrigating/aspirating u.
Fox irrigating/aspirating u.
Frigitronics cryosurgical u.
Gass irrigating/aspirating u.
Gibson
  irrigating/aspirating u.
Girard Ultrasonic u.
Hartstein
  irrigating/aspirating u.
Holzknecht u. (H)
Hyde irrigating/aspirating u.
Hyde irrigator/aspirator u.
IOLAB
  irrigating/aspirating u.
irrigating/aspirating u.
irrigation-aspiration u.
Irvine irrigating/aspirating u.
Keeler cryophake u.
Keeler cryosurgical u.
Kelman-Cavitron I/A u.

Kelman-Cavitron
  irrigating/aspirating u.
Kelman cryosurgical u.
Kelman
  irrigating/aspirating u.
Kelman
  phacoemulsification u.
u. of light
log u.'s
u. of luminous flux
u. of luminous intensity
McIntyre
  irrigating/aspirating u.
microcautery u.
Mira u.
Mira diathermy u.
N_2O cryosurgical u.
u. of ocular convergence
Ocutome vitrectomy u.
Peczon I/A u.
Peyman vitrectomy u.
Peyman vitreophage u.
Phaco Cavitron
  irrigating/aspirating u.
Pierce I/A u.
Premiere irrigation-
  aspiration u.
Rollet irrigating/aspirating u.
Schepens retinal
  detachment u.
SITE TXR 2200
  microsurgical u.
Storz-Walker retinal
  detachment u.
Surg-E-Trol System
  irrigating/aspirating u.
Svedberg u. (S)
Sylva irrigating/aspirating u.
Talbot u.
turbidity-reducing u.'s
  (TRU)
turbo-tip of
  phacoemulsification u.
underwater diathermy u.
Visitec aspiration u.
Visitec 1624
  irrigating/aspirating u.
Visitec vitrectomy u.
Vitrophage-Peyman u.
United Sonics J shock phaco fragmentor system
unity conjugacy planes

Universal
U. conformer
U. eye shield
U. shield
U. slit lamp
universale
angiokeratoma corporis
diffusum u.
University of Waterloo chart
Univis
U. bifocal
U. lens
Unna's abtropfung theory
unrefined refraction
unstained wet mount
up-and-down staircases procedure
upbeat nystagmus
updrawn pupil
up-gaze
UPOC
Ultramatic Project-O-Chart
projector
upper
u. canaliculus
u. eyelid
u. hemianopsia
u. punctum
u. retina
upside-down
u.-d. ptosis
u.-d. reversal of vision
uptake
lacrimal gland gallium u.
upward
u. gaze
u. squint
urate
u. band keratopathy
u. keratopathy
uratic
u. conjunctivitis
u. iritis
Urbach-Wiethe disease
urea
uremic
u. amaurosis
u. amblyopia
u. optic neuropathy
u. retinitis
urethane
urethritis

Uribe
U. implant
U. orbital implant
uric
u. acid crystals
u. acid metabolism
urica
keratitis u.
urinalysis
urine refractometry
urochrome
urokinase
Urrets-Zavalia retinal surgical lens
urticaria
solar u.
Usher's syndrome
uterque
oculi u.
visio oculus u.
Utrata forceps
Utrata-Kershner capsulorrhexis cystome forceps
utricular reflex
UV
UV blocking filter
UV Nova Curve lens
uvea
tunica u.
uveae
entropion u.
sarcomatosum u.
uveal
u. atrophy
u. coat
u. effusion
u. effusion syndrome
u. entropion
u. framework
u. juvenile xanthogranuloma
u. melanoma
u. metastasis
u. neurofibroma
u. nevus
u. osteoma
u. staphyloma
u. tract
u. tract hamartoma
u. tract hemangioma
uvealis
pars u.
uveitic
u. band keratopathy
u. glaucoma

uveitides
uveitis, pl. **uveitides**
    anterior u.
    aspergillosis u.
    bacterial u.
    bilateral u.
    candidal u.
    emplaced u.
    endogenous u.
    Föerster's u.
    Fuchs' u.
    fungal u.
    u. glaucoma hyphema (UGH)
    granulomatous u.
    herpes u.
    herpes simplex u.
    heterochromia u.
    heterochromic u.
    intermediate u.
    Kirisawa's u.
    lens-induced u.
    nongranulomatous u.
    parasitic u.
    peripheral u.
    phacoanaphylactic u.
    phacogenic u.
    phacolytic u.
    phacotoxic u.
    posterior u.
    protozoan u.
    sympathetic u.
    toxoplasmic u.
    tuberculous u.
    viral u.
    vitiligo u.
    Vogt-Koyanagi bilateral u.
uveitis-vitiligo-alopecia-poliosis syndrome
uveocutaneous syndrome
uveoencephalitic syndrome
uveoencephalitis
uveolabyrinthitis
uveomeningeal syndrome
uveomeningitis syndrome
uveomeningoencephalitis
uveoneuroaxitis
uveoparotid fever
uveoparotitis
uveoplasty
uveoretinitis
uveoscleral outflow
uveoscleritis
uveovertex drainage
UVEX lens
uviban
Uyemura's
    U. operation
    U. syndrome

V
 vanadium
 volt
 volume
VA
 visual acuity
  VA magnetic implant
  VA magnetic orbital
   implant
vaccination
 bacillus Calmette-Guérin v.
vaccine
 typhoid v.
vaccinia
 blepharoconjunctivitis v.
 v. gangrenosa
 generalized v.
 v. infection
 keratitis v.
 progressive v.
vaccinial keratitis
vacciniforme
 hydroa v.
vaccinulosa
 keratitis post v.
Vactro
 V. perilimbal suction
 V. perilimbal suction
  apparatus
vacuolar configuration
vacuolation
vacuole
 autophagic v.
 cortical v.
vacuuming
vaginae
 v. externa nervi optici
 v. interna nervi optici
 v. nervi optici
 v. oculi
Vaiser-Cibis muscle retractor
Vaiser sponge
validity
Valilab
 V. cautery
 V. electrocautery
Valium
valproate sodium
valproic acid
Valsalva's maneuver

value
 C v.
 DK v.
 equivalent oxygen
  percentage v.
 p v.
 predictive v.
 prismatic dioptric v.
valve
 Béraud's v.
 Bianchi's v.
 Bochdalek's v.
 Foltz's v.
 v. of Hasner
 Hasner's v.
 Huschke's v.
 Krause's v.
 Krupin v.
 v. of Rosenmüller
 Rosenmüller's v.
 Taillefer's v.
 Van Herick's v.
Van
 V. Herick's modification
 V. Herick's valve
 V. Heuven's retinopathy
 V. Lint akinesia
 V. Lint anesthesia
 V. Lint-Atkinson lid
  akinetic block
 V. Lint block
 V. Lint's flap
 V. Lint's injection
 V. Lint's modified
  technique
 V. Lint's technique
 V. Milligen's eyelid repair
  technique
 V. Milligen's operation
van
 v. der Hoeve's disease
 v. der Hoeve's syndrome
vanadium (V)
vancomycin
vanillism
Vannas
 V. capsulotomy
 V. capsulotomy scissors
 V. scissors
variable strabismus

variance
varians
    metamorphopsia v.
variation
    coefficient of v.
    diurnal v.
    v. diurnal
Vari bladebreaker
varicella
    v. iridocyclitis
    v. keratitis
    v. syndrome
varicella-zoster
    v.-z. ophthalmicus
    v.-z. virus
varices
varicoblepharon
varicose ophthalmia
varicula
Varigray
    V. implant
    V. lens
Varilux
    V. implant
    V. lens
    V. lens implant
variola
varix, pl. **varices**
    conjunctival v.
    orbital v.
vas, pl. **vasa**
    vasa sanguinea retinae
Vasco-Posada orbital retractor
vascular
    v. arcade
    v. cataract
    v. circle of optic nerve
    v. coat of eyeball
    v. filling defect
    v. fronds
    v. funnel
    v. hamartoma
    v. keratitis
    v. lamina of choroid
    v. loop
    v. network
    v. occlusion
    v. occlusive disease
    v. retinopathy
    v. supply
    v. tree
    v. trunks

    v. tumor
    v. tunic
vascularization
    corneal v.
    stromal v.
vascularized tortuosity
vasculature
    retinal v.
    spider v.
vasculitis
    obstructive retinal v.
    orbital v.
    v. retinae
    retinal v.
vasculonebulous keratitis
vasoactive amines
Vasocidin
VasoClear
VasoClear A
Vasocon-A
Vasocon Regular
vasodilation
vasodilator
vasoproliferation
vasoproliferative factor
Vasosulf
vault
    sagittal v.
vaulting of contact lens
VC
    color vision
    vital capacity
VCA
    viral capsid antigen
VDRL
    Venereal Disease Research
    Laboratory
      VDRL test
VECP
    visual evoked cortical potential
vectis
    Anis irrigating v.
    anterior chamber
      irrigating v.
    aspirating/irrigating v.
    cul-de-sac irrigating v.
    Drews-Knolle reverse
      irrigating v.
    irrigating v.
    irrigating anterior
      chamber v.
    irrigating/aspirating v.
    Look irrigating v.

Peczon I/A v.
Pierce I/A irrigating v.
Pierce irrigating v.
plastic disposable
 irrigating v.
Sheets irrigating v.
Snellen v.
vectograph chart
vectographic study
vecuronium
vegetable ophthalmia
veil
dimple v.
pigmented v.'s
Sattler's v.
vitreal v.
vitreous v.
veiling glare
vein
angular v.
antecubital v.
anterior ciliary v.
anterior conjunctival v.
aqueous v.
Ascher's v.
central v.
central retinal v. (CRV)
choroid v.
choroidovaginal v.
ciliary v.
cilioretinal v.
conjunctival v.
corticose v.
endophlebitis of retinal v.
episcleral v.
facial v.
frontal diploic v.
Galen's v.
inferior nasal v.
inferior ophthalmic v.
inferior palpebral v.
inferior temporal v.
Kuhnt's postcentral v.
lacrimal v.
muscular v.
nasofrontal v.
nicking of retinal v.
occlusion of v.
occlusion of branch v.
ophthalmic v.
ophthalmomeningeal v.
palpebral v.

posterior v.'s
posterior ciliary v.
posterior conjunctival v.
retinal v.
superior nasal v.
superior ophthalmic v.
superior palpebral v.
superior temporal v.
supraorbital v.
vortex v.
Veirs
V. cannula
V. trocar
Velcro head strap
velocardiofacial syndrome
velocity
v. error
retinal-slip v.
saccadic v.
stuttering v.'s
velonoskiascopy
velum
corneal v.
Velva Kleen
VEM
vergence eye movements
vena
v. angularis
v. centralis retinae
v. choroideae oculi
v. ciliares anteriores
v. diploica frontalis
v. facialis
v. lacrimalis
v. nasofrontalis
v. ophthalmica inferior
v. ophthalmica superior
v. ophthalmomeningea
v. vorticosae
venae
v. anteriores conjunctivales
v. conjunctivales
v. episclerale
v. palpebrales
v. palpebrales inferiores
v. palpebrales superiores
v. posteriores conjunctivales
venereal disease
Venereal Disease Research
 Laboratory (VDRL)
Venereal Disease Research
 Laboratory test

venereum
    granuloma v.
    lymphogranuloma v.
venography
    orbital v.
venomanometry
venous
    v. engorgement
    v. hemangioma
    v. laminar
    v. occlusive disease
    v. phase
    v. pulsation
    v. sheathing
    v. sheath patch
    v. sinuses
    v. stasis
    v. stasis retinopathy (VSR)
    v. stenosis retinopathy
    v. tortuosity
venter frontalis musculi
  occipitofrontalis
ventricle
    cerebral v.
ventriculography
venula, pl. **venulae**
    v. macularis inferior
    v. macularis superior
    v. medialis retinae
    v. nasalis retinae inferior
    v. nasalis retinae superior
    v. retinae medialis
    v. temporalis retinae
      inferior
    v. temporalis retinae
      superior
venule
    macular v.
    retinal v.
VEP
    visual evoked potential
VER
    visual-evoked response
vera
    polycoria v.
    polycythemia v.
    polycythemia rubra v.
verapamil
Veratrum
Verga's lacrimal groove
vergence
    ability v.
    v. eye movements (VEM)

    fusional v.
    v. of lens
    negative vertical v.
    power v.
    reduced v.
    reflux v.
    tonic v.
    vertical v.
    zero v.
Verhoeff
    V. capsule forceps
    V. expressor
    V. forceps
    V. lens expressor
    V. scissors
    V. suture
Verhoeff-Chandler
    V.-C. capsulotomy
    V.-C. operation
Verhoeff's
    V. operation
    V. stain
    V. streak
vermiform
    v. contractions
    v. movement
vermis
    cerebellar v.
Vernacel
vernal
    v. catarrh
    v. conjunctivitis
    v. keratoconjunctivitis
Vernier
    V. acuity
    V. stimulus
    V. visual acuity
verruca, pl. **verrucae**
    v. filiformis
    v. vulgaris
verrucous shape
Versed
version
    ductions and v.'s (D&V)
    v.'s and ductions
    levoversion v.
    v. movement
versions
vertebral angiography
vertebrobasilar
    v. artery
    v. system
    v. vascular abnormality

vertex
    v. of distance
    front v.
    v. of power
    v. power
    v. refractionometer
vertexmeter
vertical
    v. axis
    v. axis of eye
    v. axis of Fick
    v. comitant deviation
    v. deviation
    v. diplopia
    v. divergence
    v. divergence position
    v. ductions
    v. fusional vergence
     amplitude
    v. gaze
    v. gaze center
    v. hemianopsia
    v. illumination
    v. meridian
    v. movements
    v. nystagmus
    v. parallax
    v. phoria
    v. plane
    v. prism test
    v. retraction syndrome
    right gaze v.'s
    v. strabismus
    v. strabismus fixus
    v. stria
    v. tropia
    v. vergence
    v. vertigo
verticullata
    cornea v.
vertiginous
vertigo
    benign paroxysmal
     positional v. (BPPV)
    benign paroxysmal
     postural v.
    objective v.
    ocular v.
    sham-movement v.
    special sense v.
    subjective v.
    vertical v.
vertometer

Verwey's
    V. eyelid operation
    V. operation
vesicle
    chorionic v.
    compound v.
    lens v.
    lenticular v.
    multilocular v.
    ocular v.
    ophthalmic v.
    optic v.
    pinocytotic v.
vesicula, pl. vesiculae
    v. ophthalmica
vesicular
    v. keratitis
    v. keratopathy
vesiculation
    eyelid v.
vesiculobullous
vesiculosus linear endothelial
Vesprin
vessel
    v. abnormalities of retina
    choroidal v.
    ciliary v.
    congested v.'s
    disk neurovascular v.'s
    disk new v.'s
    episcleral blood v.
    feeder v.'s
    ghost v.
    neovascularization of
     new v.'s elsewhere (NVE)
    opticociliary v.'s
    opticociliary shunt v.'s
    orbital v.
    retinal v.
    v. sheathing
    sheathing of v.
    shunt v.'s
    silver-wire v.'s
    stromal blood v.
    succulent v.
    tensile strength of v.'s
    tortuosity of retinal v.
vestibular
    v. nystagmus
    v. pupillary reaction
    v. system
vestibulocerebellar ataxia

vestibulo-ocular
  v.-o. reflex
  v.-o. response (VOR)
vestibulopathy
VF
  visual field
V-groove gauge
VG slit lamp
VH
  vitreous hemorrhage
vibrating scissors
vibration
  photoelectric v.
vibratory nystagmus
Vickerall round ringed forceps
Vickers
  V. forceps
  V. needle holder
Vicrosurgery
Vicryl suture
VID
  visible iris diameter
vidarabine
videokeratoscope
videometer
video specular microscope
vidian
  v. nerve
  v. neuralgia
Viers
  V. erysiphake
  V. needle
  V. rod
Viers' operation
Vieth-Mueller horopter
Vieth-Muller circle
view
  axial v.
  Caldwell's v.
  Caldwell-Waters v.
  field of v.
  Waters' v.
viewing
  eccentric v.
viliginous chorioretinitis
Villasensor ultrasonic pachymeter
villi
  pectinate v.
vinyl
  v. T-tube
  v. tube
violaceous

violet
  v. haptic
  v. vision
  visual v.
Vira-A
viral
  v. blepharitis
  v. capsid antigen (VCA)
  v. conjunctivitis
  v. keratoconjunctivitis
  v. ocular disease
  v. uveitis
Virchow's corpuscle
virgin
  v. silk
  v. silk suture
viridans
  Streptococcus v.
Viroptic
virtual
  v. focus
  v. image
  v. point
virulence
virus
  cytomegalic inclusion v.
  Epstein-Barr v. (EBV)
  herpes simplex v. (HSV)
  human immunodeficiency v.
   (HIV)
  Newcastle disease v.
  type 1 herpes simplex v.
  varicella-zoster v.
Visalens
  V. contact lens cleaning
   and soaking solution
  V. Wetting
VISC
  vitreous infusion suction cutter
   OMS Machemer/Parel VISC
   VISC vitreous cutter
visceral
  v. larva migrans
  v. larva migrans syndrome
  v. myopathy
Viscoat solution
viscoelastic
VISCOFLOW cannula
Viscolens lens
viscosity
  v. agent
  blood v.
visco surgery

Viscous
 Neo-Synephrine V.
viscous
 v. fluid
 v. ochre fluid
 v. xanthochromic fluid
Visculose
visibility
 v. acuity
 v. curve
visible
 v. iris diameter (VID)
 minimum v.
 v. spectrum
VISIFLEX drape
visile
Visine
 V. A.C.
 V. Extra
 V. L.R.
visio
 v. oculus
 v. oculus dextra (vision of
  right eye) (VOD)
 v. oculus sinister (vision of
  left eye) (VOS)
 v. oculus uterque (vision of
  both eyes) (VOU)
Vision
 V. analyzer
 V. Analyzer/Overrefraction
  System
 V. Care enzymatic cleaner
 V. Tech lens
vision
 6/6 v.
 20/20 v.
 achromatic v.
 artificial v.
 best-corrected v.
 binocular v.
 binocular single v. (BSV)
 blue v.
 blurring of v.
 central v.
 central island of v.
 central keyhole of v.
 chromatic v.
 color v. (VC)
 cone v.
 day v.
 decreasing v.
 dichromatic v.

dimness of v.
direct v.
distortion of v.
double v.
eccentric v.
extramacular binocular v.
facial v.
false v.
field of v.
finger v.
form v.
foveal v.
green v.
half v.
halo v.
haploscopic v.
indirect v.
iridescent v.
keyhole v.
linear v.
loss of v.
low v.
macular binocular v.
misty v.
monocular v.
motion v.
multiple v.
naked v. (Nv.)
near v.
night v.
obscure v.
organ of v.
oscillating v.
peripheral v.
phantom v.
photopic v.
Pick's v.
pseudoscopic v.
rainbow v.
red v.
v. rod
rod v.
scoterythrous v.
scotopic v.
shaft v.
single binocular v. (SBV)
solid v.
stable v.
stereoscopic v.
subjective v.
subnormal v.
suboptimal v.
v. training

vision *(continued)*
    transient obscuration of v.
    transient obscurations of v.
    Tripier's operation v.
    triple v.
    tubular v.
    tunnel v.
    twilight v.
    upside-down reversal of v.
    violet v.
    word v.
    yellow v.
Visitec
    V. angled lens hook
    V. aspiration unit
    V. capsule polisher curette
    V. corneal shield
    V. cortex extractor
    V. cystitome
    V. double-cutting cystitome
    V. intraocular lens dialer
    V. iris retractor
    V. irrigating/aspirating
    cannula
    V. 1624 irrigating/aspirating
    cannula
    V. 1624 irrigating/aspirating
    unit
    V. lens pusher
    V. micro double iris hook
    V. micro hook
    V. micro iris hook
    V. nucleus removal loop
    V. RK zone marker
    V. straight lens hook
    V. vico manipulator
    V. vitrectomy unit
Visometer
    Lotman V.
Vistaril
Vistech 6500 contrast test
visual
    v. acuity (VA)
    v. agnosia
    v. allesthesia
    v. angle
    v. aphasia
    v. association area
    v. attentiveness
    v. axis
    v. blackout
    v. cell
    v. cone

v. confusion
v. corkscrew defects
v. cortex
v. defect
v. deprivation syndrome
v. development
v. direction
v. discrimination
v. disturbance
v. efficiency
v. evoked cortical potential
(VECP)
v. evoked potential (VEP)
v. extinction
v. field (F, VF)
v. field testing
v. function
v. function evaluation
v. hallucination
v. halo
v. image
v. inattention
v. line
v. orbicularis reflex
v. organ
v. pathway
v. perception
v. pigment
v. plane
v. point
v. preservation
v. projection
v. purple
v. radiations
v. receptor
v. sensory system
v. threshold
v. tilt
v. violet
v. white
v. yellow
v. zone
visuale
    organum v.
visual-evoked response (VER)
visualization
    contrast v.
    double-contrast v.
visualize
visually evoked potential mapping
visual-spatial agnosia
Visual-Tech machine
visual-vestibulo-ocular response

Visulab System
Visulas
    V. argon C laser
    V. argon laser
    V. argon/YAG laser
    V. Nd:YAG laser
    V. YAG C laser
    V. YAG E laser
    V. YAG S laser
visuoauditory
visuognosis
visuolexic
visuometer
visuopsychic
visuosensory
visuospatial
visus
    linea v.
    organum v.
Visuscope
    Cüppers V.
    V. motor
    V. motor test
    V. ophthalmoscope
    V. sensory test
Visuskop
Visutron
Vit-A-Drops
vital capacity (VC)
Vitallium implant
vitamin
    v. A deficiency
    v. A hypervitaminosis
    v. D hypervitaminosis
    v. D toxicity
vitamin A
vitamin A_1
vitamin A_2
vitamin B
vitamin B_6
vitamin B_{12}
vitamin C
vitamin D
vitamin E
vitamin K
vitelliform
    v. degeneration
    v. degeneration of macula
    v. dystrophy
    v. macular degeneration
    v. maculopathy
vitelline macular degeneration

vitelliruptive
    v. degeneration
    v. macular dystrophy
vitellirupture
    autosomal dominant v.
vitiligo, pl. vitiligines
    v. iridis
    v. uveitis
vitiligoidea
Vitrax
vitrea
    lamina v.
    membrana v.
vitreal
    v. bleed
    v. cells
    v. detachment
    v. hemorrhage
    v. lamina
    v. membrane
    v. veil
vitrectomy
    anterior v.
    closed-system pars plana v.
    core v.
    v. instrument
    open-sky v.
    pars plana v.
    port v.
    posterior v.
    v. sponge
    Weck-cel v.
vitrector
    Alcon v.
    Cilco v.
    CooperVision v.
    Frigitronics v.
    Kaufman v.
    Kaufman type II v.
    Microvit v.
    Peyman v.
    Storz Microvit v.
    Storz Microvit v.
vitrei
    synchesis corporis v.
vitrein
vitreitis
    idiopathic v.
vitreocapsulitis
vitreolysis
vitreophage
    Kaufman v.
vitreoretinal (VR)

vitreoretinal *(continued)*
    v. attachment
    v. choroidopathy syndrome
    v. contusion
    v. degeneration
    v. disorder
    v. dysplasia
    v. infusion cutter
    v. tag
    v. traction syndrome
    v. tuft
vitreoretinochoroidopathy
vitreoretinopathy
    closed-funnel v.
    exudative v.
    familial exudative v.
    proliferative v. (PVR)
vitreo-tapetoretinal dystrophy
vitreous
    v. abscess
    v. aspirating needle
    v. aspiration
    v. base
    v. block
    v. block glaucoma
    v. body
    v. break-through hemorrhage
    v. bulge
    v. cavity
    v. chamber
    v. chamber of eye
    v. coloboma
    v. contraction
    v. cutter
    detached v.
    v. detachment
    v. face
    v. fibers
    v. floater
    v. fluff
    v. fluorophotometry
    v. forceps
    v. foreign body
    v. foreign body forceps
    v. gel
    v. haze
    v. hemorrhage (VH)
    v. hemorrhage breakthrough
    v. hernia
    v. herniation
    v. humor
    hyperplastic v.

v. infusion suction cutter
    (VISC)
knuckle of loose v.
v. lamina
liquefied v.
liquified v.
loss of v.
v. loss
v. membrane
micelles in v.
v. neovascularization
v. opacity
organized v.
v. pencil
persistent anterior
    hyperplastic primary v.
persistent hyperplasia of
    primary v. (PHPV)
persistent hyperplastic v.
persistent hyperplastic
    primary v.
persistent posterior
    hyperplastic primary v.
primary v.
primary persistent
    hyperplastic v.
v. prolapse
puff of loose v.
v. retraction
secondary v.
v. seeding
v. separation
v. skirt
v. strands
v. strand scissors
v. stroma
v. surgery
v. sweep spatula
syneresis of v.
v. tap
tertiary v.
v. touch
v. traction
v. transplant needle
v. veil
v. wick syndrome
vitreous-aspirating cannula
vitreum
    corpus v.
    v. corpus
    stroma v.

vitrina
  v. ocularis
  v. oculi
vitritis
  idiopathic v.
  senile v.
Vitrophage-Peyman unit
vitrosi
vitrosin
V-lance
  V.-l. blade
  V.-l. blade/knife
  V.-l. Sharpoint
V-lancet knife
VOD
  visio oculus dextra (vision of
  right eye)
Vogt
  glaukomflecken of V.
  limbal girdle of V.
  V. lines
  white limbal girdle of V.
Vogt-Barraquer
  V.-B. corneal needle
  V.-B. eye needle
Vogt-Koyanagi
  V.-K. bilateral uveitis
  V.-K. syndrome
Vogt-Koyanagi-Harada
  V.-K.-H. disease
  V.-K.-H. syndrome
Vogt's
  V. cataract
  V. cornea
  V. degeneration
  V. disease
  V. limbal girdle
  V. operation
  V. syndrome
  V. white limbal girdle
Vogt-Spielmeyer
  V.-S. disease
  V.-S. syndrome
Vogt-type cataract
Volk
  V. conoid implant
  V. conoid lens implant
  V. coronoid lens
volt (V)
  electron v.
Voltaren
volume (V)

volumetric
voluntary
  v. convergence
  v. eye movement
  v. nystagmus
volvulosis
Von
  V. Ammon's operation
  V. Hippel-Lindau syndrome
  V. Hippel's internal corneal
  ulcer
von
  v. Blaskovics-Doyen
  operation
  v. Frisch's theory
  v. Gierke's disease
  v. Graefe cataract knife
  v. Graefe cautery
  v. Graefe cystitome
  v. Graefe electrocautery
  v. Graefe fixation forceps
  v. Graefe forceps
  v. Graefe hook
  v. Graefe iris forceps
  v. Graefe knife
  v. Graefe knife needle
  v. Graefe muscle hook
  v. Graefe's operation
  v. Graefe's sign
  v. Graefe's syndrome
  v. Graefe strabismus hook
  v. Graefe tissue forceps
  v. Hippel-Lindau disease
  v. Hippel's disease
  v. Hippel's operation
  v. Monakow's fiber
  v. Mondak capsule
  fragment-clot forceps
  v. Mondak forceps
  v. Noorden's incision
  v. Recklinghausen's disease
  v. Recklinghausen's
  syndrome
VOR
  vestibulo-ocular response
vortex, pl. vortices
  v. corneal dystrophy
  v. dystrophy
  Fleischer's v.
  v. keratopathy
  v. lentis
  v. pattern

vortex *(continued)*
    v. system
    v. vein
vortex-like clumps
vortices
vorticosae
    vena v.
VOS
    visio oculus sinister (vision of left eye)
Vossius
    V. lenticular ring
    V. ring
VOU
    visio oculus uterque (vision of both eyes)
V pattern
V-pattern
    V.-p. esotropia
    V.-p. exotropia

VR
    vitreoretinal
V-slit lamp
VSR
    venous stasis retinopathy
V syndrome
Vuero Meter
vulcanizing
    room temperature v. (RTV)
vulgaris
    lupus v.
    pemphigus v.
    verruca v.
Vygantas-Wilder retinal drainage probe

Waardenburg-Jonkers
    corneal dystrophy of W.-J.
    dystrophy of W.-J.
Waardenburg-Klein syndrome
Waardenburg-like syndrome
Waardenburg's syndrome
Wachendorf's membrane
Wadsworth lid forceps
Wadsworth-Todd
    W.-T. cautery
    W.-T. electrocautery
Wagener-Clay-Gipner classification
Wagener's retinitis
Wagner's
    W. disease
    W. hereditary vitreoretinal
      degeneration
    W. hyaloid retinal
      degeneration
    W. syndrome
    W. vitreoretinal dystrophy
Walnstock suturing forceps
waking ptosis
Waldeau
    W. fixation forceps
    W. forceps
Waldenström's macroglobulinemia
Waldeyer's gland
Waldhauer's operation
Walker
    W. coagulator
    W. electrode
    W. everter
    W. lid everter
    W. micro pin
    W. pin
    W. scissors
    W. trephine
Walker-Apple scissors
Walker-Atkinson scissors
Walker-Lee sclerotome
wall
    eye w.
    w. push maneuver
Wallach cryosurgical pencil
Wallenberg's
    W. lateral medullary
      syndrome
    W. syndrome
walleye

walleyed
Walser corneoscleral punch
Walter
    W. Reed implant
    W. Reed operation
    W. spud
Walton
    W. punch
    W. spud
wand
    Powell w.
wane
    wax and w.
Wang lens
Warburg syndrome
warfarin
    w. sodium
warm-same
    cold-opposite, w.-s. (COWS)
warpage
wart
    Hassall-Henle w.
    Henle's w.'s
Warthin's tumor
wartlike bodies
Wash
    Lavoptik Eye W.
    Star-Optic Eye W.
wash
    eye w.
washout
    color w.
water
    w. cell
    w. content
    w. fissures
    w. provocative test
water-drinking test
watered-silk retina
water-silk reflex
Waters' view
watery eye
Watt stave bender
Watzke
    W. band
    W. cuff
    W. forceps
    W. sleeve
    W. tire
Watzke's operation

wave
A-w.
B-w.
C-w.
D-w.
wave-edge knife
wavefront
convergent w.
waveguides
wavelength
wax and wane
waxy
w. exudate
w. tumor
W4D test
Worth's four-dot test
Wear
Enzymatic Cleaner for
Extended W.
Weaver
W. chalazion forceps
W. trocar introducer
Weber-Dubler syndrome
Weber-Elschnig
W.-E. lens
W.-E. lens loupe
W.-E. loupe
Weber knife
Weber-Rinne sign
Weber's
W. law
W. paralysis
W. sign
W. syndrome
web eye
Weck
W. astigmatism ruler
W. eye shield
W. knife
W. microscope
W. shield
W. sponge
Weck-cel
W.-c. sponge
W.-c. surgical spear
W.-c. vitrectomy
wedge
w. resection
temporal w.
Wedl cells
Weeker's operation

Weeks
W. needle
W. speculum
Weeks'
W. bacillus
W. operation
Wegener's
W. granulomatosis
W. granulomatosis
conjunctivitis
Weibel-Palade bodies
Weigert's ligament
Weil-Felix reaction
Weil lacrimal cannula
Weill-Marchesani syndrome
Weil's disease
Weisinger's operation
Weiss
W. gold dilator
W. speculum
Weiss' reflex
Welch
W. four-drop device
W. rubber bulb erysiphake
Welch-Allyn
W.-A.-Allyn Pocket scope
W.-A. ophthalmoscope
Welcker
cribra orbitalis of W.
welder's
w. conjunctivitis
w. keratoconjunctivitis
Welland's test
Wells enucleation spoon
Welsh
W. cannula
W. cortex extractor
W. cortex stripper cannula
W. erysiphake
W. flat-olive tip
W. flat olive-tip double
cannula
W. iris retractor
W. olive-tip cannula
W. pupil-spreader forceps
W. Silastic erysiphake
Wendell Hughes operation
Werb
W. right-angle probe
W. scissors
Werb's operation
Wergeland
W. double cannula

W. double needle
W. needle
Werner's
W. syndrome
W. test
Wernicke's
W. encephalopathy
W. reaction
W. sign
W. symptom
W. syndrome
W. triangle
Wesley-Jessen lens
Wessely ring
West
W. chisel
W. gouge
W. lacrimal cannula
W. lacrimal sac chisel
Westcott
W. conjunctiva scissors
W. scissors
W. stitch scissors
W. tenotomy scissors
W. utility scissors
Westcott's test
Westergren
W. method
W. sedimentation rate
Westphal-Piltz
W.-P. phenomenon
W.-P. reflex
Westphal's
W. phenomenon
W. pupillary reflex
Westphal-Strümpell disease
West's operation
Wet
Lens W.
wet
bedewing to w.
w. cell
w. dressing
w. mount
w. storage
Wet-cote
wet-field
w.-f. cautery
w.-f. electrocautery
Wet-N-Soak
W.-N.-S. Plus
Wetting
Liquifilm W.

W. & Soaking
Visalens W.
wetting
w. agent
w. angle
w. angle of contact lens
w. solution
Weve electrode
Weve's operation
Weyers-Thier syndrome
Wharton-Jones operation
Whatman filter
wheal
skin w.
Wheeler
W. blade
W. cyclodialysis system
W. cystitome
W. discission knife
W. eye sphere implant
W. implant
W. iris spatula
W. knife
W. method
W. spatula
Wheeler-Reese operation
Wheeler's
W. halving repair
W. operation
W. procedure
wheel rotation
Whipple's
W. disease
W. disk
white
w. braided silk suture
w. cells
w. cord
w. dots
w. dot syndrome
w. of eye
w. light
w. limbal girdle of Vogt
w. pupil
w. pupillary reflex
w. reflex
w. retinal necrosis
w. ring
w. ring of cornea
w. sclera
w. spot
w. stromal infiltrate
w. tunica fibrosa oculi

white *(continued)*
    visual w.
    w. without pressure
white-centered hemorrhage
White glaucoma pump shunt
whitlow
Whitnall's
    W. ligament
    W. operation
    W. sling operation
    W. tubercle
Whitney superior rectus forceps
whorl
    w. lens
    skin w.
whorl-like configuration
whorls
    ochre-colored w.
Wicherkiewicz's
    W. eyelid operation
    W. operation
wick
    filtering w.
wicking
    w. glue patch
    w. patch
wide-angle glaucoma
wide-field eyepiece
Widmark's conjunctivitis
Widowitz's sign
width
    angle w.
    orbital w.
Wieger's ligament
Wiener
    W. corneal hook
    W. hook
    W. keratome
    W. scleral hook
    W. speculum
Wiener's operation
Wies'
    W. operation
    W. procedure
    W. spot
Wies chalazion forceps
Wilbrand's prism test
Wild
    W. lens
    W. M 690 microscope
    W. operating microscope
Wilde forceps

Wilder
    W. band spreader
    W. cystitome
    W. cystitome knife
    W. dilator
    W. lacrimal dilator
    W. lens loupe
    W. scleral depressor
    W. scleral retractor
    W. scoop
Wilder's sign
Wildervanck's syndrome
Wildgen-Reck localizer
Wildgren-Reck locator
Wilkerson
    W. forceps
    W. intraocular lens-insertion
      forceps
Willebrand
    anterior knee of von W.
Williams
    W. pediatric eye speculum
    W. probe
    W. speculum
    W. syndrome
Willis
    circle of W.
Wills
    W. cautery
    W. forceps
    W. Hospital utility forceps
    W. utility eye forceps
Wilmer
    W. conjunctival scissors
    W. refractor
    W. retractor
    W. scissors
Wilmer-Bagley expressor
Wilmer's operation
Wilms' tumor
Wilson's
    W. degeneration
    W. disease
    W. syndrome
Wincor enucleation scissors
window defect
windows
    clear w.
windshield wiper syndrome
wing cell
winking
    jaw w.
    w. spasm

wink reflex
Winslow's star
Wintersteiner rosettes
wipe-out syndrome
wire
    cheese w.
    w. enucleation snare
    w. frame spectacles
    Kirschner w.
    w. lid speculum
    w. mesh implant
wire-loop keratoscope
Wirt's
    W. stereopsis test
    W. stereo test
    W. stereo test
    W. vision test
Wise
    W. iridotomy laser lens
    W. iridotomy-sphincterotomy
    laser lens
Wiskott-Aldrich syndrome
with
    w. correction (cc)
    w. motion
without correction (sc)
with-the-rule astigmatism
Wolfe forceps
Wolfe's
    W. graft
    W. method
    W. operation
    W. ptosis operation
Wolff-Eisner
    W.-E. prism
    W.-E. test
Wolfring
    gland of W.
Wolfring's
    W. gland
    W. lacrimal gland
Wolf's syndrome
Wollaston's
    W. doublet
    W. theory
Woods'
    W. light examination
    W. sign

Woods Concept lens
wool saturated in saline dressing
Wooten needle
word
    w. blindness
    w. vision
Worksheet
    Thill Aniseikonia W.
Worst
    W. corneal bur
    W. goniotomy lens
    W. Medallion lens
    W. needle
    W. pigtail probe
    W. Platina iris-fixated lens
    W. probe
    W. suture
Worst's operation
Worth
    W. amblyoscope
    W. forceps
    W. strabismus forceps
Worth's
    W. concept of fusion
    W. four-dot test (W4D test)
    W. operation
    W. ptosis operation
wound
    w. closure
    puncture w.
WR-77913
Wrattan filter
Wright
    W fascia needle
    W. needle
    W. ophthalmic needle
Wright's operation
wrinkling
    macular surface w.
    w. membrane
Wucherer's conjunctivitis
Wullstein-House cup forceps
Wundt-Lamansky law
Wyburn-Mason syndrome
Wydase

χ^2 **test**

X

exophoria

x

axis of cylindric lens

xanthelasma

x. around eyelid

xanthelasmatosis

x. bulbi

x. iridis

xanthism

xanthochromic fluid

xanthocyanopsia

xanthogranuloma

juvenile x. (JXG)

juvenile iris x.

necrobiotic x.

uveal juvenile x.

xanthogranulomatosis

xanthokyanopy

xanthoma, pl. xanthomata

x. elasticum

x. palpebrarum

x. planum

tonofibrils tendinous x.

tonofibrils tuberous x.

xanthomatosis

x. bulbi

cerbrotendinous x.

essential

hypercholesterolemic x.

familial

hypercholesterolemic x.

hypercholesterolemic x.

x. iridis

xanthophane

xanthophyll

x. pigment

xanthopsia, xanthopia

xanthopsin

x axis

X cell

X chrom contact lens

X chrom lens

X chromosome

xenon

x. arc

x. arc photocoagulation

x. arc photocoagulator

x. photocoagulator

xenophthalmia

xeroderma

x. of Kaposi

x. pigmentosum

xerodermatic

xeroma

xeromycteria

xeronosus

xerophthalmia

xerophthalmic ulcer

xerophthalmicus

fundus x.

xerophthalmus

xerosis

x. conjunctivae

conjunctival x.

x. of cornea

corneal x.

x. parenchymatosus

x. superficialis

xerostomia

xerotic

x. degeneration

x. keratitis

X-linked

X.-l. achromatopsia

X.-l. blue cone
monochromatism

X.-l. disease

X.-l. dominant disorder

X.-l.
hypogammaglobulinemia

X.-l. inheritance

X.-l. juvenile retinopathy

X.-l. juvenile retinoschisis

X.-l. recessive disease

X.-l. recessive disorder

X.-l. retinoschisis

x-ray

x.-r. cataract

polytome x.-r.

x-ray-induced cataract

XT

exotropia

X(T)

intermittent exotropia

XXXXX syndrome

XXXXY syndrome

XXXY syndrome

Xylocaine
    X. with epinephrine

xylonite frame

YAG
    YAG cyclocryotherapy
    YAG laser
Yale
    Y. Luer-Lok
    Y. Luer-Lok needle
    Y. Luer-Lok syringe
Yannuzzi
    Y. fundus laser lens
    Y. lens
yaws
y axis
Yazujian bur
Y cells
Y chromosome
yellow
    y. blindness
    indicator y.
    y. light reflex
    y. mercuric oxide
    y. point

    y. reflex
    y. spot
    y. spot of retina
    y. vision
    visual y.
yellow-mutant oculocutaneous albinism
yellow-ochre hemorrhage
Y hook
yoked muscle
yoke movement
Youens lens
Young-Helmholtz theory of color vision
Young's
    Y. operation
    Y. theory of light
Y suture
yttrium-aluminum-garnet laser (YAG laser)

Z

Z axis of Fick
Z band
Zeeman's effect
Zeis
    gland of Z.
    Z. glands
zeisian
    z. gland
    z. sty
Zeiss
    Z. carbon arc slit lamp
    Z. cine adaptor
    Z. colposcope
    Z. Fiber Optic Illumination
     System
    Z. fundus camera
    Z. goniolens
    Z. gonioscope
    Z. lamp
    Z. lens
    Z. lens loupe
    Z. microscope
    Z. operating field loupe
    Z. operating microscope
    Z. ophthalmoscope
    Z. photocoagulator
    Z. slit lamp
    Z. slit-lamp series
    Z. vertex refractionometer
Zeiss-Barraquer
    Z. B. cine microscope
    Z.-B. surgical microscope
Zeiss-Comberg slit lamp
Zeiss-Gullstrand
    Z.-G. lens
    Z.-G. loupe
Zeiss-Nordenson fundus camera
Zellballen pattern
Zellweger's syndrome
Zephiran
zero
    z. optical power
    z. power lenses
    z. vergence
zeta sedimentation rate
zidovudine
Ziegler
    Z. blade
    Z. cautery
    Z. cilia forceps

    Z. dilator
    Z. electrocautery
    Z. forceps
    Z. iris knife-needle
    Z. knife
    Z. knife-needle
    Z. lacrimal dilator
    Z. probe
    Z. speculum
Ziegler's
    Z. operation
    Z. puncture
zinc
    bacitracin z.
    z. bacitracin
    z. incrustations
    z. sulfate
    z. sulfate solution
Zincfrin
Zinn
    annulus of Z.
    zone of Z.
    zonule of Z.
Zinn-Haller arterial circle
zinnii
    annulus z.
    circulus z.
Zinn's
    Z. circle
    Z. circlet
    Z. corona
    Z. ligament
    Z. membrane
    Z. ring
    Z. tendon
    Z. zonule
zipped angle
zipper stitch
Z marginal tenotomy
Z myotomy
Zöllner's
    Z. figure
    Z. line
Zolyse
zona, pl. zonae
    z. ciliaris
    z. ophthalmica
zone
    anterior optical z. (AOZ)
    apical z.

zone *(continued)*
    blur z.
    Bowman's z.
    Boyd's z.
    ciliary z.
    z. of contact lens
    z. of discontinuity
    z.'s of discontinuity
    extravisual z.
    fissure z.
    foveal avascular z.
    interpalpebral z.
    junctional z.
    limbal z.
    markers for z.
    neutral z.
    nuclear z.
    null z.
    optical z.
    posterior optical z. (POZ)
    pupillary z.
    retinal z.
    transition z.
    transitional z.
    visual z.
    z. of Zinn
zonula, pl. **zonulae**
    z. adherens
    z. ciliaris
    z. occludens
zonular
    z. attachment
    z. band
    z. cataract
    z. fiber
    z. keratitis
    z. pulverulent cataract
    z. scotoma
    z. spaces
    z. stripper
    z. tension
    z. tetany
zonulares
    fibrae z.
zonularia
    spatia z.
zonular-traction retinal tuft
zonule
    ciliary z.
    lens z.

    z. stripper
    z. of Zinn
    Zinn's z.
zonulitis
zonulolysis, zonulysis
    Barraquer's z.
    enzymatic z.
zonulotomy
zoom system
zoonoses
zoster
    herpes z.
    z. ophthalmicus
    z. sine eruptio
Zostrix
Zovirax
Z-plasty
    Spencer-Watson Z.-p.
Z tenotomy
Zuckerkandl's dehiscence
zygoma
zygomatic
    z. bone
    z. foramen
    z. foramen of Arnold
    z. fracture
    z. nerve
zygomatici
    facies orbitalis ossis z.
    processus frontosphenoidalis ossis z.
zygomaticofacial
    z. canal
    z. foramen
zygomatico-orbital
    z.-o. artery
    z.-o. foramen
    z.-o. process
    z.-o. process of the maxilla
zygomatico-orbitale
    foramen z.-o.
zygomaticotemporal
    z. canal
    z. foramen
zygomaticus
    nervus z.
zyl frame
Zylik's operation
zylonite frame

Appendix 1
Cataract Extraction

AMO intraocular lens
Anis forceps
anterior capsulotomy
Beaver blade
bridle suture
cannula
capsular bag
capsulorrhexis forceps
Cavitron I/A handpiece
Cilco intraocular lens
Coburn intraocular lens
collagen shield
collar button
CooperVision I/A machine
cystotome
ECCE — extracapsular cataract
  extraction
eraser cautery
extracapsular cataract extraction
  (ECCE)
Fox shield
Geuder implanter
Grieshaber blade
Honan balloon
intraocular lens
intraocular lens implant
IOLAB intraocular lens
Ioptex intraocular lens
Jaffe lid speculum
jeweler forceps

Kelman-McPherson forceps
keratome
Kratz polisher
McPherson forceps
mosquito clamp
muscle hook
MVR blade
ORC intraocular lens
pencil cautery
phacoemulsification
Pharmacia intraocular lens
Schiötz tonometer
Sheets glide
Shepard forceps
Simcoe upeop
Sinskey hook
SITE irrigating/aspirating needle
SITE macrobore needle
SITE macrobore plus needle
SITE TXR phacoemulsification
  system
Steri-Strips
Utrata forceps
Vicryl suture
Weck sponge
Westcott scissors
wet-field cautery
Wheeler blade
Y hook